Infection Control in the Community

For Churchill Livingstone:

Senior Commissioning Editor: Ninette Premdas
Project Development Manager: Dinah Thom
Project Manager: Gail Wright
Designer: Judith Wright

Infection Control in the Community

Edited by

Jean Lawrence RGN ONC ENB 329, 910, 934
Senior Nurse Infection Control, Leeds Mental Health Teaching NHS Trust, Leeds, UK

Dee May RGN DMS
Clinical Director, Infection Management Ltd, Wembley, UK

Foreword by

Jennie Wilson BSc(Hons) RGN MPH DFPHM
Senior Nurse Manager and Surveillance Coordinator, Nosocomial Infection Surveillance Unit,
Public Health Laboratory, London, UK

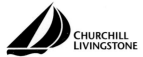

CHURCHILL LIVINGSTONE

Edinburgh   London   New York   Oxford   Philadelphia   St Louis   Sydney   Toronto

CHURCHILL LIVINGSTONE
An imprint of Elsevier Science Limited

First published 2003

ISBN 0 443 06406 7

British Library Cataloguing in Publication Data
A catalogue record for this book is available from the British Library

Library of Congress Cataloging in Publication Data
A catalog record for this book is available from the Library of Congress

Notice
Medical knowledge is constantly changing. Standard safety precautions
must be followed, but as new research and clinical experience broaden
our knowledge, changes in treatment and drug therapy may become
necessary or appropriate. Readers are advised to check the most
current product information provided by the manufacturer of each
drug to be administered to verify the recommended dose, the method
and duration of administration, and contraindications. It is the
responsibility of the practitioner, relying on experience and knowledge
of the patient, to determine dosages and the best treatment for each
individual patient. Neither the Publisher nor the authors assume any
liability for any injury and/or damage to persons or property arising
from this publication

The Publisher

ELSEVIER SCIENCE
your source for books,
journals and multimedia
in the health sciences
www.elsevierhealth.com

The
publisher's
policy is to use
**paper manufactured
from sustainable forests**

Printed in China by RDC Group Limited

Contents

keeping and reporting; Infection control risk assessment in studios and guidance for 'best practice'; Notes on acupuncture and electrolysis.

Contributors

John Babb FIBMS
Formerly Laboratory Manager, Hospital
Infection Research Laboratory, City Hospital
NHS Trust, Birmingham, UK

Michelle Briggs RGN BSc MSc CIM
Research Fellow, Centre for the Analysis of
Nursing Practice, Leeds Mental Health Teaching
NHS Trust, Leeds, UK

Carole Fry RN RM
Nursing Officer Communicable Diseases,
Department of Health, London, UK

Alison Fuller RGN ENB 329, 870 BSc Hons
(HealthStudies)
Public House/Infection Control Nurse,
Bradford South and West Primary Care Trust,
Bradford, UK

Kim Gunn RGN MPH ENB 329, 934 C&G 7306
Public Health Specialist, Communicable Disease
and Infection Control, North Staffordshire
Health Authority, Stoke-on-Trent, UK

Janet Howard RN RM DipHV DipInfCont
DipFoodHyg DipMan Module
Community Infection Control Nurse,
Shrewsbury, UK

Debra Khan RGN ENB 329 CertInfCont MPH(Birm)
Public Health Specialist – Health Protection
Department of Public Health, Warwickshire
Health Protection Unit, North Warwickshire
PCT, UK

Jean Lawrence RGN ONC ENB 329, 910, 934
Senior Nurse Infection Control, Leeds Mental
Health Teaching NHS Trust, Leeds, UK

Sharon Lowe RGN SCM BA(HealthStudies)
District Infection Control Nurse for Public
Health, Liverpool, UK

Gillian Manojlovic RGN ENB 264, 998 DipInfCont
Senior Nurse Infection Control (Community),
Calderdale and Huddersfield NHS Trust,
Halifax, UK

Dee May RGN DMS ENB 329, 934 FETC 730
Clinical Director, Infection Management Ltd,
Wembley, UK

Lynn Parker RN MSc(NursStudies) CertEd(Nurses)
ENB 329
Clinical Nurse Specialist in Infection
Control, Sheffield Teaching Hospitals
NHS Trust, Sheffield, UK

Sue Ross RGN ONC BSc DipInfCont PGCE
Senior Nurse Infection Control, Wakefield and
Pontefract Community NHS Trust, Bradford, UK

Elizabeth Scanlon RGN RM CertDN MSc
Nurse Consultant Tissue Viability,
North West Primary Care Trust, Leeds, UK

Alyson Smith RGN MPH ENB 329
DipCommNursStud Hon MFPHM
Nurse Consultant Public Health (Health
Protection), Buckinghamshire Health Protection,
Vale of Aylesbury Primary Care Trust,
Aylesbury, UK

Mary Steen RGN RM BHSc PGCRM MCGI
Community Midwife/Research Fellow,
Leeds Teaching Hospitals NHS Trust, Leeds, UK

Maggie Whitlock RGN
Public Health Nurse Specialist/Infection
Control, East Riding Health Authority,
Willerby, UK

Gladys Xavier RGN Dip(N) CIIN BSc(Hons)
Nurse Consultant/Communicable Disease/
Public Health, Redbridge and Waltham
Forest Primary Care Trust, Ilford, UK

Foreword

I am delighted to have been given the opportunity to write the foreword for this exciting new textbook on infection control in the community. There has long been a call for such a book and I am pleased to see that two such eminently qualified infection control specialists as Jean Lawrence and Dee May have been able to address this need. When I began my career in infection control in the early 1980s, infection control nurses (ICNs) based in the community were a rarity. Advice to community staff tended to be provided, in an *ad hoc* way, by over-stretched hospital ICNs who had limited knowledge of the particular problems faced by those working in community settings. Fortunately, this has now begun to change and the needs of community staff have been recognized with the appointment of many more community-based ICNs.

The importance of infection control in hospitals has been recognized for many years and was highlighted recently with the National Audit Office report on *The Management and Control of Hospital Acquired Infection in Acute NHS Trusts in England*. However, enormous changes over the last decade have greatly affected the way that healthcare is both managed and delivered. There has been both a shift towards early discharge from hospital into the community and an increasing emphasis on managing the elderly and disabled in their own homes for as long as possible. As a result, community staff are now involved in the management of a wide range of invasive devices, with their attendant infection control risks, in the patients' own home. *Shifting the Balance of Power,*

Securing Delivery (Department of Health 2001) has signalled the formal devolution of power to local communities, transferring responsibility for the commissioning of local services to Primary Care Trusts. Demand for treatment locally has seen the growth of minor surgery or other invasive treatments being performed in health centres and general practice surgeries. At the same time concern about the risk of infection, especially from blood-borne viruses, has increased and the need for good infection control practice has become of paramount importance. In addition, the development of partnership working with local authorities has opened up new areas where infection control is an issue, such as homes for the elderly, schools and nurseries. The recent publication of *Getting Ahead of the Curve* (Department of Health 2002) focuses specifically on the future strategy for preventing and controlling infectious disease and recognizes the importance of establishing structures within which infection control expertise can operate at a community level. The changes outlined in this document are likely to continue to increase the profile of community-based infection control services in the future. Thus the control of infection in community settings has acquired a whole new significance and the need for specific information and advice has become essential.

Reading this book one cannot help but be struck by the huge diversity of settings within the community that have implications for infection control. The focus of the chapters ranges from general practice to tattooing and the homeless.

Whilst the principles of infection control should be applicable to any setting, the community environment often makes their implementation in practice problematic, and decisions about what is, or is not, important can be difficult to make. Hospital staff can solve most of their decontamination problems by simply dispatching equipment to the central sterile supplies department, or deal with patients with communicable disease by moving them into a side room. Things are never quite so simple in a general practice, dental surgeries or residential homes, yet the risks of cross infection through inadequately decontaminated equipment in a surgery or person-to-person spread in a residential home are just as real.

As the editors point out in their introductory chapter, community healthcare staff have limited access to training or advice in infection control. This book is set to become an important source of information and a tool for making decisions for many such staff, helping to improve their knowledge and providing a community focus to infection control issues. It brings together expertise from a wide range of different specialist areas and sets infection control in context in each. There is an excellent balance between enabling chapters to be read alone and avoiding too much repetition between them. The comprehensive chapters on some of the basic issues such as decontamination and wound care will be of particular value to a wide range of staff. This book will also be an invaluable aid to community ICNs through helping to transfer the principles of infection control from the more familiar hospital environment to the community setting. Its publication is to be greatly welcomed.

Jennie Wilson

Preface

Over the past decade, many questions have been raised regarding infection control and prevention in very diverse community settings. This book has been written in response to those questions, ranging from situations in a patient's home to tattooing and piercing establishments. The authors are all highly experienced in their field.

The primary care teams of today deal with procedures previously carried out in hospitals, for example minor surgery. This book provides a resource for primary care staff to ensure that evidence based practice is being applied with control of infection practice and procedures. This textbook is aimed primarily at nurses, midwives and health visitors working in the community. It will also provide reference material for students in training where an infection control module is part of the learning process. Those working in the professions allied to medicine will find it of value for infection control aspects of their particular specialism, for example podiatry within health centres, physiotherapy issues and equipment, and dental treatment. Professionals in the areas of communicable disease and public health should find it a good reference source for day-to-day infection control problems in particular settings such as among the homeless, in prisons, and in nurseries and schools.

A chapter on basic microbiology is included to allow the reader to underpin practice, and the chapter on immunosuppressive diseases will give the reader an understanding of the immune system in relation to the prevention and control of infection. The standard infection control precautions are applied to each setting within the individual chapters to make it easier for the reader to refer to within the setting context. For example, the application of precautions in a patient's home will differ to their application in a prison or health centre.

Some chapters give practice points, figures, photographs and examples of practice to focus on infection control practice for the particular setting. References are at the end of each chapter, and further practical information on specific topics is included in the appendices. To facilitate reading, a glossary of terms is included.

It is hoped that this book will provide practical advice on infection control for everyday practice to maintain a high standard in the prevention and control of infection.

Jean Lawrence
Dee May

Leeds and Wembley 2002

Abbreviations

ACDP	Advisory Committee on Dangerous Pathogens	MAF	Macrophage activation factor
BSG	British Society of Gastroenterology	MDA	Medical Devices Agency
CAI	Community-acquired infection	MDRTB	Multi-drug resistant tuberculosis
CCDC	Consultant in Communicable Disease Control	MEL	Maximum exposure limit
CDC	Centers for Disease Control, Atlanta, GA	MIF	Migratory inhibition factor
		MMWR	Morbidity and Mortality Weekly Report (CDC, Atlanta)
CDSC	Communicable Disease Surveillance Centre	MNPS	Mononuclear phagocyte system
CMO	Chief Medical Officer	MOEH	Medical Officer for Environmental Health
COSHH	Control of Substances Hazardous to Health	MOH	Medical Officer of Health
DoH	Department of Health	MPI	Micro-pigmentation
DOT	Directly-observed therapy	ONS	Office for National Statistics (formerly OPCS)
DTB	Drug and Therapeutics Bulletin	PEP	Post-exposure prophylaxis
EHO	Environmental Health Officer	PHLS	Public Health Laboratory Service
HAI	Hospital-acquired infection	PMN	Polymorphonuclear neutrophils
HBV	Hepatitis B virus	PPE	Personal protective equipment
HPV	Human papillomavirus	SEAC	Spongiform Encephalopathies Advisory Committee
HSG	Health Service Guidelines	SICP	Standard Infection Control Precautions
HTM	Health Technical Memo		
ICC	Infection Control Committee	SRSV	Small, round structured virus
ICN	Infection control nurse	SSD	Sterile Services Department
ICT	Infection Control Team	TPN	Total parenteral nutrition
ISSM	Institute of Sterile Services Management	TWA	Time-weighted average
		UICP	Universal Infection Control Precautions
LMF	Lymphocytic mitogenic factor		
LT	Lymphotoxin		

1

Introduction

J. Lawrence
D. May

Risks relating to the spread of infection have led to many initiatives over the past two decades aimed at controlling or eliminating those risks. During this time, a number of significant incidents have occurred, which have ultimately influenced the development of these initiatives.

Probably the major influence on risk reduction during this time has been the emergence of the Human Immunodeficiency Virus (HIV) as a human pathogen. This micro-organism had the potential to infect healthcare workers as a result of injuries at work, such as a needlestick injury. As a result of the need to protect both the healthcare worker and the confidentiality and rights of the patient, universal precautions were introduced in 1985 as a mechanism of risk reduction used for *all* patients at *all* times.

Two significant outbreaks of infection in the mid 1980s – salmonella food poisoning at Stanley Royd Hospital and Legionnaires' disease at Stafford Hospital – led to public inquiries which criticized infection control standards. This in turn prompted the Department of Health to commission a report into infection control arrangements in England – the so-called Cooke Report (named after the Report's Chair, Dr Mary Cooke) which resulted in recommendations being made that all acute hospitals employ infection control doctors supported by infection control nurses (ICNs). However, at this stage, few hospitals employed more than one ICN and some – including major teaching hospitals – employed none!

The removal of Crown Immunity from healthcare premises in the late 1980s ushered in a new era of accountability for managers, with hospitals no longer able to ignore their liability for incidents such as outbreaks of infection.

And finally, more recently the emergence of epidemic strains of methicillin-resistant *Staphylococcus aureus* (MRSA), new diseases such as variant Creutzfeldt–Jakob disease (vCJD) and Hepatitis C, together with the re-emergence of diseases such as pulmonary tuberculosis (TB), have seen healthcare face an unprecedented challenge in communicable disease control.

The introduction of the NHS Reforms in the early 1990s, together with increasing public expectation, advances in medical technology, an ageing population and an increasingly litigious society have fundamentally re-focused the delivery of healthcare over the last decade. Clinical care is now delivered within the structured framework of clinical governance that is itself firmly embedded in an environment of managed risk. In addition, the focus of healthcare delivery has shifted from a predominantly hospital-based service to one now firmly rooted in the community, both commissioned and, increasingly, delivered by Primary Care Trusts.

In order for patients and staff to be managed safely, risks must be eliminated, reduced or effectively managed. One key element of risk management is the prevention and control of infection. Infection is one of the most significant causes of morbidity and mortality. The specialism of infection control in the UK is grounded in medical microbiology and has rapidly developed in recent years, more or less in tandem with the changes in healthcare delivery. However, infection control services in community settings have, historically, been less comprehensive than in hospitals. Many community healthcare staff do not receive regular infection control training and many more do not have access to up-to-date comprehensive policies and procedures to support their practice. In some community settings, access to infection control advice is also limited. In order to effectively manage the infection risks of healthcare delivered in a wide array of community settings – health centres, GP practices, nursing and residential homes, patients' own homes, etc. – clinical staff must have a working knowledge of the principles of infection control, firmly supported by a team of specialist professionals for expert guidance. The infection control problems faced by staff in community settings have historically been perceived as being different and somehow less significant than those occurring within the hospital environment, probably because most significant healthcare interventions were traditionally undertaken within a hospital setting. However, as more and more patients receive their healthcare in community settings, this can no longer be deemed to be the case. A wide range of significant clinical interventions takes place in community settings, including minor surgery, the management of long-term ventilated patients, the care and management of central and tunnelled lines for parenteral nutrition, to name but three. The knowledge base of community staff managing these patients is required to be comprehensive and broad. Accessing evidence-based information to support practice in community settings is both time-consuming and fragmented. Texts such as this should make that process a little less fraught.

SOME SIGNIFICANT EVENTS IN INFECTION CONTROL

1959 First infection control nurse appointed in Torquay
1984 Stanley Royd Hospital outbreak of salmonella food poisoning
1985 Stafford Hospital outbreak of Legionnaires' disease
1985 Universal precautions introduced for protection against HIV
1987 Cooke Report into hospital infection control management
1988 Control of Substances Hazardous to Health (COSHH) Regulations
1988 Public Health (Communicable Diseases) Regulations (creation of CCDC)
1988 Removal of Crown Immunity from healthcare premises
1992 Personal Protective Equipment Regulations
1994 First epidemic strains of MRSA reported
1995 Revised Cooke Report published

1995 Community management of MRSA guidelines published

1996 Second national prevalence survey of hospital-acquired infection

1997 National Nosocomial Infection Surveillance (NNIS) scheme launched

1997 House of Lords Select Committee Enquiry into antimicrobial resistance

1998 Revised MRSA guidelines in hospital published

1999 Major review of hospital decontamination arrangements announced in response to concerns regarding vCJD

2000 UK Health Departments' antimicrobial strategy issued

2000 Socio-economic Burden of Hospital Infection Report published

2000 National Audit Office (NAO) Report on Management Arrangements for Hospital-acquired Infection published

2000 Health Services Circular 2000/002 – management arrangements for infection control issued by the Department of Health

2000 Controls Assurance standards (including infection control) first published

2001 Public Accounts Committee response to the NAO report published

2001 Environmental standards for hygiene in hospitals launched and PEAT teams created in acute NHS trusts to monitor the patient environment

2001 Controls assurance standards for infection control in primary care published

2002 Creation of the Health Protection Agency announced

2002 Creation of Strategic Health Authorities and subsequent re-focusing of community infection control

2002 Re-structuring of the public health and communicable disease function with the creation of Strategic Health Authorities

2

Basic microbiology

L. Parker

INTRODUCTION

Safe infection control practice requires knowledge of micro-organisms, the diseases they cause and how they spread between humans. This chapter attempts to provide an introduction to the subject, outlining their basic properties and characteristics.

Microbes (micro-organisms) are believed to have been the first living organisms, and can be found from the coldest surface areas to the hottest core of the planet. They survive in all habitats, however extreme, in soil, water and air, food and clothes, on the surface of the body and within it. Some are visible with an ordinary microscope, but viruses require an electron microscope. Micro-organisms are useful to humans in many respects, performing beneficial functions in the ecological chain, including the breakdown of dead plant and animal matter. They are also used in biotechnology and in food production in the dairy, brewing and bakery industries.

This book is concerned with pathogenic organisms which can be subdivided into bacteria, rickettsiae and chlamydia, viruses, fungi and protozoa.

HISTORICAL PERSPECTIVE

For centuries before scientific discoveries were made, common sense suggested that there was a connection between dirt and disease but it was not possible to explain what the link could be. Popular explanations included miasma or bad air, in which the poisonous fumes from decaying waste were

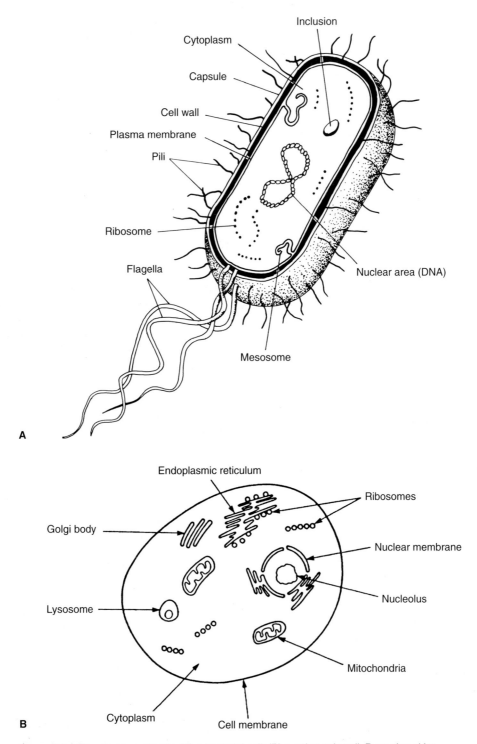

Figure 2.1 The structure of cells. (A) a bacterial cell; (B) a eukaryotic cell. Reproduced by permission from Wilson J 2001 *Infection Control in Clinical Practice,* 2nd edn. Baillière Tindall, Edinburgh.

blown by the wind from one place to another. In London during the Plague of 1665 people carried bunches of strong-smelling herbs to protect them from the fumes thought to spread the disease. But it was not until the late seventeenth century when the Dutch amateur scientist Antoni van Leewenhoek invented a microscope and described the small creatures he found in water, food and human excreta, that a connection was made. He even described them in the scrapings from his teeth, calling the organisms 'animalcules', and presented his findings in a series of 200 papers to the Royal Society of London (Wilson 2001).

Van Leewenhoek's discoveries encouraged other scientists, including the chemist Louis Pasteur. In the 1850s Pasteur became interested in microbes when asked to help a brewing company discover why their vats of alcohol were going bad. Through his experiments he found that microbes were responsible for spoiling many types of foods, and published his germ theory. He hypothesized that if wines and beer could be changed by germs, then the same could happen in humans and animals. A German doctor, Robert Koch, who applied Pasteur's theory to human disease, completed the final link in the chain. After conducting a series of experiments he proved that specific microbes caused specific diseases. This process is known as Koch's postulates.

BASIC CELL STRUCTURE

All living cells are composed of two distinct cell types, called **prokaryotic** or **eukaryotic** (Fig. 2.1). A cell is the basis of all living structures, and consists of a nucleus and cytoplasm within a semi-permeable membrane. In some instances they also have an outer cell wall.

Eukaryotic cells are found in plants, animals, protozoa, fungi and algae. Prokaryotic cells are less complex, forming single-celled organisms including all bacteria: see Box 2.1.

Capsules

These are found in most bacteria and form a loose layer of gelatinous material outside the cell wall.

Box 2.1 Basic cell types

Eukaryotic	**Prokaryotic**
Algae	Bacteria
Fungi	Mycoplasma
Protozoa	Rickettsiae
	Chlamydia

- Enclosed by a membrane rather than cell wall
- Cell walls, when present, are simple structures made of sugars or cellulose in algae and plants

- Rigid cell wall made of network of carbohydrates and amino acids

---

Spores and cysts

Some bacteria form spores when environmental conditions are not suitable, that is, when they have no food, water, oxygen or the temperature is too hot or too cold. Spores can survive for a long time in the environment until the conditions start to improve, when they start to germinate and the cells begin to multiply again. Examples of organisms that form spores are *Clostridium difficile*, responsible for antibiotic-associated diarrhoeal infections.

Certain protozoa have the ability to form cysts, allowing them to survive for long periods outside the host; examples include giardia and entamoeba.

Cytoplasm

Within the cytoplasm of the cell, biochemical reactions take place that maintain the cell and enable it to reproduce. Eukaryotic cells have a complex cytoplasm reflecting the amount of cellular activity taking place. The cytoplasm of prokaryotic cells is by comparison simpler, as these cells are unicellular and do not require the same complex transport mechanism.

Nucleus

Eukaryotic cells have a nucleus that contains more than one chromosome and is surrounded by a nuclear membrane. Prokaryotic cells contain only one chromosome, that lies free within the cytoplasm.

CLASSIFICATION OF MICROBES

Over the years a system has evolved for identifying individual organisms by placing them into groups according to their similarities in structure. Two names are given to an organism: **genus**, which identifies the group it belongs to, and **species**, which is its specific name within the group. An example of this is:

Genus: Staphylococcus
Species: *S. aureus, S. epidermidis, S. saprophyticus.*

As scientific knowledge advances and more is discovered about microbes, they can be reclassified and moved into other groupings.

Bacteria

Bacteria are usually unicellular, appear in a variety of shapes (Fig. 2.2) and are capable of different metabolic activities to grow and reproduce. Individual cells range from 0.5–1 μm (micrometre) and consist of a semi-solid **cytoplasm** surrounded by a **cytoplasmic membrane** contained normally in a rigid **cell wall**. DNA and RNA (deoxyribonucleic acid and ribonucleic acid) are found in the cytoplasm, with most of the DNA in one part of the cell in a ring or loop making the **nucleus**. The rigidity of the cell wall is due to a complex of aminosugars and polypeptides. Reproduction is by **binary fission** (see Genetics section on reproduction, below). Some bacteria form **capsules**, usually made of polysaccharide, outside their cell walls, with some forming **flagella** organs of movement and others forming **spores**.

As Figure 2.2 illustrates, **cocci** are round, and normally grouped together in pairs called diplococci (for example *Neisseria meningitidis* causing bacterial meningitis). Repeated division produces chains, and when occurring at right angles produces packets of four, eight or more. Elongated cylindrical forms are called **bacilli** or rods that are straight or slightly curved (such as *Listeria monocytogenes* responsible for causing listeriosis). Those definitely curved are called **vibrios** (for example *Vibrio cholerae* that causes cholera), and **spirochaetes** are corkscrew-like spirals (examples are *Treponema pallidum* causing syphilis and *Borrelia burgdorferi* responsible for Lyme disease).

Resembling bacteria and containing both DNA and RNA, **chlamydia** and **rickettsiae** are both obligate intracellular organisms. They reproduce by binary fission but are nearer in size to viruses than to bacteria, with diameters 0.25–0.5 μm. Like viruses they can only reproduce within the host's cells. They are susceptible to antimicrobial drugs.

Rickettsiae are pathogenic to humans, and can survive at normal temperatures outside their hosts. Patients with rickettsial infections form species-specific and strain-specific antibodies, making possible a serological diagnosis. Epidemic typhus is particular to humans, caused by *Rickettsia prowazeki* and transmitted by the human body louse. It cannot be transmitted directly from person to person. Epidemics are often associated with wars and famines, when the washing of clothing cannot be done on a regular basis.

Chlamydia cannot live independently of the host. Chlamydiae of the psittacosis group are bird

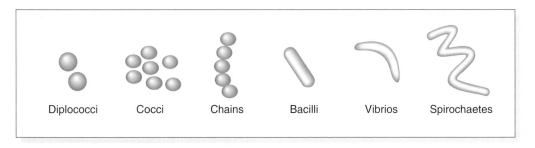

Diplococci   Cocci   Chains   Bacilli   Vibrios   Spirochaetes

Figure 2.2 Bacteria: the variety of types. Reproduced by permission from Horton R, Parker L 2002 *Informed Infection Control*, 2nd edn. Churchill Livingstone, Edinburgh.

pathogens found in parrots. In humans they are responsible for causing respiratory tract infections by inhalation of contaminated dust containing dried droppings from infected birds. Illness ranges from a mild influenza to a severe and sometimes fatal pneumonia.

Chlamydia trachomatis is responsible for causing trachoma, a form of conjunctivitis. Its primary habitat is the human genital tract, where carriage is usually asymptomatic, though it can cause urethritis and other genital infections. Neonatal conjunctivitis and pneumonia are acquired during delivery from the mother's genital tract.

Classification of bacteria

The most important characteristic for classification is shape and reaction to staining.

Gram-staining was first developed by the Danish physician Hans Christian Gram in 1884, to differentiate pneumococci from *Klebsiella pneumoniae*. The process colours cells with a violet dye, then a pink counter-stain. Gram-positive bacteria retain purple dye when treated with the decolorizing agent, but Gram-negative bacteria do not retain the blue stain; when counter-stained they take up the pink colour. The reason for the take-up of colour is not really understood but is thought to be due to the acidic nature of the organism or the permeability of the cell walls. Gram-staining and microscopic examination provide an initial identification, after which specimens are cultured to identify the organism. Those bacteria that normally live on the human body or cause disease in humans grow best in a medium that mimics body secretions and tissues. But it can take between 24 and 48 hours before there are enough cells to enable further testing and to provide test results. For mycobacterial species, acid-fast stains such as Ziehl–Neelsen are used; for spirochaetes, the most useful methods are either dark-ground illumination microscopy or a silver stain under the light microscope (Shanson 1999).

Fungi

Fungi are eukaryotic cells, more complex than bacteria. They may be described as **moulds** or **yeasts**, growth being dependent upon the temperature, availability of oxygen and nutrients. They reproduce sexually or by formation of spores. Diseases caused by fungi are **mycoses**, and are divided into those causing superficial or deep infections. Superficial infections such as ringworm affect only the skin. Deep ones affect the whole body, causing systemic infections; one example is aspergillus, which is usually an opportunistic organism that takes advantage of a person's lowered immune response.

Protozoa

These are eukaryotic, relatively large, single-celled microbes and more complex than bacteria. Instead of a cell wall, the tough outer cell membrane of protozoa can ingest solid particles to obtain nutrients. Protozoa are considered to be the lowest form of animal life. Those that cause disease in humans include:

- *Plasmodium* spp. (malaria)
- *Entamoeba histolytica* (amoebic dysentery)
- *Cryptosporidium parvum* (diarrhoeal diseases)
- *Pneumocystis carinii* (opportunistic lung disease)
- *Toxoplasma gondii* (congenital infection).

Prions

Prions are thought to be found in the central nervous system and also in other tissues such as the lymph glands, and particularly the tonsils. Intensive research into prions continues: they are believed to be the cause of transmissible spongiform encephalopathies (TSE). Normal prions (PrP) are made almost entirely from proteins.

Abnormal PrP^{sc} (scrapie) has the same sequence of amino acids but it is thought that they are folded differently so they have a different secondary structure that is protease-resistant and insoluble. They cause a build-up in the brain, forming fibrils and plaques with a lack of immune response from the body. Abnormal prions latch on to the normal prion protein, causing it to change its shape. So the normal becomes abnormal, causing disease. During the 1980s new types of prion evolved in the UK, causing bovine spongiform encephalopathy (BSE) in cattle, resulting in variant Creutzfeldt–Jakob disease (vCJD) in humans.

Viruses

Viruses attack a wide range of organisms in the microbial, plant and animal kingdom. They consist of a single type of nucleic acid in a protein coat called a **capsid**. Inside the human cell the virus takes over the cellular metabolism to make new **virons** (Shanson 1999).

Identification of viruses is by growing in tissue culture, by special staining techniques or by electron microscope (Horton and Parker 2002). The central nucleic acid core of RNA or DNA is surrounded by the protein coat or capsid made of capsomeres (nucleo-capsid). The purpose of the capsid is to give protection to the virus and to assist the virus to attach to the targeted host cell. Some viruses, including the herpes virus, have another covering called an **envelope**, while those without envelopes are called **naked** viruses.

Viruses replicate inside living cells and recognize the protein receptors of the target (host) cells that they then attach to. The nucleic acid of the virus is injected into the host cell and then uses the DNA of the cell to make new virus particles. The host cell in effect becomes a factory to produce new viruses, usually destroying itself in the process. Viruses do not survive long outside a living cell, but some, like rhinoviruses, do survive for short periods on equipment and the hands of individuals. Rhinoviruses are spread more commonly on hands than by sneezing, and are responsible for the common cold.

While many viruses are harmless to humans, they are prolific and can be found everywhere, and certain viruses cause a wide range of infections and diseases. They can be said to cause three different effects on the host cells:

- The infection kills the cell (cytopathic effect).
- The virus stays within the body and may recur later (latency, e.g. shingles).
- The virus transforms the cell, causing malignancy (Hep B and C in the liver).

Table 2.1 Viruses responsible for common infections

Group of infections	Suspected viruses
Skin vesicles	Herpes simplex Varicella zoster
Respiratory infections	Influenza virus Para-influenza virus Respiratory syncytial virus Rhinoviruses Adenoviruses
Childhood infections	Measles Mumps Chickenpox
Gastroenteritis	Rotavirus Small round structured viruses
Hepatitis	Hepatitis A, B, C, D, E, G
Congenital infections	Cytomegalovirus Rubella
Aseptic meningitis	Enteroviruses Mumps
Eye infections	Herpes simplex Adenoviruses

Examples of viruses that are responsible for common infections are listed in Table 2.1.

CELL PHYSIOLOGY

Because of their diverse shape, size, structure and varied environment, microbes differ widely in their physiology. The following section refers mainly to bacteria. For viruses, rickettsiae and protozoa their requirements are inextricably intertwined with those of their host cells.

Metabolic needs

The bacterial cell is a complex structure of protein, nucleic acids, polysaccharides, lipids and derivatives. The main activity of bacteria is to reproduce, and under ideal conditions some species divide by binary fission every twenty minutes. So a single bacterium can convert itself overnight into a colony with a population of millions. Such an amount of activity requires an adequate supply of energy and raw materials, with appropriate environmental conditions. The precise needs of a particular organism depend upon its enzymes.

The majority of microbes, including those important in medicine, are **chemotrophs** and get their energy from the oxidation of chemical compounds.

Water

Bacteria need water to grow, and most die rapidly in its absence, with some bacteria more resistant to drying than others, such as *Staphylococcus aureus*. Other bacteria have the ability to form **spores** (*Clostridium difficile*), surviving for hours or even months until their water supply is resumed and they can start to replicate again.

Oxygen

Those microbes that grow (increase in numbers) in the presence of air are described as **aerobes**, such as pseudomonas species. **Obligatory aerobes** need free oxygen to grow, but most bacteria are known as **facultative aerobes**, such as *Staphylococcus aureus* or *Escherichia coli*, and are able to grow in the absence of oxygen but less vigorously.

Carbon dioxide

This is probably necessary in small amounts, as is present in the atmosphere. Some species improve their growth with a higher concentration of 5–10% carbon dioxide, for example *Neisseria gonorrhoeae*.

Raw materials

There are some bacteria that can grow in simple inorganic solutions, such as *E. coli*, whilst those at the other end of the scale cannot be cultivated in non-living media, such as the leprosy bacillus and the spirochaetes of syphilis. This difference in the individual growth requirements of organisms helps medical microbiologists in their choice of culture media when receiving specimens for investigation, thus emphasizing the need for adequate clinical details to enable the correct choices to be made.

Temperature

The majority of bacteria, including all those that are parasitic on humans, require optimal growth temperatures somewhere between 20 and 40°C but are best suited by temperatures around 37°C. Many will multiply at 20°C or less (*Listeria monocytogenes* can multiply at 5°C) but there are few that grow at more than 45°C. *N. gonorrhoeae* for example grows only in a narrow temperature range of 30–39°C.

pH

This is an abbreviation for the term 'potential hydrogen', which is a scale representing the relative acidity or alkalinity of a solution. Neutral pH is 7.0; numbers lower than this are considered acid and higher numbers as alkaline. Most bacteria prefer a neutral solution but there are a few that can survive in a very acidic environment. Unusual among the bacterial flora in humans are lactobacilli, found in the adult vagina, producing lactic acid which keeps the vaginal secretions too acidic for the growth of most other organisms. Again at the other end of the scale *Vibrio cholerae* grows best at around pH 8.5.

Metabolic products

The most important end result of bacterial metabolism is more bacteria, but other by-products also occur: toxins, extracellular enzymes, pigments and other products.

Toxins

Bacteria produce powerful poisons whilst growing in the tissues of their hosts. **Exotoxins** liberated by the living bacteria are produced mainly by Gram-positive bacteria. They are proteins and relatively easily inactivated by heat. Examples of organisms that produce these exotoxins are *Clostridium botulinum* responsible for botulism, *Clostridium tetani* causing tetanus, and *Corynebacterium diphtheriae* causing diphtheria. When bacteria die, **endotoxins** are released into the body and are mainly connected with Gram-negative organisms such as *Salmonella typhi* or *Escherichia coli*. Endotoxins are relatively heat-stable, and considered less potent than exotoxins.

Extracellular enzymes

Bacteria produce a variety of enzymes that assist them in a number of ways. Some enzymes contribute to the pathogenicity of the organisms. Staphylococci produce **coagulase**, which gives protection by coating the organism with fibrin. Other enzymes destroy toxic substances in the bacterial cell; one that is important to medicine is the production of **penicillinase** by a number of bacteria, mainly Gram-negative organisms like coliforms and pseudomonads.

Finally, extracellular enzymes can assist in cell nutrition by breaking down nutrients small enough to pass through their cytoplasmic membrane.

Pigments

Some bacteria and many moulds contain pigments of a variety of colours that can aid in their identification. An example of one such pigment is the characteristic green colour of pseudomonas seen when cultured in the laboratory.

Other products

It is important to remember that a number of essential vitamins are synthesized by the normal flora found in the gut, such as vitamins B and K.

CELL GENETICS AND REPRODUCTION

Reproduction

Reproduction generally takes place by simple fission of the micro-organism, dividing one cell into two, or by a sexual process where genetic material from two or more cells is pooled and redistributed. Protozoa like Plasmodium, causing malaria, have life cycles including both sexual and asexual phases. Fungi of interest in medicine have no sexual phase but form asexual reproductive spores.

A bacterium that replicates by simple binary fission as described earlier produces two identical organisms, with constant repetition of this process producing a population of identical organisms. Changing the genetic composition can occur in a number of ways (Fig. 2.3).

Mutation

Mutation happens within a single cell, whereas the other three methods described involve the movement of genetic material from one cell to another. The nucleus of a chromosome of the bacterium consists of a double strand of DNA, which is found in the form of a closed loop. The two strands are not identical but complementary, consisting of deoxyribose component and projecting nitrogenous base component. When the cell is about to divide, the two strands separate, each acting as a template for the construction of its new partner. So two new double-stranded molecules are formed, each identical to the original. In the majority of cases all goes well, but occasionally the process is interrupted and the strands are broken or errors occur in the copying and consequently change the code. The altered pattern is then reproduced and passed on to later generations. Spontaneous mutation is rare.

Transformation

This is where free DNA of the same or a closely-related species is absorbed through the cell wall, where it is taken up by and incorporated into the genetic make-up of the cell.

Transduction

When a bacteriophage or bacterial virus infects a cell, it brings with it DNA from a previous host cell. As it uses the host DNA to replicate, sometimes this DNA gets transmitted into the new host. It is by this method that antibiotic resistance can happen in some species.

Conjugation

In some bacteria extra DNA as free units is found in the plasma, known as **plasmids** or **episomes**, and replicates independently of the nucleus. Plasmids contain genes that are not essential to

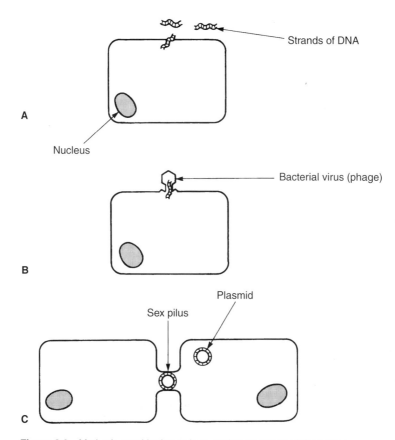

Figure 2.3   Methods used by bacteria to exchange genetic information. (A) Transformation, (B) Transduction, (C) Conjugation. Reproduced by permission from Wilson J 2001 *Infection Control in Clinical Practice*, 2nd edn. Baillière Tindall, Edinburgh.

the survival of the bacterium. They give the cell the ability to join to other bacteria by a fine tube or **sex pilus** linking the cytoplasm together. Through the tube genetic material is exchanged and incorporated into the cell. Unlike transformation or transduction, this form of genetic transfer does not depend upon the two bacteria being of the same species. This is important in medicine as antibiotic resistance from harmless bacteria can, by plasma transfer, be incorporated into the genetic make-up of pathogenic bacteria that were previously antibiotic-sensitive.

PATHOGENICITY

Pathogenicity is the ability of a microbe to invade and cause disease. Some microbes are not pathogenic at all, whilst others are highly pathogenic. The differences in pathogenicity are due to a number of closely related factors. These are:

- **Infectivity** – the capacity of the organism to spread from one host to another.
- **Toxigenicity** – the ability to produce toxins that damage the tissues of the host.
- **Invasiveness** – the capacity of the organism to invade the tissues of the host and to multiply and spread within the host.

Sometimes the word **virulence** is used to mean the combined effect of toxigenicity and invasiveness. These closely-related factors could best be considered when we know that certain microorganisms are responsible for specific diseases, such as *Clostridium tetani* causing tetanus, whereas other microbes like *Staphylococcus aureus* can cause a number of different forms of disease from impetigo to wound infections and toxic shock syndrome.

There are a few generalizations that can be made about pathogenic organisms, as stated above. A microbe can remain near the surface of the host, like ringworm, or *N. meningitidis* in the pharynx. Similarly to allow the organism to multiply in the host, it needs appropriate nutrients from the host tissues, and suitable atmospheric conditions and temperature. Abnormal conditions in the host may be the reason that the organism is able to thrive. Hence an anaerobic organism such as Clostridium responsible for gas-gangrene occurs in tissues that have lost their blood supply. Finally, pathogenic organisms damage the tissues of the host. This happens in a number of ways: malarial parasites multiply inside the red blood cells and burst them, causing anaemia. Viruses take over a host cell and use its chemical and genetic make-up to produce more viruses. The host cell then dies when the viruses burst out of it to search for other cells to infect in the body.

NORMAL FLORA

A small minority of microbes live parasitic lives inside or on the surfaces of other living organisms. Such organisms live on the human body and can be referred to as **commensal**, **symbiotic** or **pathogenic** micro-organisms. Pathogenicity is covered in the previous section. **Commensals** take their nourishment from the host and give nothing back. Examples can be found on the skin and mucous membranes, such as staphylococci (mainly *Staphylococcus epidermidis*) and diphtheroid bacilli. **Symbionts** live in partnership with the host, taking nutrients from the host and giving a service in return: an example is the vitamin-synthesizing bacteria in the intestine.

It must be remembered that pathogenicity reflects the susceptibility of the host to disease as much as it does the ability of an organism to cause that disease.

Colonization describes the presence of microbes on or in the body, growing and multiplying without invading the surrounding tissues or causing damage: an example is normal skin, colonized by a stable population of microbes that help the body's natural defence against infection (see the list in Table 2.2). This begins at birth and continues throughout environmental and personal contact to establish the delicate balance of 'normal flora'. Microbes are defined as **resident** or **transient** flora, depending on the length of time they co-exist with the body. **Resident** flora are found in certain areas of the body on a regular basis, such as coliforms in the small bowel, Lactobacillus sp. and yeasts in the vagina, and Staphylococcus sp. on the skin. Table 2.2 gives further examples of where commensal organisms are found, and pathogens of greatest significance.

Transient flora, as their name suggests, inhabit the body only for hours, days or weeks. They survive and multiply until removed, for example by hand washing. They do not normally cause disease in the host but are responsible for much cross-infection in healthcare settings. Methicillin-resistant *Staphylococcus aureus* (MRSA) is frequently found on the hands of healthcare workers, and it is easily passed on unwashed hands between patients. Viruses are easily acquired and passed on unwashed hands, such as when changing nappies and emptying bedpans.

Other terms used to describe colonization of the body by microbes are **intermittent** and **chronic** carriage. Intermittent carriage occurs when microbes colonize the body for longer than transient flora, then disappear and recur at a later date. For some patients MRSA can be considered as causing intermittent carriage, being found on various body sites such as the nose for months after the initial colonization. Chronic carriage is the persistent carriage of a pathogenic organism without causing illness in the host, as with salmonella in the gut.

INFECTION

To a certain extent all disease in humans comes from microbes that are opportunistic in nature, as disease is not the normal state of being. Micro-organisms causing infections are referred to as

Table 2.2 Normal flora: site, specimen taken, common pathogens

Site	Normal flora	Specimen	Common pathogens
Central nervous system	Normally sterile	CSF	Strep. pneumoniae N. meningitidis H. influenzae Other Gram-negative rods
Bladder and urinary tract	Normally sterile	Urine	E. coli Ent. faecalis M. tuberculosis
Lower respiratory tract	Normally sterile	Sputum	Strep. pneumoniae H. influenzae M. tuberculosis Viruses
Upper respiratory tract	S. epidermidis S. aureus H. influenzae Bacteroides	Throat swab	Strep. pyogenes Viruses
Skin and hair	S. epidermidis S. aureus Diphtheroides	Swab from wound lesions	S. aureus Strep. pyogenes
Perianal skin	Ent. faecalis Bacteroides fragilis Yeasts	Swab from wound lesions	Gram-negative rods Anaerobic Gram-negative rods Dermatophytes
Small bowel and colon	Ent. faecalis C. perfringens Coliforms Yeasts Bacteroides sp.	Faeces	Shigella sp. Salmonella sp. Campylobacter sp. Yersinia sp. Ova, cysts, parasites, viruses
Vagina (adult)	Lactobacillus sp. S. epidermidis Group B Streptococcus Yeasts Gram-negative rods	HVS	N. gonorrhoeae T. vaginalis Candida albicans Gardnerella sp.

being **pathogenic** or **opportunistic**. Pathogenic organisms are those that specifically cause infections, such as salmonella responsible for food poisoning. The term opportunistic can be considered in three different ways:

- Those organisms that rarely cause disease in people who are healthy.
- Common organisms that cause an unusual infection, rarely seen in those who are vulnerable to infections.
- Disease that is caused by an individual's own endogenous normal flora, usually when introduced to another part of the body where it is not normally found (E. coli in the gut causing urinary tract infection).

It is impossible to determine from clinical specimens whether an individual has an infection or is merely colonized by the organism isolated in the laboratory, especially if the organism is one that would be considered as part of the normal flora such as Staphylococcus aureus. In these circumstances the clinical conditions of the patient must determine whether an individual has an infection or not:

- Are there visible signs of infection present in the patient?
- Has the patient appropriate symptoms of pain, pyrexia, dysuria, purulent sputum, presence of pus, etc.?
- Are the bacteria reported on the laboratory form significant?

- Do other investigations support the diagnosis of infection, e.g. X-ray, haematology results?
- What was the quality of the specimen sent to the laboratory?

PATIENT SUSCEPTIBILITY

It is the vulnerability of the human host to the micro-organism that finally determines whether an individual will succumb to an infection. It is for this reason that healthcare workers need to undertake a risk assessment of a patient's vulnerability to infection. Factors to be considered (as set out in Horton and Parker 2002) are:

- Extremes of age – the very young and the old are more likely to acquire infections.
- Underlying diseases such as diabetes, chronic obstructive pulmonary disease and blood disorders.
- Those having therapy for disorders requiring chemotherapy, radiotherapy, steroids and antimicrobials. These all affect the individual's host defences by reducing their natural immunity or removing beneficial bacteria.
- Treatments and procedures being carried out, especially invasive techniques such as surgery, urinary catheterization and intravenous therapy.
- Smoking, substance abuse and nutritional status can also play a part in reducing an individual's ability to resist infection.

When considering the sources of micro-organisms that cause infection they are often described as being **endogenous** or **exogenous** in nature. **Endogenous** organisms are those that reside on or in the body, resulting in self-infection. Organisms that are normally found in a specific part of the body can cause infection for different reasons: for example, Gram-negative bacilli can cause wound infections following abdominal surgery; *E. coli* usually found in the gut is often responsible for causing urinary tract infections, especially in women due to the close proximity of the rectum and the urethra. **Exogenous** or **cross-infection** is when micro-organisms are transferred to a patient from an external source. This can be from another person, as with colds and flu, or via shared equipment such as multi-use vials of drugs like heparin, or via invasive devices that become contaminated, as with nebulizers, intravascular and urinary catheters, wound drains and nasogastric feeding tubes.

BREAKING THE CHAIN OF INFECTION

There is considered to be a number of interconnecting factors that come together, resulting in an individual acquiring an infection. Figure 2.4 demonstrates how they link together and the practices that can be considered to help break the chain.

Infectious agent

Here it is important that there is rapid identification of the micro-organism likely to cause an infection. Healthcare workers need to understand and interpret the results given on laboratory report forms. It is important to remember that this needs to be linked to the patient's symptoms, so that it is the patient and not the laboratory form that is treated.

Reservoir

Once the micro-organism has been identified we are able to consider where it is normally found. As described earlier, micro-organisms can be found in the environment, on people and the equipment we use. Regulation and legislation, expert opinion and research all provide guidance for the prevention of transmission of infection. It is for this purpose that policies exist on infection control, especially those for cleaning, disinfection and sterilization processes.

Portal of exit

These are exit routes by which micro-organisms can leave their reservoir, either by excretions and secretions of body fluids, in droplets or on the skin. Thus consideration needs to be given to the wearing of appropriate personal protective equipment by staff, and the safe disposal of clinical waste and laundry.

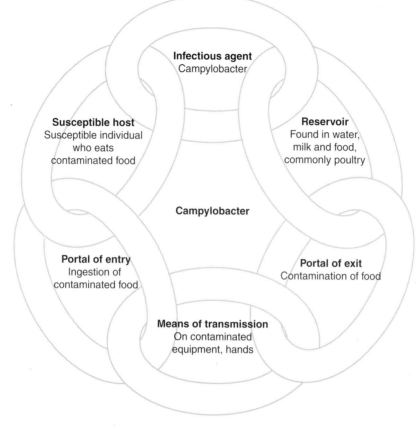

Figure 2.4 The chain of infection.

Means of transmission

Once a micro-organism exits from the reservoir, it requires a means of transmission to the susceptible host. This can be in a number of ways, as illustrated in the chain of infection. Emphasis is given to prevention of these means of transmission by advocating the importance of, for example, hand washing, safe disposal of sharps, controls for ventilation, water temperature and food hygiene.

Portal of entry

Micro-organisms enter the host through the gastrointestinal, respiratory and urinary tracts of the body. They can also enter the body through broken skin and contact with mucous membranes.

Attention is needed to the importance of the principles of asepsis, for example during surgery, and the management of invasive devices such as intravenous devices and urinary catheters.

Susceptible host

There are certain groups of people who are considered to be more susceptible to infections than others. These groups include neonates and the elderly, those with underlying diseases, such as diabetics, and the immunosuppressed. It is important that healthcare workers assess their patients for the risk of acquiring an infection. Consideration needs to be given to the appropriate placement of these patients and the treatments they are given that could contribute to their acquiring an infection, such as chemotherapy.

THE INFECTIOUS PROCESS

An example of the chain of infection in action can be used when considering an organism such as Campylobacter. Using the chain of infection we can identify how the organism can be transmitted and identify the areas of practice that can be improved, thus breaking the links in the chain.

The application of effective measures to control and prevent the spread of infection requires healthcare workers to plan a strategy for preventing infection. Three questions need to be asked:

1. What is the source of the infection?
2. Who or what is the susceptible host?
3. What is the means of transmission?

Disruption of the method of spread stops the progress of microbes. If a micro-organism is denied its normal mode of spread it will be unable to achieve its aim of causing infection. Once an individual understands how micro-organisms behave and function, the control and prevention of infection is possible.

REFERENCES

Benenson A S (ed.) 1995 Control of Communicable Diseases Manual, 16th edn. American Public Health Association, Washington DC

Horton R, Parker L 2002 Informed Infection Control, 2nd edn. Churchill Livingstone, Edinburgh

Shanson D C 1999 Microbiology in Clinical Practice, 3rd edn. Butterworth-Heinemann, Oxford

Wilson J 2001 Infection Control in Clinical Practice, 2nd edn. Baillière Tindall, Edinburgh

3

Public Health function

J. Howard

INTRODUCTION

Community Nurses who view infection control from a Public Health perspective can make an enormous contribution to the prevention and control of cross infection.

This chapter is concerned with Public Health from the perspective of infectious disease and infection control. The nature of Public Health practice is discussed briefly and related to infection control practice, but the main concern is to explain the function and the role of the Communicable Disease team as a core service within Public Health.

At the time of writing, the Department of Health, in a document entitled *Shifting the Balance of Power, Securing Delivery* (DoH 2001) has set out development of the National Health Service in England. There will be fundamental changes in organizational structures from April 2002 and the overall aim is to devolve the power base of the NHS from government to the local NHS services, thus enabling local people, both patients and professionals, to have more influence over the services to be delivered.

Primary Care Trusts will undertake most of the duties currently performed by Health Authorities. The number of Health Authorities will be reduced by two thirds, and they will then become known as Strategic Health Authorities with a responsibility for the performance management of Primary Care Trusts, Acute Trusts, and Care Trusts.

Nine Regional Offices will be retained, but they will be directly accountable to the Department of

Health and the Strategic Health Authorities will undertake some of their current duties.

The publication in January 2002 by the Chief Medical Officer for England of *Getting Ahead of the Curve: A Strategy for Combating Infectious Diseases* (including other aspects of health protection) (DoH 2002) makes it clear that Health Protection Functions (communicable disease/ infection control, non-infectious hazard control and emergency planning) will be undertaken within the Primary Care Trusts. However, the proposal is for Consultants in Communicable Disease Control and their teams, including the nurses, to be placed with local Health Protection Units, which will be part of a new agency to be established from April 2003 called The Health Protection Agency.

There is now a Director of Public Health on the Board of each Primary Care Trust. It is presumed that the communicable disease/infection control specialists will continue to work at a local level with the new Primary Care Trusts and that service level agreements will ensure they continue to support and be supported by the overall Public Health structures within these Trusts.

It is unclear at the time of writing how these services will be structured in Wales, Scotland and Northern Ireland.

WHAT IS PUBLIC HEALTH?

Public Health is widely defined as 'the science and art of preventing disease, prolonging life and promoting health through organised efforts of society' (Acheson 1988).

Acheson then goes on to summarize Public Health activities as follows:

- Monitoring and describing the health of the population
- Identifying those groups most in need of healthcare of all kinds and most likely to benefit from healthcare
- Identifying social, economic, environmental factors that impinge on health
- Taking action to promote and improve health
- Assessing the impact of healthcare and other interventions on the health of the population.

Public Health work involves action at a population or community level. This action is aimed at addressing the root causes of ill health rather than responding to the individual needs of those who are in ill health. In other words, a creative vision of Public Health does not start or end with the provision of health services (Caraher and McNab 1997). There are still many questions about the different perspectives of Public Health practice, but the one important point to emphasize is that Public Health is not an activity that takes place solely within the Public Health Department of a Primary Health Care Trust.

Two main types of activity are involved in Public Health practice:

- *Public Health as a resource*: This covers the activities of information gathering, i.e. surveillance and epidemiology, then using such information to underpin health service planning and activities to improve health generally (see Chapter 4).
- *Public Health action*: This covers the actual activities which promote health, prevent disease and maximize the benefits of clinical services. It should involve the actions of local authorities, Primary Care Trusts, NHS Trusts, community health services, business enterprises, community groups, voluntary groups and of course families and individuals (Peckham, Taylor and Turton 1998).

PUBLIC HEALTH STRATEGY

The White Paper *The New NHS, Modern and Dependable* (DoH 1997) sets out a new vision for the NHS based on collaboration rather than competition. The central themes of a Public Health approach to healthcare, that is, working in partnership and tackling inequalities, are very much in evidence in this vision for a new NHS. This approach was further strengthened by the publication of *Saving Lives: Our Healthier Nation* (DoH 1999a) and a government strategy for public health which advocates bringing together all the other government departments and assessing the impact on health of other policy decisions.

There are essentially three key points to this strategy:

- Concerted government action, i.e. intersectoral working between government departments
- Individual responsibility and partnership with government, i.e. local communities and individuals working together to deal with issues such as poor housing, social exclusion, poverty, and to improve health-related opportunities
- Enabling actions which allow individuals the opportunity to realize their own potential and influence their health (Whitehorn 1997).

The ultimate objective of this practice is a Public Health programme to improve the quality of life for the individual and the community.

This programme is called a Health Improvement Programme. The Health Authority role, as set out in *Delivering the Agenda* (DoH 1998) was one of strategic leadership, and they were given lead responsibility for ensuring that the programme was developed in partnership with the communities the particular Health Authority served. They were also responsible for ensuring that the programme was implemented and delivered within available resources.

Primary Care Trusts have now taken over this responsibility.

Local Authorities also produce a plan, which sets out their contribution to the health of the community. The Duty of Partnership is one of the most important aspects of a 'New NHS, Modern and Dependable', and it places an onus on all these different organizations to work together, thus preventing duplication of effort. The control of communicable diseases and non-infectious environmental hazards is central to this public health activity (DoH 1999b).

THE EVOLUTION OF PUBLIC HEALTH

The study of medicine is ancient and dates back more than 5000 years to the civilization of Egypt. It was based very much on the perceived pharmacological effects of plants on human diseases. The concept of prevention was not appreciated at that time.

Some of the first evidence of preventative health measures is to be found during the period of Brahmanism in India (600–500 BC). They describe the need for personal cleanliness and the need to keep public areas free of human excrement (Jepson 1997).

However, hygiene as a component of prevention was not truly recognized as a part of medicine until Pasteur, Semmelweis, Koch and Lister demonstrated the presence of living organisms and proved their ability to spread disease. This acceptance occurred relatively recently, 200 years ago (Gould 1987).

The conflict and dilemma between prevention and treatment has its roots in Ancient Greek beliefs, which centred on the worship of the Greek goddess Hygieia and the God of Medicine, Asklepios. Hygieia was associated with health, and people believed they would remain healthy if they lived life without excess or indulgence. Asklepios was probably a real doctor, and did not promote health as an art but as a practical issue of cure using herbal remedies and surgery. Consequently people perceived the concept of prevention, that is, hygiene, as an art and medicine as a science. Medicine had a much higher profile; its impact was more visible, and consequently hygiene – the preventative measure – was considered inferior.

At the end of the nineteenth and during the early twentieth century the understanding of hygiene was still strongly influenced by the Greek concept of clean living, and still today many infections continue to be associated with 'dirty living', particularly the parasitic and sexually-transmitted infections.

Today, the conflict still remains – prevention or cure? In Great Britain the National Health Service has finite resources. Difficult decisions have to be made when allocating resources to balance the funding of both the art and the science of modern medicine, the ultimate aim being to improve the public's health.

The first wave of public health action in the United Kingdom involved the far-reaching sanitary reforms of the mid 1800s. These involved measures to ensure bacteriologically safe water supplies and safe disposal of sewage. Diseases such as cholera, typhoid, and smallpox were causing severe morbidity and as medical science developed it became clear that concerted effort and political action were required to prevent and control these infectious diseases (see Box 3.1).

In Britain today the modern epidemics are linked to lifestyle choices, for example lung cancer and smoking. Nevertheless the infectious diseases remain important, still cause significant ill health and account for numerous visits to doctors and admissions to hospital. Antibiotics remain the most frequently prescribed medicines and infections account for economic losses as a result of absence from work (Plowman et al 2000).

McKeown (1979) argues in his book *The Role of Medicine* that it was the opportunities for employment, improved income and the environmental reforms which led to improvements in nutrition, hygiene and education and thus to an improvement in the health of the nation in the nineteenth and early twentieth centuries. Today where these opportunities do not exist, or exist in a limited form (including the UK), mortality and morbidity rates are higher. In many developing countries some infectious diseases are at epidemic level. Tuberculosis for example has been declared a global emergency by the World Health Organization (WHO 1996).

THE PUBLIC HEALTH AGENDA AND COMMUNICABLE DISEASE CONTROL

There are no explicit targets for the prevention and control of infectious disease in *Our Healthier Nation: a Contrary Opinion* (Mortimer 1998); however, a number of reports have served to emphasize that communicable disease control and infection control are important to the protection of the public health and to the provision of safe, effective healthcare services. These reports and health services circulars are listed in Box 3.2.

Box 3.2 Reports emphasizing need for prevention and control of infectious and communicable disease

1) Communicable Disease Surveillance Centre 1997 *A Survey of the Communicable Disease Control Function in England*. CDSC, London
2) Acheson D (Chair) 1998 *Public Health in England – Report on the enquiry into the future development of the Public Health function*. HMSO, London
3) House of Lords Select Committee on Science and Technology 1998 *Resistance to Antibiotics and other Antimicrobial agents*. HMSO, London
4) *Resistance to Antibiotics and other Antimicrobial Agents*, Health Service Circular 1999/049 – Action for NHS. DoH, London
5) Plowman R, Graves N, Griffin M et al (2000) *Socio-economic Burden of Hospital Acquired Infection*. Public Health Laboratory Service, London
6) National Audit Office February 2000 *The Management and Control of Hospital Acquired Infection in Acute NHS Trusts in England*, HC 230. National Audit Office, London

---

Box 3.1 Some historical perspectives of infectious disease prevention (source: DoH 1989)

1875 The first measures were introduced to prevent a person from knowingly infecting others.
1907 The first measures were introduced to ensure people did not work with a notifiable disease (powers allowing Local Authorities to compensate for loss of earnings appeared in 1961).
1907 The first restrictions on children to prevent the spread of disease were introduced.
1907 First legislation concerning the disposal and disinfection of infected articles.
1875 First measures to deal with infected premises and letting of rooms in a hotel or inn before disinfection had taken place.

1875 Measures to prevent an infected person using public transport. The infected person could be liable for the cost of disinfecting the vehicle.
1875 Provision appeared to ensure notification of infection in any lodging houses, and magistrates were given powers to close premises down.
1875 Measures were brought in covering the movement of bodies following death due to infection.
1907 Legislation disallowing wakes following death due to a notifiable disease.
1925 Persons in charge of premises were bound by law to restrict other people from coming into contact with an infected body following a death due to a notifiable disease.

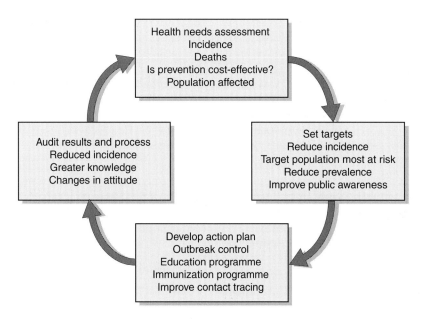

Figure 3.1 A health gain cycle – communicable disease.

The health protection agenda is central to any Health Improvement programme. This is realized for infectious disease by ensuring that Communicable Disease Control remains a core function of the Primary Care Trust Public Health department, as emphasized in government policy documents (NHSE 1997, 1999, DoH 2001, 2002). A communicable disease/infection control programme should be planned and delivered as a core public health function, aiming to:

- prevent and control infection by policy development, infection control audit, training and risk management
- ensure facilities are available to undertake surveillance and detection of communicable disease and infections
- advise on effective antibiotic policy treatment and care
- prevent and control infection by ensuring prompt contact tracing where applicable and follow-up of notifications of infectious diseases
- manage outbreaks effectively
- promote immunization programmes
- raise public awareness.

Box 3.3 Health needs assessment: the three elements*

1) Epidemiological – incidence, prevalence, natural history of infection, effectiveness of interventions
2) Comparative – i.e. how the situation compares with national or regional situations
3) Pragmatic – incorporating professional judgement of the situation and the views of others involved, including the public

*Adapted from Annual Report of the Director of Public Health, Shropshire Health Authority 1994

Programme development and decision-making processes are influenced throughout by adopting an epidemiological approach (see Chapter 4).

To achieve the aims of the programme on a population basis, a health gain cycle and health needs assessment are used (see Figure 3.1 and Box 3.3).

THE ROLE OF THE CONSULTANT IN COMMUNICABLE DISEASE CONTROL

Traditionally it was the Medical Officer of Health (MOH) who was responsible for all medical advice to the local authority on environmental and other issues including infection. The post of MOH disappeared during 1974 when local authority responsibilities for personal health were transferred to area health authorities. A Medical Officer for Environmental Health (MOEH) was now responsible for advice about infection; however, most were expected to combine the role with District Medical Officer. Much concern was expressed about this dual role and it was considered in the Acheson Report (1988) to be a significant factor during the investigation into deaths at Stanley Royd Hospital in August 1984 (see Chapter 4, Epidemiology and Surveillance).

Acheson recommended the appointment of a named leader for public health, that is, the Director of Public Health. Consequently the MOEH post was abolished and health authorities were to assign executive responsibility for necessary action on communicable disease and infection control to a district control of infection officer, subsequently known as Consultant in Communicable Disease Control (CCDC). This post is directly accountable to the Director of Public Health.

The CCDC is responsible for ensuring that the requirements under current legislation relating to infectious disease are met. There are four key legislative areas (see Appendix C at the end of this volume):

- Public Health
- Port Health
- Food Law
- Health and Safety.

The role is supported and undertaken by other public health specialists such as community infection control nurses, communicable disease nurses, HIV workers, immunization specialists, research analysts, data clerks and administrators. Immunization co-ordination, and overall co-ordination of HIV/AIDS services including ensuring treatment, care and prevention services, are usually part of the role. Other non-infectious disease responsibilities include emergency planning and environmental hazard protection.

Good working relationships and communication are essential between the CCDC team and local hospital and community trusts, local authority organizations, primary care groups/trusts and the private sector.

Nationally and regionally there is communication with other organizations such as the Public Health Laboratory Service and Communicable Disease Surveillance Centre. This is central to the effective surveillance, prevention and control of infectious disease (see Chapter 4, Epidemiology and Surveillance).

External agencies in collaboration include Department of the Environment, Food and Rural Affairs, veterinary laboratories, water companies, private food analysis laboratories and the Environment Agency.

COMMUNICABLE DISEASE CONTROL

Box 3.4 sets out the elements to the control of communicable disease.

The executive responsibilities of the CCDC can be divided into two broad categories, operational and strategic.

Operational responsibilities

- Managing outbreaks in the community and in hospitals if there are implications to the community as a whole
- A reactive advice service to the population
- Teaching and education
- Monitoring health of immigrants.

Strategic responsibilities

- The surveillance of communicable disease
- Policy development

Box 3.4 Control of communicable disease: the three elements

- Knowing and appreciating the causative agent, its mode of transmission, risk to public health and relevant control measures
- Knowledge of the environment to enable effective management of the situation
- Deciding the appropriate method of investigations based on social/epidemiological strategies.

- Developing outbreak plans
- Preventative services
- Immunization co-ordination
- Advice service – to all organizations in the community
- Liaison with other groups such as local authorities, public health laboratories, hospital infection control teams, veterinary groups
- Audit and research
- Advice on services required to Primary Care Trusts and NHS Trusts.

THE PROPER OFFICER AND THE NOTIFICATION SYSTEM

A number of communicable diseases are notifiable (see Box 3.5).

Clinicians are paid a small fee for each notification form sent in to the Proper Officer. Doctors in England and Wales have a statutory duty to notify to the Proper Officer of the Local Authority (usually the Consultant in Communicable Disease Control) cases of certain infectious diseases. This statutory requirement began over one hundred years ago and is now a legal requirement under the Public Health (Control of Disease) Act 1984 (HMSO 1984) and the Public Health (Infectious Diseases) Regulations 1988 (HMSO 1988a) (McCormick 1993).

McCormick highlights five important points, which must be made clear within the infectious diseases notification system. These are set out in Box 3.6.

The Proper Officer is appointed by the Local Authority to be the designated person to receive notifications (under Section 101 of Local Government Act 1972) (Meredith Davies 1983). The Proper Officer also receives information from food- and milk-producing premises if someone is known to be suffering from specific conditions or carrying an infection such as typhoid or salmonella.

Because the Proper Officer is usually the CCDC (i.e. the named individual within the Primary Care Trust responsible for communicable disease and infection control), then prompt action can be taken to prevent further infection. These actions include surveillance (see Chapter 4, Epidemiology and Surveillance):

- Ongoing surveillance of trends in infectious disease locally
- National surveillance because under current law the Proper Officer is required to send the Office of National Census weekly returns of the number of cases of disease notified

---

Box 3.5 Notifiable diseases

Diseases notifiable under the Public Health (Control of Disease) Act 1984

Cholera	Smallpox
Plague	Typhus
Relapsing fever	Food poisoning

Diseases notifiable under the Public Health (Infectious Diseases) Regulation 1988

Acute encephalitis	Ophthalmia
Anthrax	neonatorum
Acute poliomyelitis	Paratyphoid fever
Diphtheria	Rabies
Dysentery (amoebic or bacillary)	Rubella
Leprosy	Scarlet fever
Leptospirosis	Tetanus
Malaria	Tuberculosis
Measles	Typhoid fever
Meningitis	Viral haemorrhagic
Meningococcal	fever
septicaemia	Viral hepatitis
(without meningitis)	Whooping cough
Mumps	Yellow fever

Food poisoning is also notifiable and subject to certain controls under the various food hygiene regulations and laws.

AIDS is not strictly notifiable but is covered by separate legislation – the AIDS Control Act 1989.

Box 3.6 Requirements of the notification system

- Who is notifying – should be the doctor attending the patient when diagnosed
- What is the infection – any clinically manifested disease on notifiable list
- When is it notified – date infection is suspected or diagnosed
- How is it notified – on designated form available from Proper Officer (usually a CCDC) or by telephone if urgent action required
- To whom is it notified – Proper Officer (usually CCDC) of the local authority district where patient is diagnosed

- Regional surveillance; information on each disease notified is sent (usually electronically) to the Regional Epidemiologist of the Communicable Disease Surveillance Centre (CDSC), then forwarded to CDSC London to be collated nationally.

Prompt action to control the disease is particularly important where it is known contacts can become symptomless carriers or the case is working in at-risk situations or a patient in a hospital or nursing home.

CONTACT TRACING

For certain infectious diseases, contact tracing is an important preventative activity. A contact is defined as someone who has had contact with the infected person during the time they were thought to be infectious. The precise nature of the contact depends on the infectious disease concerned. Contact tracing is commonly undertaken for tuberculosis, meningitis, sexually-transmitted diseases, gastrointestinal infections, Hepatitis B and C, scabies and headlice.

There are broad aims in identifying contacts:

- to screen contacts to identify if cross infection has occurred
- to offer prompt prophylaxis if appropriate
- to offer prompt treatment to infected contacts
- to prevent further spread of the disease.

A contact tracing service should offer information to the person involved and be available to offer support and advice and allay anxiety about the nature of the infection. An effective service requires the co-operation of primary care, general practitioners and hospital physicians to implement.

The CCDC is responsible for ensuring policies and protocols are available to guide the contact tracing activity, and subsequent administration of prophylaxis, screening or treatment facilities.

IMMUNIZATION

Edward H. Jenner (1749–1823) first recorded his observations in 1796 that people previously inoculated with cowpox were protected against smallpox. However, it took nearly 200 years for smallpox to be eradicated as the result of a world-wide immunization programme (Parker 1990).

Today, the Immunization Co-ordinator is responsible for ensuring a complete immunization service is available: this involves strategic planning and cross-agency co-operation. Comprehensive information on vaccination schedules, indications and contraindications is available (DoH 1996).

A comprehensive immunization service encompasses:

- a neonatal immunization programme
- a childhood immunization programme (Box 3.7)
- an adult immunization programme for adults in special risk situations, e.g. healthcare workers, flu vaccine for the over 75 s
- access to immunizations needed for travel to at-risk countries
- access to prophylactic immunization following exposure to certain infectious diseases, e.g. chickenpox, Hepatitis B, Hepatitis A

Box 3.7 Primary immunization programme in the United Kingdom (source: DoH 1996)

Full implementation of this programme will ensure children will have received the following vaccines:

• By age of 6 months – 3 doses of	diphtheria pertussis tetanus polio haemophilus influenzae B meningitis C
• By age 15 months	measles/mumps/rubella
• By school entry, 4th dose	diphtheria pertussis polio tetanus
and 2nd dose	measles/mumps/rubella
• Between age 10 and 14 years	BCG
• Before leaving school, 5th dose	polio tetanus diphtheria

- capacity to deliver immunization following an outbreak, e.g. meningitis C
- capacity to respond to national calls for a mass immunization programme, e.g. measles/rubella campaign (1995) and meningitis C campaign (1999–2000).

With the exception of the childhood immunization programme and mass immunization programmes, the other centrally-led immunization programmes are based on various risk assessment processes.

At patient level criteria set out in the Immunization Against Infectious Diseases information (DoH 1996) guide individual risk assessment and the immunizing nurse is responsible for ensuring that there are no contraindications and that informed consent is obtained.

The role of the immunization co-ordinator is one of policy development and strategic leadership. They work with the immunizing personnel to ensure educational opportunities are available to maintain competencies.

Figures for uptake of the childhood immunization programme are collated nationally and distributed as a percentage uptake locally. Uptake must remain above certain percentages to retain herd immunity and prevent re-emergence of infections. If a fall in uptake occurs locally, the Immunization Co-ordinator is responsible for investigating possible causes and negotiating initiatives to improve uptake, such as evening clinics, vaccination in the home and public awareness campaigns. The challenge is now to ensure immunization uptake levels remain high enough to retain herd immunity.

In the UK today there is an active anti-immunization lobby. An anti-vaccination lobby was known to exist in 1802 against smallpox vaccine (DoH 1996). Legislation to make vaccination enforceable had been tried initially in 1842; this was very unpopular and finally withdrawn in 1948.

If vaccine uptake does fall, community practitioners will be seeing cases of measles, mumps, rubella or whooping cough in increasing numbers and for many it will be their first experience of supporting families when these infections cause serious complications or even death.

PUBLIC HEALTH AND PORT HEALTH

Many CsCDC undertake the role of Port Medical Inspectors. For more detail on this role and the link with the control of communicable diseases, see Chapter 17, Prisoners, travellers, the homeless and refugees.

THE ROLE OF THE ENVIRONMENTAL HEALTH OFFICER

Environmental health is defined by the World Health Organization (WHO) in the *Report of the Committee of Enquiry into the Future Development of the Public Health Function* as being 'the control of all those factors in man's physical environment which exercise, or may exercise, a deleterious effect on his physical development, health or survival' (HMSO 1988b). This is a broad concept and forms one important facet of Public Health practice. The objective of the environmental health organization as a whole is to prevent, detect and control environmental hazards which affect human health. To do this, Environmental Health Officers are involved together with other agencies in the following:

- waste management
- food control
- housing
- epidemiological control
- air quality management
- occupational health and safety
- water resource management
- noise control
- protection of recreational environment
- radiation protection
- port health, immigration issues, asylum seekers
- educational activities.

Within all these areas there is a clear law-enforcement role as well as education and prevention roles. It must be emphasized that the Environmental Health Officer (EHO) role also encompasses the promotion of environmental health, quality standards and the education of the public and industry in safe practices as they relate to the relevant areas listed.

In addition, collaborative work with other agencies is undertaken locally, nationally and internationally to study the effects of environmental hazards and to assess the environmental impact of such hazards.

The EHO works closely with members of the Public Health Department, particularly those responsible for communicable diseases and environmental hazard control (WHO 1987). A professional profile for EHOs emphasizes that environmental health is very much a team concept and cannot be successful without good liaison. The EHO is trained as a generalist across the areas previously listed, although many specialize and develop expertise in particular areas of practice such as food safety, waste management or water resources. When a particular problem needs to be managed, the EHO brings an understanding of the environmental aspects of the actual problem and the environmental context within which a solution can be found.

THE ROLE OF THE COMMUNITY INFECTION CONTROL NURSE (CICN)

The nurse provides a specialized service which enables others (including nurses) to prevent and control infection. The CICN may work in a Public Health Department as part of the CCDC team; the membership of the team varies depending on where the nurse is employed. A key element of the role is to work in partnership (see Box 3.8). Partners include professionals, outside agencies, outside organizations, multidisciplinary groups and the public. Change of practice and changes in perception are frequently necessary to ensure adequate infection control across a given population, therefore effective working relationships across a range of agencies as outlined in Box 3.8 are essential to the role. CICNs employed by Community and Primary Care Trusts should be the key contact for all issues relating to infection control within that Trust, as they are usually the only member of the infection control team employed full-time in the speciality. Their role encompasses all the services within the Trust, and community nurses should attempt to involve them where new services are being developed, new premises designed or old premises rebuilt. Early advice about infection control issues can frequently stem serious problems at a later time. The role bears similarities to that of an ICN working in an acute hospital trust, but the settings and cross infection risks are different, as the chapters in this book emphasize.

INCORPORATING PUBLIC HEALTH APPROACHES WITHIN THE NURSING ROLE

Cowley (1999) explores the theoretical framework and the concept of moving Public Health in practice from population to people and states:

Activities are justified as public health interventions if their main purpose is to contribute to the health of

---

Box 3.8 Potential partners for the Community Infection Control Nurse

- The public
- Public Health Laboratory Service
- Department of Microbiology
- AIDS Co-ordinator
- Environmental Health Departments (local authority)
- Occupational Health Departments (NHS and private)
- Staff of all Directorates
- Health and Safety Advisers (NHS and private)
- School of Health Studies, University
- Local Education Establishments/Colleges
- Environment Agency
- Department of the Environment, Food and Rural Affairs
- Veterinary services
- Local prisons
- Public Health Department
- CCDC

- Infection Control Nurses – Trusts
- Consultant Microbiologists
- Nurse Executives
- Commission for Care Standards
- Department Public Health Medicine
- Infection Control Nursing Association
- Professional Nursing Bodies
- UKCC
- Community Practitioner and Health Visitor Association
- Royal College of Nursing
- Local Authority Education Department
- Social Services Department
- Community Health Trust
- Private/Voluntary sector care
- Mental Health Trust
- General medical practices
- General dental practices

the whole population they serve, even though they meet the immediate health needs of individuals and families along the way.

The Budapest Declaration of Health Promoting Hospitals (WHO 1991) discusses the role of nurses in hospitals in relation to Public Health. *Making it Happen* (SNMAC 1995) set out a clear role for nurses in Public Health, and finally *Saving Lives: Our Healthier Nation* (DoH 1999a) has reinforced this role for community nurses.

The Royal College of Nursing (1994) describes three levels at which Public Health approaches are incorporated within nursing practice. These are:

- individual level
- total population, group or community level
- policy level, national and/or local campaign level.

Infection Control Nurses often carry out these three levels of Public Health activity simultaneously.

A Public Health approach must stem from a collective overview and population-based health analysis, so for example the health professional who advises an informal carer in the home to hand wash correctly is undertaking a Public Health role, as this advice stems from a collective overview of all the evidence available on the role of hands in spreading infection and will, if implemented, protect the social circle (i.e. the population base).

Community Nurse specialists who will now be prescribing from the Nurses' National Formulary will need to take this collective overview before prescribing to treat scabies or headlice, as outbreaks of these two infections often involve an extensive Public Health approach to affect control and containment.

Nurses who take a wider view when considering infection control issues affecting an individual will perform a series of tasks.

Undertaking analysis

- How is the problem affecting the individual and family?
- Is the problem isolated?
- Is the problem part of a wider infection control issue?

Centralizing the problem in relation to research findings

- Consider the epidemiology of the infection.
- Assess the risks in the current situation.

Planning

- Nursing intervention
- Infection control interventions, e.g. use of protective clothing, clinical waste disposal.

Networking

- Training programmes for significant others, e.g. respite carers
- Inform relevant departments
- Inform relevant others, e.g. family, informal carers.

Embracing multidisciplinary working

- Involve relevant others, e.g. HIV nurse specialist, Environmental Health Officer, Infection Control Nurse, TB nurse.

Undertaking development work

- Especially enabling strategies, e.g. information to help relatives or carers cope with infection
- Information to alleviate fears
- Pragmatic solutions to infection control problems which enable patients to maximize all care and opportunities.

Teaching

- Implement education/training programmes for carers, informal carers, respite carers – this does not need to be extensive and can involve simple activities such as reading an information leaflet together, answering queries, etc. Structures to support all community nurses in taking this wider view include:
  — infection control guidelines and protocols
  — an infection control link nurse network
  — community ICN (in some areas)
  — public health on-call services
  — microbiology on-call service.

Selecting the most appropriate method to initiate Public Health action depends upon the health area targeted, and this may be best undertaken through individual interactions (RCN 1994). It must however be emphasized that nurses, midwives and health visitors are not only hands-on professionals delivering care to individuals but have also an important strategic role to play in the development and implementation of local health improvement initiatives (Cornish and Knight 2000) including those which prevent and control communicable disease and infectious disease.

REFERENCES

Acheson D 1988 Public Health in England. HMSO, London

Caraher M, McNab M 1997 Using lessons from health visiting past to inform the public health role. Health Visitor 70(10): 380–384

Cornish Y, Knight T 2000 Exploring Public Health Career Paths, Joint Report SE Institute of Public Health, University of Birmingham Health Service Management Centre and NHS Executive, London

Cowley S 1999 From Population to People, Public Health in Practice. Community Practitioner 72(4): April

Department of Health 1989 Review of the law on infectious disease control, Consultative Document. DoH, London

Department of Health 1996 Immunization against infectious diseases. HMSO, London

Department of Health 1997 The New NHS, Modern and Dependable. The Stationery Office, London

Department of Health 1998 Delivering the Agenda. National Health Service Executive, London

Department of Health 1999a Saving Lives: Our Healthier Nation. The Stationery Office, London

Department of Health 1999b HSC 999, Leadership for Health. National Health Service Executive, London

Department of Health 2001 Shifting the Balance of Power, Securing Delivery. The Stationery Office, London

Department of Health 2002 Getting Ahead of the Curve. A strategy for combating infectious diseases (including other aspects of health protection). A Report by the Chief Medical Officer for England. Department of Health, London

Gould D 1987 Infection and Patient Care: A Guide for Nurses. Heinemann, London

HMSO 1984 Public Health (Control of Disease) Act 1984. HMSO, London

HMSO 1988a The Public Health (Infectious Diseases) Regulations 1988. HMSO, London

HMSO 1988b Report of the Committee of Enquiry into the Future Development of the Public Health Function, Cmmd. 289. HMSO, London

Jepson O B 1997 Worldwide importance of infection control, cited in Research and Clinical Forums 19(6)

McCormick A 1993 The notification of infectious diseases in England and Wales. Communicable Disease Report 3(2): 29 Jan 1993

McKeown T 1979 The Role of Medicine. Blackwell, Oxford

Meredith Davies J B 1983 Community Health, Preventative Medicine and Social Services. Baillière Tindall, London

Mortimer P 1998 Our Healthier Nation: a contrary opinion. Communicable Disease and Public Health 1: 3

National Health Service Executive 1997 Public health: responsibilities of the NHS and the roles of others. HSG (93), 56. NHSE, Leeds

National Health Service Executive 1999 Resistance to Antibiotics and other Antimicrobial Agents, NHSE, Leeds

Parker L 1990 From Pestilence to Asepsis. Journal of Infection Control Nursing, NT (86): 49, Dec 5

Peckham S, Taylor P, Turton, P 1998 A public health model of primary care – from concept to reality. A research document. Public Health Alliance, 138 Digbeth, Birmingham, B5 6DR

Plowman R, Graves N, Griffin M 2000 The socio-economic burden of hospital acquired infection. Public Health Laboratory Service, London

Royal College of Nursing 1994 Public Health Nursing Rises to the Challenge. Royal College of Nursing, London

SNMAC (Standing Nursing and Midwifery Advisory Committee) 1995 Making it Happen – Public Health, the contribution, role and development of nurses, midwives and health visitors. Department of Health, London

Whitehorn K 1997 Health of the Nation – A prescription to tackle all of society's ills. The Observer, London, May 11 1997

World Health Organization 1987 Development of Environmental Health Manpower, EH series 18. WHO Regional Offices for Europe, Copenhagen

World Health Organization 1991 The Budapest Declaration of Health Promoting Hospitals. WHO, Copenhagen

World Health Organization 1996 Fighting Disease, Fostering Development. Report of the Director General. WHO, Geneva

4

Epidemiology and surveillance

J. Howard

INTRODUCTION

The word 'epidemiology' is derived from the Greek and means 'studies upon people'. It has been further defined as 'the study of the distribution and determinants of health and disease frequencies in populations for the purpose of promoting wellness and preventing disease' (McMahon and Pugh 1970).

Epidemiology became an established scientific discipline in the twentieth century, although epidemiological reasoning goes back to ancient times. Hippocrates in his writings on Airs, Waters and Places commented that the physician should investigate matters such as the climate and geographical situation of a locality, the waters used by the inhabitants and 'the mode in which inhabitants live and what their pursuits, whether they are fond of excess and given to indolence or are fond of exercise and labour' (Friedman 1985).

Like all scientific disciplines, epidemiology has its own techniques for collection and interpretation of data, and uses specific technical terms (see Glossary). The epidemiologist is concerned with the diagnosis and treatment of disease at a whole population level rather than at an individual level. Epidemiological studies place the role of medicine and nursing as practised at an individual level into a wider perspective.

An American Public Health Nurse (Valanis 1986) describes epidemiology thus:

… in practice terms (epidemiology) is the study of how various states of health are distributed in the population and what environmental conditions, life styles, or other circumstances are associated with the presence or absence of disease. Epidemiologists are essentially medical detectives concerned with the who, what, where, when and how of disease causation. By searching to find who does and who does not get sick with a particular disease and determining where the illness is and is not found, under what particular circumstances, epidemiologists narrow down the suspected causal agents. When an agent is finally identified, public health officials can take steps to prevent or control the occurrence of the disease.

The epidemiological approach underlines the fact that improvements in health result from a wide range of interventions:

• changes in personal behaviour
• effective medicine and care
• changes in the physical and psychosocial environment.

The science of epidemiology is the cornerstone of public health policy and preventative medicine, and also makes a contribution to clinical medicine (Stolley and Laskey 1995). It has become known as a medical speciality, although it is now increasingly carried out by non-medical personnel including medical scientists, statisticians, medical geographers, nurses, professions allied to medicine and environmental health officers.

THE HISTORICAL PERSPECTIVE

During a cholera epidemic in London in 1848–9, the London Epidemiological Society was founded and John Snow was a member.

Snow subsequently investigated this cholera outbreak and published a clear description of his activities in 1854, 'On the Mode of Communication of Cholera'.

He reasoned that spread followed international trade routes. He also reasoned in this publication that 'diseases which are communicated from person to person are caused by some material which passes from the sick to the healthy'. Using classic epidemiological techniques he formed an hypothesis, that cholera occurred when water contaminated with infected human faeces was consumed. To this end he described outbreaks of cholera

associated with a contaminated well on Thomas Street, a burst drain in Albion Terrace and finally among the persons drinking water from the Broad Street pump. Here the people who died of cholera had all consumed water from this pump. He used mapping techniques to demonstrate this by removing the pump handle, which resulted in a decline in the number of cholera cases. The handle was later reinstated, and not finally removed until 1856 when a number of other contaminated wells were also closed. Snow expanded his hypothesis to include the distribution of cholera via all water systems where the water companies used contaminated supplies.

William Farr's statistical work supported Snow's hypothesis, and during another cholera outbreak in 1853 Snow tested this hypothesis in what he describes as an 'experiment'. This experiment involved ascertaining the water supply company that each cholera victim used. He found that mortality in persons consuming water supplied by the Southwark and Vauxhall Company was ten times higher compared to that supplied by the Lambeth Company and five times higher than the rest.

Snow was a methodical and accurate worker, and his example provided an example for future workers although a structured approach to epidemiology did not emerge until the 1930s.

Snow's original hypothesis about cholera being caused by contaminated water was proven when in 1882 Koch isolated the organism *Vibrio cholerae* (Stolley and Laskey 1995).

The main objective of epidemiology in the late nineteenth and early twentieth century was the investigation, study and control of infectious diseases. Today it is also used to investigate the modern epidemics such as coronary heart disease, drug abuse, suicides and child abuse, and the efficiency of screening programmes, and therapeutic regimes.

THE EPIDEMIOLOGICAL APPROACH

This approach accepts that very few diseases, including infectious diseases, have one single cause. Most are the result of a complex set of circumstances which underlie or exacerbate the

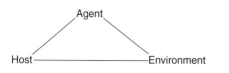

Figure 4.1   The causes of disease (Robinson and Elkan 1996).

cause of the disease. As Figure 4.1 shows, this complexity can be viewed in the form of a triangle.

This concept is of particular importance to infectious disease, as not everyone exposed to an infectious agent will develop disease.

- The agent is the organism, for example bacterium, virus, parasite or fungus.
- The host is the susceptible individual or population. Susceptibility is linked to factors such as herd immunity, heredity, immunity and predisposing disease.
- The environmental factors are the wider determinants of health such as poverty, living conditions, social exclusion, and access to healthcare.

Increasingly factors such as climate change and demographic changes are influencing the environment and in many areas of the world civil strife and forced movements of peoples are important factors in the epidemiology of infectious diseases.

SURVEILLANCE IN COMMUNICABLE DISEASE AND INFECTION CONTROL

Surveillance has been defined as:

1. The systemic, active, ongoing observation of the occurrence and distribution of disease in a population. It is important to recognize that the definition also includes analysis of data and dissemination of results so that appropriate action can be taken (Hughes 1987).

2. The continued watchfulness over the distribution and trends of incidence through the systematic collection, consolidation and evaluation of morbidity and mortality reports and other relevant data (Langmuir 1963).

A well-defined existing methodology should be used so that the actual process of surveillance can contribute to the epidemiological function as a whole.

The overall objectives of an infectious disease surveillance programme are:

- to facilitate the early recognition of changes in the pattern of any disease
- to identify any changes in environmental and host factors that may lead to an increase in the frequency of disease
- to monitor the safety and effectiveness of preventative and control measures
- to provide information to clinicians on prevalent infections so that action can be taken
- to collect data on rare diseases for epidemiological studies
- to evaluate actions taken for effectiveness.

Box 4.1 gives an early example and a more recent example of surveillance in practice.

PATTERNS OF COMMUNICABLE DISEASE AND INFORMATION SOURCES

Patterns of communicable disease are continuously changing, and any assessment of the risk they pose to a given population may become dated in a relatively short period of time. The factors which influence these changes are complex. They include:

- genetic changes in microbiological agents
- global changes in climate
- movements of populations
- discovery of new antibiotics
- development of new vaccines
- changes in socioeconomic/psychosocial status of populations due to war, famine, poverty, environmental disaster
- changes in patterns of healthcare delivery
- demographic changes in population, e.g. increase in elderly population.

It therefore follows that a wide variety of information sources are required to inform communicable

---

Box 4.1 Early and recent examples of surveillance in practice

In London during the sixteenth century a scheme began to monitor plague. Its aim was to inform the Royal Court when to leave London to avoid the disease.

Parish burial registers were first kept in 1538, at first only sporadically during plague years. By the seventeenth century in London, regular weekly burial returns were being submitted to the Hall of the Parish Clerks Company where death statistics for the City of London were compiled and issued as a 'bill of mortality' so that people were aware of plague in particular and could leave the city.

This early system embodies the principles of modern surveillance systems, i.e. data collection, analysis to produce statistics, interpretation to provide information and dissemination to inform action (Galbraith 1982).

A more recent example demonstrates the relevance of surveillance data to one aspect of the 1999/2000 Meningitis C vaccination programme undertaken in the United Kingdom.

Established routine surveillance data collected via the Statutory Notification System (see Chapter 3) formed the basis for decision making about how the programme was to be introduced. Population age groups shown to be most at risk of contracting Meningitis C were targeted first, and the remaining age groups were then targeted during the year-long programme in risk order.

Using surveillance data in this way enabled a planned approach based on risk assessment which was manageable and justifiable given the large number of children to be vaccinated within the time scale. Continued surveillance of cases of serogroup C meningococcal infection saw a fall of 75% in the number of reported cases in the initial age groups vaccinated (PHLS 2000).

Box 4.2 Information sources: general

Demographic data http://www.ons.gov.uk (Office of National Censuses)
Vital statistics, e.g. death rate
Performance Assessment data – http://www.doh.gov.uk/indicat/media.pdf
Hospital Activity data – via information department of the Health Authority
Deprivation indicators – Townsend and Jarman Scores, Department of Environment, Z Score. Available from local health authority information departments and local authority departments
Annual Report, Director of Public Health
Annual Report, Chief Medical Officer – http://www.doh.gov.uk/cmo/execsum
Survey data – local public health department
Survey data – Cabinet Office, People Panel – http://www.cabinet-office.gov.uk/servicefirst/index/pphome.htm
Local authority data, including:
    General population data
    Social services data
    Leisure data
    Education/Schoolchildren data
    Housing information
    Transport information
    Environmental Health data

Box 4.3 Information sources: Communicable Disease and Infection Control

Statutory notification of infectious diseases
Non-statutory notification of infections, e.g. the school notification system
Reports from microbiology laboratory
In-patient activity data
Cause of death registrations
Birth registrations
Prescribing information in Primary Care
Vaccine coverage figures
International surveillance systems
Primary care diagnoses notification via designated GP practices (Spotter Practices)
Reported outbreaks and incidents
Diagnoses of sexually transmitted diseases
Submission of food and water specimens for analysis
National enhanced surveillance systems for specific diseases, e.g. tuberculosis, E. coli 0157

---

disease control and infection control. These are illustrated in Boxes 4.2 and 4.3. It is essential to be able to access information in this way because of the complexities of infectious disease causation.

The data sources listed also provide key information about the wider determinants of health such as housing, sanitation, clean water or clean air. McKeown (1979) felt that improvements in these wider determinants of health were hugely significant in reducing mortality and morbidity rates due to infectious disease in the United Kingdom during the nineteenth and twentieth centuries, and they continue to influence the prevalence and control of infection today.

The collection of data and analysis is of very little practical use to those attempting to control infection unless there is a mechanism for feeding the collated information back. Box 4.4 lists some of these feedback mechanisms.

Box 4.4 Feedback and information from collated data

The Public Health Laboratory Service has its own web site (www.phls.co.uk) where electronic versions of the Communicable Disease Report and the journal *Communicable Disease and Public Health* are available.
Other sources include:

- Electronic bulletin *Eurosurveillance Weekly* (www.eurosurv.org)
- *Eurosurveillance Monthly* (paper copy and www.ceses.org/eurosurv)
- *Morbidity and Mortality Weekly Report* (www.cdc.gov/)
- World Health Organisation's Weekly Epidemiological Record (www.who.ch/wer/wer-home.htm)

Box 4.5 An example of an epidemiological description

- Campylobacter spp. is found in the intestines of most animals and is part of their normal flora
- May cause disease in sheep
- Transmission to humans occurs via food or via contamination of the environment
- Common infection world-wide
- Incidence is seasonal with a rise in cases during summer months
- Large outbreaks may be due to contamination of water or milk with animal faeces
- Undercooked poultry is regularly associated with infection
- In families the presence of a kitten or puppy with diarrhoea may cause infection
- It is unusual for the infected person to spread the infection
- The infected person may carry the organism for some weeks
- See also Chin 2000, Cruikshank 1992

INVESTIGATING AND CONTROLLING AN OUTBREAK OF INFECTIOUS DISEASE

The recognized definition of an outbreak is two or more linked cases of infection, which suggest a common source or person-to-person spread (Cruikshank 1992).

Clearly an outbreak involving a food-related organism linked to a particular venue, that is, a local outbreak, is relatively easy to recognize, investigate and control using standard epidemiological techniques. A disseminated outbreak across a region or country is much more difficult to recognize and it is here that the processing and interpretation of routine surveillance data plays such an important part in the initial recognition of the problem.

The notification system and the communication systems which extend from local to international are discussed in Chapter 3, and practice points in Chapter 16 give some indication of how infection can spread both locally and nationally.

Although food-related infections are used for illustration purposes in both this chapter and Chapter 16, the principles remain the same for any infection.

Investigating an outbreak will draw on available routine surveillance data, medical knowledge, and follow standard epidemiological techniques.

Descriptive epidemiology as used in outbreak control demonstrates associations which help form an opinion or judgement about causality, but does not claim to prove this causality. Box 4.5 is an example of an epidemiological description.

Precise analytical studies can be undertaken to confirm the cause or causes of the outbreak (see Further Reading section). A combination between microbiology and epidemiology is usually the accepted way forward. For example, legionella isolated in water systems may only be colonizing the system, not causing a health problem. However, epidemiological evidence will provide any link between the contaminated water and incidence of disease.

It must be remembered that epidemiological findings can have major political, economic and social implications, and can therefore be affected by prevailing attitudes and the major issues that are of current concern to society. This makes it essential for the epidemiologist to adopt a robust scientific approach. The key advantages of adopting a structured scientific approach when attempting to control outbreaks of infectious disease can be summarized as follows (Stolley and Laskey 1995):

- It brings reason to bear where there is human suffering.
- It combats the myths and superstitions which still abound concerning the transmission of infection.

- It helps alleviate public fears quickly.
- During large outbreaks or epidemics it can help prevent social disruption.
- It structures the search for a cause.

THE OUTBREAK TEAM

Comprehensive investigation will involve the formation of an outbreak team by the Consultant in Communicable Disease Control (CCDC). Composition of this team will depend on the type of outbreak under investigation and may include:

- Consultant in Communicable Disease Control – Chairperson
- Consultant Microbiologist
- Community Infection Control Nurse
- Environmental Health Officer
- Statisticians
- Veterinarian
- Other clinicians
- Representatives of organizations where the outbreak is occurring, e.g. a school or nursing home
- Other clinical experts
- Regional or national experts.

Other relevant persons may be invited to join the team as the initial investigation progresses and outbreak control measures are agreed.

There are a number of key steps undertaken by the outbreak team during the investigation and control of an outbreak. These steps may be undertaken in sequence but usually a number will be happening simultaneously; therefore frequent meetings of the outbreak team are crucial to ensure co-ordination and that everyone is clear about their role.

KEY STAGES IN THE INVESTIGATION AND CONTROL OF AN OUTBREAK

Task of the initial enquiry

- Confirm that the reports of an outbreak are true.
- Establish a diagnosis based on clinical information and microbiological findings.
- Set out a case definition of the disease.

— A case definition may be based on microbiological or serological findings or on a particular set of signs and symptoms presenting in the affected person within a defined time period.
- The above information together with information from the affected persons, their carers, if relevant, or family members, should allow the outbreak team to form a possible hypothesis as to the sources and route of spread of the infection (see Box 4.6).

Box 4.6 Summary of a preliminary investigation of an outbreak of diarrhoea and vomiting using a descriptive epidemiological methodology

Evening wedding reception at anonymous public house – Saturday
Also lunch time reception at same hotel – only 2 of those who were ill went to both
Approximately 80 people attended evening reception
So far contacted 46 (know of another 9)
33/46 ill
Most people had nausea and either vomiting (violent) or diarrhoea or both by early Monday morning–late Monday
Also aching, stomach cramps, fever, malaise. Lasted approximately 24 hours
No secondary cases so far
No one ill at reception
Those who didn't eat didn't become ill
Landlord – prepared food for 80 people with one assistant
Beef and pork sandwiches – beef cooked and used on carvery previous Sunday then frozen
Pork prepared same way
Egg sandwiches – hard boiled and with bought mayonnaise
Vol au vent – frozen bought-in cases; bought in pâté filling
Sausage roll and scotch egg frozen bought-in
Landlord ill 2 days before reception
Assistant ill 2 days before reception
No food available for sampling
Stool specimens × 4 sent for analysis including specimens from landlord and assistant

Actions:

1) Pursue microbiology – food handlers and guests
2) Obtain guest list from bridegroom
3) Questionnaire – prepare and send to all guests
4) Premises to be visited by environmental health officers
5) Landlord and assistant excluded from preparing food, which in effect closes the public house

Tentative hypothesis – illness resulted from consumption of food at evening wedding party. Landlord and assistant possibly source of infection when preparing food

• Tentative infection control measures are implemented – the aim being to interrupt the spread of infection as soon as possible.

Further management of an outbreak

Further management of the outbreak will depend on the findings at preliminary enquiry. Epidemiological fieldwork will continue using descriptive epidemiological techniques. These include:

• describing the disease in detail from its mildest to most severe form
• describing the natural history of the disease, e.g. if left untreated does it resolve?
• describing characteristics of the affected persons (e.g. age, gender, employment, residence) and looking for commonality
• searching for additional cases which may not have been recognized or reported
• mapping the distribution of cases
• calculating an attack rate (number of cases plotted against time)
• refining the case definition as necessary
• formulating questionnaires, which will identify factors and activities associated with the outbreak (Fig. 4.2).

As the investigation progresses infection control measures can be modified, and the implementation monitored.

Throughout the process all communications with the press, public and other professionals are issued via the outbreak team. Usually the CCDC has the final say on content.

This structured approach to an outbreak is vital. To illustrate this, Box 4.7 briefly outlines the course of the now famous outbreak at the Stanley Royd Hospital in 1985 and the subsequent death of 19 patients. Lack of prompt action and lack of leadership were all identified as contributing factors to the disastrous consequences of this outbreak.

Sir Donald Acheson (1988) headed the enquiry into the circumstances of the outbreak. Current organizational structures for the control of communicable disease as discussed in Chapter 3 are the result of the recommendations made following this enquiry.

A GLOBAL VIEW OF INFECTIOUS DISEASE CONTROL

Globally there are still 21 million deaths per year among those aged under 50 years; most of them are due to infections and many are preventable (WHO 1996). Interventions such as immunization, personal hygiene, public health and sanitation practices and the safe processing, preparation and handling of food would do much to reduce this death toll.

Some infections once believed to be all but conquered are returning, and others have developed resistance to antibiotics. Pockets of poverty exist all over the world and they have become the breeding grounds for many infections (WHO 1996). Increasing international travel and huge population movements due to war and internal conflicts are two of the factors influencing an upsurge in food-borne infection as a major threat to population health (WHO 1998).

In developed countries physicians are now treating patients with antibiotic-resistant infections using increasingly expensive or toxic drugs (WHO 1995). Antibiotics are used to either treat or prevent infection, and 50% of antibiotics prescribed are used by humans with the remaining 50% being used in animal health (WHO 1996). The NHS Executive recommends (NHSE 1999):

• a reduced use of antibiotics
• effective surveillance systems to monitor antibiotic-resistant infections
• an emphasis on infection control measures to prevent the spread of infection (both resistant and non-resistant).

Cohen (1997) makes the important point that complacency has led to breakdowns in public health measures at a time when technology and advanced treatments are resulting in a rise in susceptible patients.

Global travel enhances the potential for international spread of both non-resistant and resistant infection (Cohen 1997, WHO 1996, 1998).

In addition the population is ageing, with the percentage of people requiring support from adults of working age increasing from 10.5% in 1955 to 12.3% in 1995, to a predicted 17.2% in

---

ANONYMOUS HEALTH AUTHORITY

Outbreak of Gastro-enteritis

1. Personal details

Surname _____

First names _____

Address _____

_____ Postcode _____

Phone number _____ Occupation _____

Date of Birth _____ \ _____ \ _____   Age _____   Sex M/F
                                                                                                            (Please circle M or F)

Name and address of GP _____

_____

2. Details of illness

Please put a circle round Y if answer is Yes, N if answer is No

a) Have you had a tummy upset or bowel infection since [date]?   **Y/N**

   (If the answer is no, go to question 3 (food history). If yes, please complete the rest of this question.)

b) Date of onset of illness _____ \ _____ \ _____   Time of onset _____ AM/PM (e.g. 2 p.m.)

c) Which of the following symptoms do/did you have? (You may have suffered more than one symptom)

   i. Diarrhoea (3 or more loose stools in 24 hours)   **Y/N**

      If yes, maximum number of stools in 24 hours

   ii. Blood in stools   **Y/N**

   iii. Vomiting   **Y/N**

   iv. Tummy pain   **Y/N**

   v. Fever   **Y/N**

d) How long were you ill (hours)?

e) Were you admitted to hospital?   **Y/N**

   If yes, name of hospital _____

f) Have you seen your GP regarding this illness?   **Y/N**

3. Food history

a) Did you attend the evening wedding reception at the hotel on [date]?   **Y/N**

b) Did you **eat** at the hotel, [time or date]?   **Y/N**

   (If you did, please indicate which foods you ate out of the choices below. If no, please go to question 4.)

   **Circle Y if you ate the food, circle N if you did not and circle Unsure if you cannot remember.
   Please circle one for every food item.**

   Beef sandwich   **Y/N/Unsure**

   Pork sandwich   **Y/N/Unsure**

   Egg mayonnaise sandwich   **Y/N/Unsure**

   Cheese sandwich   **Y/N/Unsure**

Figure 4.2 A questionnaire used as part of an investigation.

Pizza	**Y/N/Unsure**
Vol-au-vent	**Y/N/Unsure**
Sausage roll	**Y/N/Unsure**
Scotch eggs	**Y/N/Unsure**
Crisps	**Y/N/Unsure**
Nuts	**Y/N/Unsure**
Other food	**Y/N/Unsure**

c) If you ate other foods at the reception, please indicate what you ate _____

_____

4. Other relevant information

a) Have you, or any of your family or close contacts, had a similar illness in the week
   before [date]? **Y/N/Unsure**

   If yes, please give details: _____

   _____

b) Were you unwell DURING the evening reception at the hotel on [date]?
   Please note this only applies to illness at the reception itself. **Y/N/Unsure**

   If yes, did you:

   Vomit? **Y/N**

   Have diarrhoea? **Y/N**

   Have other symptoms? **Y/N**

   If yes, please describe: _____

   _____   _____

c) Have you been abroad in the 3 weeks before your illness began? **Y/N**

Many thanks for your cooperation
Please return the questionnaire in the freepost envelope provided –
to Anonymous Health Authority

THANK YOU

Figure 4.2 (*continued*).

Box 4.7   The outbreak at the Stanley Royd Hospital 1985

The outbreak began over a bank holiday weekend. There was a rapid onset.

First morning – 7.00 a.m. – first patient ill
                9.00 a.m. – 36 patients over 8 wards
At the end of first day – 94 patients were ill and 1 died
At the end of outbreak – 400 patients and staff affected and 19 patients died

Causative organism was identified as salmonella. Transmission of salmonella occurred from uncooked chicken to cooked beef which was served for the evening meal prior to the first case becoming ill.

Mode of transmission probably kitchen knives or staff hands.
Catering management heavily criticized.
Senior nurse manager heavily criticized for lack of action and leadership.
Public health involvement also lacked clarity and leadership.
NB – there were very few secondary cases of infection, which means the nurses on the wards, although under tremendous pressure, did not spread the infection to patients who had not consumed the beef and were therefore not ill.

2025 (WHO 1998). Many of these people are cared for in institutions where the risk of cross infection is high.

Reducing morbidity and mortality from infectious disease requires both political will and commitment from individual governments. Health has become a global issue and will have to be recognized as such in the globalization process that is reshaping the world today. Many of the policies influencing the shape of public health in Great Britain are influenced by the World Health Organization's vision of a partnership for health based on social justice, equity and solidarity.

Increasingly health professionals everywhere will find that global communications, information technology and global surveillance systems will detect the problems and provide the knowledge which will help them implement infection control strategies or communicable disease strategies at the earliest stage.

REFERENCES

Acheson D 1988 Public Health in England. HMSO, London
Chin J (ed.) 2000 Control of Communicable Disease, 17th edn. American Public Health Association, Washington DC
Cohen M L 1997 Epidemiological factors influencing the emergence of antimicrobial resistance. Cited in Antibiotic Resistance: Origins, Evolution, Selection and Spread, Ciba Foundation Symposium 207. Wiley, Chichester, 223–237
Cruikshank J 1992 Foodborne disease, Ch. 16. In: Clay's Handbook of Environmental Health, 16th edn. Chapman & Hall, London
Friedman G D 1985 Epidemiology. In: Kuper A, Kuper J (eds) The Social Science Encyclopaedia. Routledge, London
Galbraith N S 1982 Communicable disease surveillance. In: Smith A (ed.) Recent Advances in Community Medicine. Churchill Livingstone, London
HMSO 1988 Report of the Committee of Enquiry into the Future Development of the Public Health, Function Cmmd, 289. HMSO, London
Hughes J M 1987 Infection Surveillance in the United States: Historical Perspective. Infection Control 8: 450–453. Cited in Pugh P 1999 An appraisal of the use of surveillance to promote the control of infection. British Journal of Infection Control, May 1999

Langmuir A D 1963 The surveillance of communicable diseases of national importance. New England Journal of Medicine 268: 182–192
McKeown T 1979 The Role of Medicine. Blackwell, Oxford
McMahon B, Pugh T F 1970 Epidemiology, Principles and Methods. Little, Brown, Boston. Cited in Robinson J, Elkan R 1996 Health Needs Assessment, Theory and Practice. Churchill Livingstone, London
NHS Executive 1999 Resistance to Antibiotics and other Antimicrobial Agents. NHSE, Leeds
Public Health Laboratory Service 2000 Meningococcal disease falls in vaccine recipients. Communicable Disease Report 10(15)
Robinson J, Elkan R 1996 Health Needs Assessment, Theory and Practice. Churchill Livingstone, London
Stolley P, Laskey T 1995 Investigating Disease Patterns. Scientific American Library
Valanis B 1986 Epidemiology in Nursing and Health Care. Appleton and Lange, Norwalk, CT, 3
World Health Organization 1995 Scientific Working Group on Monitoring and Management of Bacterial Resistance to Antimicrobial Agents. WHO, Geneva
World Health Organization 1996 Fighting disease, fostering development. The World Health Report. WHO, Geneva
World Health Organization 1998 Life in the 21st Century, A Vision for All. WHO, Geneva

FURTHER READING

Beaglehole R, Borita R, Kjellstrom T 1993 Basic Epidemiology. WHO, Geneva
Farmer R, Miller D 1991 Lecture notes on Epidemiology and Public Health Medicine. Blackwell Science, Oxford

Unwin N, Carr S, Leeson J, Pless-Mulloli J 1997 An Introductory Study Guide to Public Health and Epidemiology. Open University Press, Buckingham
Webster C (ed.) 1993 Caring for Health, History and Diversity. Open University Press, Buckingham

5

Cleaning, disinfection and sterilization

J. Babb
S. Lowe

INTRODUCTION

Surveys of decontamination practice in the late 1980s (Hoffman et al 1988, Farrow et al 1988 and Morgan et al 1990) indicated that hot water disinfectors (boilers) and chemical disinfectants were widely used for processing instruments and that the practice nurses, general practitioners and receptionists who were largely responsible for decontamination had 'uncertain' knowledge of dealing with blood and other body fluid spillages. Hot air sterilizers were often used for sterilization processes and these were poorly maintained and validated. Those responsible for surveys concluded that in almost half of the general practices surveyed, sterilization procedures were of doubtful efficacy or were unsatisfactory. A comprehensive central code of practice was therefore required for the control of infection and decontamination in the community. The British Medical Association responded with the publication of their guidelines in 1989 (BMA 1989).

As a result of changes in the organization of primary healthcare services, the number of minor operations and screening procedures performed by general practitioners has risen with a corresponding increase in infection risk. There has also been an increase in people infected with HIV, hepatitis B and C, tuberculosis, cytomegalovirus and human papillomavirus.

The introduction of the Control of Substances Hazardous to Health (COSHH) regulations in 1988 (HSC 1998) has placed a responsibility on general practitioners and other community employers to assess risks to health in the workplace and implement effective but safe decontamination practices. There is therefore a greater need for the implementation of rigorous and safe infection control and decontamination procedures. Subsequent surveys (White and Smith 1995, Sneddon et al 1997) have shown an improvement in decontamination since the implementation of the BMA and other guidelines, but the need for documented policy, professional guidance and staff training is still apparent.

Cleaning, disinfection and sterilization are processes which remove or destroy micro-organisms. Most infections are acquired by contact between a susceptible site, such as a wound, and potentially pathogenic micro-organisms present on equipment, instruments, environmental surfaces and the hands of healthcare staff. The method of decontamination used will depend on the nature of the micro-organisms present and the infection risk associated with the surface, procedure or device. In this chapter prominence will be given to a review of the decontamination procedures likely to be undertaken by nurses and other healthcare workers within the community.

Decontamination

Decontamination is a term now widely used (Medical Devices Agency 1993/96) to collectively describe the processes of cleaning, disinfection and sterilization. Simply, it refers to the elimination of 'contaminants', which include micro-organisms and other unwanted material which would otherwise be conveyed to a susceptible site and cause infection or some other harmful response.

Sterilization

This is a process which destroys or removes all living micro-organisms, including bacterial spores. It renders medical devices free from viable micro-organisms and is recommended for items penetrating intact skin or mucous membranes or entering sterile body cavities. Many instruments and other invasive items are packaged or contained before sterilization to protect them from recontamination on removal from the sterilizer or whilst being stored for reuse.

Disinfection

This reduces the number of viable micro-organisms but may not inactivate some bacterial spores. Disinfection may not achieve the same reduction in microbial contamination levels as sterilization but it is a process widely used to make items free of infection risk and safe to handle. Disinfection is normally used for instruments, equipment and surfaces which are not intentionally invasive but are in contact with mucous membranes, blood, body fluids and other potentially infectious material. Although not the preferred option, this process may also be used for invasive items if no practical means of sterilization is available, for example for heat-sensitive items.

Cleaning

Cleaning physically removes micro-organisms and the organic material on which they thrive. It is therefore an essential pre-requisite to disinfection and sterilization. Exposure to disinfectants and heat are unlikely to be effective unless body fluids and other protective material are removed first. Cleaning also removes other contaminants, such as chemical residues, degradation products, pyrogens, soil and dust, which may otherwise jeopardize the safe performance of the device.

CHOICE OF DECONTAMINATION METHOD

The choice as to which of the numerous methods available for cleaning, disinfection and sterilization will depend on many factors. These include:

- infection risk
- the nature of contamination
- the time available for processing
- the heat, pressure, moisture and chemical tolerance of the item
- the availability of suitable processing equipment
- the risks to processing staff.

A requirement of the Medical Devices Directive (93/42/EEC) is that the manufacturers of reusable medical devices must state appropriate methods of cleaning and be able to identify those methods of disinfection or sterilization which are compatible with the components of their device. If they are unable to do this, the item should not be purchased.

INFECTION RISK ASSESSMENT

To obtain a consistently sterile environment would be prohibitively expensive, impractical

and unnecessary. Even if this were momentarily achieved, it could not be sustained with persons present as these are the principal source of micro-organisms. There is little point in destroying micro-organisms, many of which are beneficial, if this is not associated with preventing or reducing infection risk.

The nature of the decontamination process chosen will depend primarily on the item's intended use and the nature of micro-organisms present. If it penetrates intact skin or mucous membranes or enters an otherwise sterile body cavity, it is considered high risk and should be clean and free of all viable micro-organisms, in other words sterile (see Table 5.1). The process used should ensure that even the most heat- and chemically-resistant spores, such as the clostridial spores responsible for tetanus, gas gangrene and food poisoning, are destroyed.

Process-resistant spores are not a problem on surfaces or instruments which are not intentionally invasive, such as those in contact with intact skin and mucous membranes. These are considered an intermediate risk. Disinfection, or the elimination of non-sporing pathogens, that is, bacteria, viruses and fungi, is the requirement for these (see Table 5.1). However, if it is safer and more cost-effective to use a single use item, or to use a sterilized device, it would seem more logical to do so. A good example of this is a vaginal speculum. It is not intentionally invasive and therefore requires cleaning and disinfection but if it is heat-tolerant and can be more effectively and safely steam sterilized than disinfected by immersing in hot/boiling water or disinfectants, you should do so. This is quite clearly stated in the Safety Action Bulletin SAB(94)22 from the Department of Health.

Unfortunately there are some heat-sensitive items, such as flexible endoscopes, which may be used for an invasive procedure which cannot be effectively sterilized with the equipment available in the community. The only practical option is to disinfect by immersion in a suitable disinfectant.

Similarly, low-cost items which are heat-sensitive and difficult to clean are often purchased as single use, for example syringes, needles, scalpels, stitch cutters, specula, proctoscopes, thermometers, tongue depressors and forceps.

Table 5.1 Classification of equipment in relation to risk (based on risk assessment by Ayliffe et al 1993)

Risk	Method of decontamination	Process options	Examples
HIGH In contact with a break in the skin or mucous membranes. Entry into sterile body cavities or vascular systems	**Cleaning and sterilization or single use**	1) Autoclave 2) Hot air oven (no longer recommended) 3) Pre-sterilized single use 4) Low temperature sterilization options available in some Sterile Service Departments, e.g. ethylene oxide, low-temperature steam and formaldehyde, gas plasma	Surgical instruments Surgical scissors and forceps Stitch cutters Tenaculums Intrauterine device sets Uterine sounds Neurological examination pins Vaginal specula (for inserting IUCDs) Sutures and needles Hypodermic needles and syringes Surgical dressings Cryoprobes Cautery probes
INTERMEDIATE In contact with intact mucous membranes and body fluids	**Cleaning and disinfection** or **cleaning and sterilization or single use**	All the above plus 1) Boiling 2) Washer disinfectors (thermal and chemical) 3) Disinfectants	Vaginal speculae (for vaginal examinations) Ring pessaries Fitting rings/diaphragms Nasal speculae Tongue depressors Laryngeal mirrors Oral/rectal thermometers Resuscitation equipment Brushes; cleaning/nail Proctoscopes, sigmoidoscopes Gastrointestinal endoscopes Peakflow meter mouthpieces Auroscope nozzles
LOW In contact with intact healthy skin	**Cleaning only** **Disinfection if known infection risk**, e.g. MRSA patient	All the above plus Manual or automated cleaning with detergent	Ear syringe nozzles Skin thermometers Stethoscopes Face masks (inhalers, nebulizers) ECG pads Toys Commodes

Applying this risk assessment to the skin, for example prior to an invasive procedure such as surgery, the preferred option would be to sterilize. However, this is impractical and in these circumstances the less rigorous process of disinfection would apply.

Cleaning is an essential prerequisite for effective disinfection and sterilization, and yet cleaning alone may be sufficient for many low-risk items and surfaces, particularly those in contact with normal, healthy skin or remote from the patient (see Table 5.1). However, some patients are carriers of multi-resistant or problematic micro-organisms such as methicillin-resistant *Staphylococcus aureus* (MRSA) and, although their skin is healthy, it would be advisable to disinfect surfaces and equipment in contact with their skin before the item is used by others, for instance baths, hoists, commodes and linen. Disinfection is also advised for some items which are in contact with severely immunocompromised patients if there is an identifiable risk.

The importance of cleaning should also be emphasized to protect the quality of diagnostic samples. For example, if reusable endoscopic biopsy forceps are not thoroughly cleaned before they are sterilized or disinfected using heat or a disinfectant, the tissue sample may become fixed to the jaws of forceps. When the instrument is next used these tissue residues may still be present and this could lead to misdiagnosis, with serious implications for both patients and staff. In addition, cleaning is essential to remove material which may otherwise block lumens or cause friction and wear. This is particularly important when processing dental handpieces or hinged instruments.

Cleaning is also important from an aesthetic standpoint. Patients are unlikely to have confidence in community-based medicine if this is done in an untidy and dirty environment.

Table 5.1 shows a classification of equipment in relation to risk. It is based upon that of Ayliffe, Coates and Hoffman (1993) and gives examples of process options and the range of instruments and equipment used and processed within the community. Similar advice is produced in the British Medical Association guidelines 1989, and British Dental Association Advice Sheet A12 (2000).

STERILE SERVICES FOR THE COMMUNITY

Most large and District General hospitals have a Sterile Services Department (SSD) which supplies a range of pre-sterilized items to theatres, wards and other healthcare establishments including those which are community-based, such as general practice, chiropody and dentistry. SSDs are able to provide a much wider range of process options than those normally encountered in the community.

The decontamination processes used are closely monitored by the SSD manager and staff who are advised by the Infection Control Doctor or Consultant Microbiologist. Great care is taken to ensure that all protocols for the handling and processing of instruments and equipment meet quality and good practice standards and guidelines (Institute of Sterile Services Management (ISSM) 1998a, NHS Estates 1994/95 Health Technical Memorandum 2010 and 1995 HTM 2030). Records are kept of all decontamination efficacy tests and these are identified with the packs or instrument

sets issued to users. In recent years, SSDs have rationalized their function and now obtain a large range of sterile procedure packs, dressings and single-use supplementary instruments from commercial sources at a competitive price (ISSM Resource Manual 1998b).

Wherever it is cost-effective and logistically viable to use SSDs to supply prepacked sterilized instruments and procedure packs, you are advised to do so. Sterile Service Departments offer a far wider range of processing options, particularly for heat-sensitive items, and the processes are automated and more effectively controlled.

Medical devices, in general, are covered by Directive 93/42/EEC implemented into UK law by the Medical Device Regulations 1994 (with a four-year transition period to July 1998). The Directive provides a legal definition of a 'medical device', which may be an instrument, apparatus, appliance, material or other article intended for use on human beings for one of four purposes:

- diagnosis, prevention, monitoring, treatment or alleviation of disease
- diagnosis, monitoring of treatment of injury or handicap
- control of conception
- investigation, replacement or modification of the anatomy or a physiological process.

The Medical Devices regulations (Directive 93/42/EEC) also apply to accessories used with the above items.

The European Commission proposes that commercial activities undertaken by healthcare providers, which fall within the definition of placing on the market, should be regulated by the Medical Devices Directive. Hence, if an SSD supplies to a general practitioner, this constitutes placing on the market and would therefore be regulated and must comply with the Directive. However, devices processed by the community for its own exclusive use do not have to comply with these regulations.

The cost of upgrading many SSDs to comply with design and quality standards required by the Directive has reduced the number of hospital establishments prepared to offer instrument sets and procedure packs to community establishments. Many infection-control practitioners have expressed concern over this as the processing facilities in most community healthcare establishments are less well regulated and controlled. The range of surgical and investigative procedures now carried out in the community is also much wider than it was a decade or more ago.

POLICY FORMULATION

Role of infection control team/committee

It is the responsibility of the Chief Executive in hospitals to ensure that effective infection control arrangements are instigated and monitored. The usual process for managing this is by setting up an Infection Control Committee (ICC) and Team (ICT). The ICC is responsible for producing an Infection Control Procedure Manual, which includes decontamination, and the ICT for formulating and overseeing policy implementation. In the community the composition of the ICC and ICT is less clear. Those with specialist knowledge of decontamination and infection control are: Infection Control Nurses, Control of Communicable Diseases Consultants (CCDCs) and Medical Microbiologists. Where possible, policy is based on national 'good practice' guidelines, such as Medical Devices Agency 1993/96, BMA 1989 and BDA 2000. Many decontamination guidelines are 'consensus' opinion rather than 'evidence-based'. The latter are preferred by Professional Societies and the Medical Devices Agency (DoH).

Sources of information

Infection control practitioners are strongly advised to seek information on suitable methods of cleaning, disinfection and sterilization before formulating a decontamination policy for the community. Several possible sources of information are available and these are given in Box 5.1.

Decontamination policy

Those responsible for formulating and implementing policy are strongly advised to follow the national good practice guidelines. The process

---

Box 5.1 Sources of information for decontamination policy

The Department of Health
NHS Estates, e.g. Health Technical Memoranda: HTM 2030 Washer Disinfectors, HTM 2010 Sterilizers
Medical Devices Agency, Device Bulletins e.g. DB 9607 Endoscopes, DB 9605, DB 9804, DB 2000(5) Benchtop Sterilizers
Microbiology Advisory Committee to MDA, Dept. of Health, Decontamination of Medical Devices

Professional Societies, e.g. Hospital Infection Society, Infection Control Nurses Association, British Medical Association, British Dental Association

Reference Centres (WHO collaborating laboratories in Infection Control), e.g. Central Public Health Laboratory, Colindale, London and Hospital Infection Research Laboratory, City Hospital, Birmingham

Books, Working Party Reports and peer reviewed articles (see reference list/bibliography)

British, European and International Standards, e.g. BSI, CEN, ISO

The manufacturers of instruments, equipment, sterilizers, washer disinfectors and disinfectants

---

options selected are dependent on the infection risk, nature of contamination, the time, safety, cost and availability of processing methods and the heat, pressure, moisture and chemical tolerance of the item (Ayliffe et al 2000, Ayliffe, Babb and Taylor 1999). Heat sterilization or disinfection is preferred but if the item is heat-sensitive, disinfectants or single-use items may have to be used. It is essential that the process is effective against patient-associated micro-organisms and opportunistic pathogens present in the environment. Validated automated processes are the safest, most reliable options but these are often expensive and not always available in the community. Processes must be monitored and equipment satisfactorily maintained. Many disinfectants and heat processes are potentially hazardous, and staff must be suitably protected and trained. Invasive items should preferably be packaged before sterilization to prevent environmental contamination after processing. This can only be done in a vacuum steam sterilizer (see Steam sterilization, below).

Before deciding on a particular method of decontamination, the factors set out in Box 5.2 should be considered.

Box 5.2   Factors in deciding method of decontamination

- Ensure that the item is intended for reuse
- For what purpose is the device used? Is it invasive, in contact with body fluids or potentially infectious material?
- How do the manufacturers recommend it is decontaminated?
- Can it be disassembled to facilitate cleaning?
- Is decontamination necessary at the point of use?
- Is an SSD tray service appropriate?
- Will it withstand an automated cleansing process?
- Is it heat-tolerant?
- How can it be disinfected or sterilized, do you have the facility?
- Can it be immersed in fluids?
- How soon will it be needed?
- Can it be wrapped to protect it from recontamination?
- How many times can it be reprocessed?
- Does processing constitute a hazard to patients and staff? If so, is Health and Safety data available and has a COSHH assessment been performed?
- What personal protective equipment is required?

Box 5.3   Selection of disinfectants for heat-sensitive equipment, environmental surfaces and skin

---

• Range of activity	Is the disinfectant effective against pathogenic micro-organisms including spores, mycobacteria and other vegetative bacteria, fungi and viruses?
• Rate of kill	How quickly does it work at use dilution? A rapidly effective agent is required for environmental surfaces and the skin
• Toxicity	Is it irritant to the skin, eyes and respiratory tract?
• Surface compatibility	Is it corrosive or damaging to the surface or device?
• Inactivation	Is it inactivated by organic matter, e.g. spillage, detergents or hard water, etc.?
• Stability	How often should it be prepared and how long should it be stored or used?
• Cost	How much does the disinfectant, processing equipment, protective clothing and disposal cost?

Automated cleaning followed by steam sterilization or thermal disinfection is the preferred option. However, the only practical method of disinfecting heat-sensitive items in the community is to use disinfectants. Wherever possible, community healthcare establishments are encouraged to use a centralized Sterile Service Department (SSD) (see Sterile services for the community, above).

Disinfectant policy

The properties set out in Box 5.3 should be considered when selecting disinfectants for heat-sensitive equipment, environmental surfaces and the skin (Ayliffe, Coates and Hoffman 1993, Babb 1996).

The properties of several widely-used disinfectants are shown in Table 5.2.

Policy audit

For a decontamination policy to be effective, procedures must be suitably monitored and audited. A trained infection control nurse is most suited to this task. Changes will be necessary as new products and procedures emerge and the merits and disadvantages of current processing options become more widely known.

DECONTAMINATION PRIOR TO INSPECTION, SERVICE AND REPAIR

Equipment which has been contaminated with blood or body fluids, or exposed to patients with known infectious diseases, must not be supplied to third parties without first being decontaminated. It will require cleaning and disinfection or sterilization using one of the methods described in the Summary following this chapter. A declaration of contamination status should be provided to the third party in accordance with HSG (93) 26 (NHS Management Executive 1993). If the equipment has not been in contact with blood, body fluids or infectious material, for instance items in contact with intact healthy skin, cleaning with detergent will suffice (see Table 5.1). If the equipment is complex, the user or processor may not be able to decontaminate the device without it first being dismantled by a competent engineer. In this event the equipment should be suitably contained and a biohazard label attached. A clearance certificate should be completed

Table 5.2 Instrument and environmental disinfectants: microbicidal activity (varies with concentration)

	Spores	Mycobacteria	Bacteria	Viruses		Stability	Inactivation by organic matter	Corrosive/ damaging	Irritant(I)/ sensitizing(S)
				Enveloped	Non-enveloped				
Glutaraldehyde (2%)	Good (slow)	Good (slow)	Good	Good	Good	Moderate (14–28 days)	No	No	Yes (I/S)
Peracetic acid (0.2–3.5%)	Good	Good	Good	Good	Good	No (1 day)	No	Slight	Yes (I)
Alcohol (60–80%)	None	Good	Good	Good	Moderate	Yes	Yes	Slight (lens cements)	No (flammable)
Chlorine-releasing agents (>1000 ppm)	Good	Good	Good	Good	Good	No (1 day)	Yes	Yes	Yes (I)
Clear soluble phenolics (0.6–2%)	None	Good	Good	Poor	None	Yes	No	Yes	Yes (I)
Quaternary ammonium compounds* e.g. Dettol ED, Sactimed Sinald	None	Poor	Good	Good	Poor	Yes	Yes	No	No
Peroxygen compounds (1–3%)	None	Poor	Good	Good	Moderate	Moderate	Yes	Slight	No

accordingly and staff advised on the protective measures required.

Equipment loan store

Many community healthcare premises are now served by equipment loan stores with facilities for the collection, decontamination, maintenance, calibration, storage and dispatch of loan equipment (Medical Devices Agency DB 9801, 1998a). These are equipped with manual and automated cleaning, disinfection and sterilization facilities. Thermal decontamination procedures are preferred but disinfectants are sometimes required for bulky or heat-sensitive items. Washer disinfectors are used for human waste receptacles, glassware, respiratory equipment, mattress covers and linen. High pressure jet washing or steam lances are also available for use in protective booths. Heat-sensitive equipment may be covered with, or immersed in, a suitable disinfectant such as a chlorine-releasing agent, or alcohol (see section on Disinfectants for instruments and equipment, below). Large sinks for immersing items, jet washing equipment and drying cabinets should also be available within the unit.

PROCESS OPTIONS: MOIST HEAT STERILIZATION

Reusable invasive items should be thoroughly cleaned, dried, preferably packaged and sterilized using an autoclave or benchtop steam sterilizer.

Steam sterilization (autoclave)

Steam under pressure at the highest temperature compatible with the product is the preferred method of sterilizing medical devices. Sterilization requires direct contact between dry, saturated, steam and all surfaces of the load at a specified temperature and pressure for a specified time. Examples of cycle parameters are shown in Table 5.3.

Direct contact between steam and microorganisms may be prevented if blood, mucus and tissue deposits are present on load items, or if air is present within the chamber or load.

Wherever practicable and cost-effective to do so, sterile items should be obtained from a Sterile Services Department (see Sterile services for the community, above) which has suitable processing equipment, tracking systems and expertise. If this service is not available locally or is logistically impractical, a suitable benchtop steam sterilizer may be used provided it is properly validated for the intended load.

Benchtop steam sterilizers

Minor surgical procedures are being performed increasingly by general practitioners, dentists and chiropodists. If it is impractical to acquire pre-sterilized instruments and procedure packs from an SSD, which is the preferred option, a benchtop autoclave may be used. The use of these necessitates strict adherence to a wide range of operational checks to ensure optimum performance.

Benchtop or transportable steam sterilizers (see Fig. 5.1) all have fully automatic, predetermined cycles, are electrically heated and generate steam internally by boiling water. They also have

Table 5.3 Sterilization temperature bands, holding times and pressure

Sterilization temperature range (°C)	Pressure (bar)	Minimum hold time (min)
134–137	2.25	3
126–129	1.50	10
121–124	1.15	15

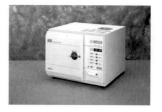

Figure 5.1 Transportable (benchtop) steam sterilizer suitable for the sterilization of unwrapped instruments, utensils and other items for immediate use. A vacuum sterilizer must be used for packaged, porous and lumened items. © Eschmann Holdings Limited. Reproduced by kind permission of Eschmann Holdings Ltd., Peter Road, Lancing BN15 8TJ, UK.

a single manually-operated door. The safe and efficient operation of these sterilizers is dependent on training and a sound knowledge of the sterilizer and its function. Professional advice on the selection, purchase and testing of sterilizers may be obtained from an 'Authorized Person (sterilizers)' – see brief section at the end of this chapter. Advice on the selection, purchase, safe use, validation and periodic testing of such sterilizers may be found in Device Bulletins DB 9605 (1997), DB 9804 (1998b) and DB 2000(05) (2000a) published by the Medical Devices Agency.

In a benchtop or transportable steam sterilizer (autoclave) the air is displaced by steam generated by boiling water. This type of sterilizer is only suitable for processing instruments that are unwrapped, non-porous and non-lumened (Medical Devices Agency DB 9605 1997). There is, however, a new range of benchtop autoclaves which are equipped with an active vacuum air removal system which operates prior to the sterilizing stage. These remove trapped air from wrapped, porous and lumened devices. Vacuum benchtop sterilizers also have a post-sterilization drying stage and, although smaller, mimic the cycle parameters of the much larger SSD porous load sterilizers widely used in hospitals. The drying stage is included to reduce the moisture content of packages and porous materials, which may otherwise compromise the protective quality of the material from a bacteriological standpoint. These vacuum benchtop sterilizers are preferred because of their suitability for a much wider range of load items (MDA DB 9804 (1998b), DB 2000(05) (2000a)). Also, the packaging can incorporate a process indicator and a label showing the contents. This will assist with tracking should an adverse incident occur.

Managers and users of benchtop steam sterilizers must ensure that they are installed and maintained appropriately and that they are validated and routinely tested. Sterilization cannot be confirmed by inspection of the load. Successful sterilization will depend on the consistent reproducibility of sterilizing conditions. Sterilizers have therefore to be validated before use, their performance monitored routinely and the equipment properly maintained (NHS Estates 1994/5 HTM 2010).

It is essential that wrapped instruments are not processed in a 'displacement' (non-vacuum) steam sterilizer. Vacuum-assisted air removal is recommended for packaged, lumened and porous loads.

Safety

All sterilizers, including benchtop autoclaves, are potentially dangerous as they include pressure vessels, and must therefore comply with 'the pressure systems and transportable gas container regulations'. Under these regulations all steam sterilizers are subject to periodic inspection by a competent person. It is the responsibility of the owner of the sterilizer to make sure it is not used until there is a written procedure for this inspection and that the sterilizer is properly maintained and in good repair. The Authorized Person (see section at the end of this chapter) will give advice on this if required. The Medical Devices Agency (DoH) now recommend that only sterilizers bearing the European Commission CE mark are purchased and used. These comply with European Safety and Medical Device Regulations (93/42 EEC 1998).

Testing of benchtop sterilizers

After installation the sterilizer must be validated prior to use. The validation procedure is complex and requires the specialized skills of a trained 'Test Person' familiar with the procedures outlined in NHS Estates 1994/5 HTM 2010 Part 3, and BS EN 554 1994. Validation is a documented procedure which consists of commissioning and performance qualification tests. All records of the validation must be kept by the owner or user of the sterilizer for future inspection.

Periodic tests

A series of periodic tests follows the initial validation. This must be agreed between the test person and owner or user of the benchtop sterilizer after discussion with the manufacturer. If these periodic tests and maintenance are not carried out it could compromise the safe use of the sterilizer. This may have legal and insurance implications for the user or owner of the sterilizer. The schedule of periodic tests should provide details of daily, quarterly and yearly testing. Each sterilizer should have a log book which details all maintenance, tests, faults and modifications for future reference. Details of test procedures may be found in NHS Estates 1994/5 HTM 2010 Part 4.

Daily tests (user)

The owner or user of the sterilizer is responsible for daily tests, and consequently this is dealt with in greater detail. As with other periodic tests, details must be kept in the log book. Daily tests are designed to show that the operating cycle functions correctly as shown by the cycle variables indicated and recorded by the instruments fitted to the sterilizer. Daily tests are as follows:

- A normal (warm up) cycle is operated with the chamber empty (with shelves if fitted).
- A record is kept in the log book of elapsed time, indicated temperature and pressure shown on dials or displays. At each stage of the cycle the maximum temperature and pressure should be recorded.
- In addition, if the sterilizer is fitted with a temperature and pressure recorder, the printout should be compared with previous records and retained for further inspection.
- Daily tests can be considered satisfactory if the following apply:
  — a visual display of cycle complete is indicated
  — the values of the cycle variables are within the limits established as satisfactory by the manufacturers
  — the sterilization time is not less than that given in the table, i.e. 3 minutes (134–137°C), 15 minutes (121–124°C), etc.
  — the temperatures during the hold time are within the temperature band specified by the manufacturer
  — the door cannot be opened until the cycle is complete
  — no mechanical or other abnormality is observed
  — where the sterilizer is fitted with a temperature and pressure recorder, then during the plateau period, a) the indicated and recorded temperatures are within the appropriate temperature band (see Table 5.3), b) the difference between the indicated and recorded temperature does not exceed 2°C, c) the difference between the indicated and recorded pressures does not exceed 0.1 bar.

Weekly tests (user or test person)

If the sterilizer does not meet these requirements or those of other periodic tests, it should be withdrawn from service and advice sought from the manufacturer or service contractor.

These weekly tests may be carried out by the user in agreement with the Test Person (sterilizers) or contractor.

- Automatic control tests as described in daily tests section, above.
- Additional tests for vacuum benchtop steam sterilizers:
  — air leakage test (automatic)
  — automatic air detection system function test
  — steam penetration test (Bowie and Dick type testing – see Fig. 5.2).
- Safety checks:
  — examine door seal
  — check security and performance of door safety devices
  — check safety valves or other pressure limiting devices are free to operate – make any check required by the competent person in connection with the written scheme for examination of the pressure vessel.

Quarterly and annual tests

These tests require specific skills and specialized equipment. They should be done by a qualified Test Person (sterilizers). Guidance on quarterly and annual testing can be sought from the Authorized Person or the sterilizer manufacturer.

Maintenance

Owners of benchtop steam sterilizers are required to ensure that the sterilizer is subject to a planned, documented schedule of preventative

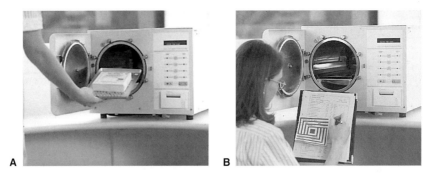

Figure 5.2 Steam penetration test (Bowie and Dick type) for vacuum transportable steam sterilizers. (A) Wrapped test piece. (B) Recording results. © Eschmann Holdings Limited. Reproduced by kind permission of Eschmann Holdings Ltd., Peter Road, Lancing BN15 8TJ, UK.

maintenance. The manufacturer's programme should be followed. Guidance is given in HTM 2010 Parts 1 and 4. Guidance is also available from Authorized Persons. Many manufacturers offer a maintenance contract.

PROCESS OPTIONS: DRY HEAT STERILIZATION

Dry heat is less efficient in destroying microorganisms than moist heat, and longer exposure times and higher temperatures are required, that is, 160°C for 2 hours, 170°C for 1 hour or 180°C for 30 minutes.

Hot air ovens, although widely used for sterilizing instruments in the community several years ago, are now rarely used and are not recommended. Processing times are lengthy, as the oven and its contents must reach sterilizing temperatures before the hold time commences. Also, the load must cool before it can be removed. Steam sterilization is a much shorter process and is therefore the preferred option for heat-tolerant items. Several surveys of community sterilization processes have shown that sterilization temperatures and times are rarely achieved using hot air ovens; thus the process is unreliable and should be avoided.

Hot air ovens

Sterilizing ovens are electrically heated boxes controlled by an adjustable thermostat. A fan is fitted to circulate hot air, ensuring an even temperature throughout the processing chamber. A timer is included and, in modern ovens, the door automatically locks on commencing a cycle to ensure items are not removed until sterilization is complete. Also, the chamber temperature is indicated and recorded.

Hot air ovens are most suited to sterilizing solids and non-aqueous fluids (such as oils, waxes, powders), glassware (including reusable glass syringes) and delicate metal instruments that may be blunted or damaged by moist heat (MDA/MAC 1993/96). Such items are rarely used in community healthcare establishments.

Items to be sterilized should be clean and dry and packaged in kraft paper or metal foil. Alternatively, metal containers may be used. Packaged items should be placed on shelves within the processing chamber which allow the hot air to circulate freely.

Glass bead sterilizers

Glass bead sterilizers are available which are small electrically heated pots containing glass beads. These are heated to temperatures in excess of 300°C. Glass bead sterilizers have been used to sterilize the cutting or piercing surfaces of metal instruments used for example in body piercing, acupuncture or tattooing, etc. which are plunged into the glass beads. However, the process is poorly controlled and burn accidents could easily occur if the sterilizer is knocked over. The process is not included in national good practice guidelines or HTM 2010, and should be avoided.

PROCESS OPTIONS FOR STERILIZING HEAT-SENSITIVE DEVICES

Many heat-sensitive items purchased for use in the community are manufactured as single use, for instance needles, syringes, scalpel blades, vaginal specula, forceps, stitch cutters and scalpels, and these should not be reused (MDA 2000b). However, there are some reusable items which are expensive and which will not tolerate the high temperatures associated with steam sterilization, such as flexible endoscopes, transducers, cryo and cautery probes. These should be processed using low temperature or chemical processing techniques.

Low-temperature sterilization technologies

Ethylene oxide, low temperature steam and formaldehyde and gas plasma are all low temperature processing technologies used for sterilizing heat-sensitive instruments and other devices in the Sterile Services Departments of some large District Hospitals. The processing equipment used is complex, costly and requires measurers and expertise unlikely to be found in the community. These processes often involve the use of hazardous chemicals such as ethylene oxide and formaldehyde, the use of which involves strict process and environmental controls. A description of these processes is not, therefore, included in this chapter but may be found elsewhere (MDA 1993/96). Irradiation is an entirely industrial process and is particularly suited to sterilizing large batches of packaged single use devices. Sterilization is achieved using gamma rays or accelerated electron beams.

Filtration, unlike other methods of sterilization, does not involve killing micro-organisms but their removal. It is particularly useful for sterilizing heat-sensitive fluids and gases, including air. Micro-organisms and particles are removed by passage through fibrous, granular or synthetic membrane filters. Micro-organisms are trapped either on or within the filter. Pore sizes of $0.2–0.45\mu$ should entrap bacteria. Bacteria-retaining filters are now incorporated in endoscope washer disinfectors to remove micro-organisms from the water used to rinse away toxic residues of disinfectant. Gaseous filters are used on some respiratory equipment.

Sporicidal disinfectants

Some disinfectants are capable of destroying a wide range of micro-organisms, including the more resistant bacterial spores. These are referred to as sterilants or sporicidal disinfectants (see Table 5.4). Immersion for a suitable period in these agents is often referred to as 'cold sterilization' and may be the only practical means of processing some heat-sensitive instruments and equipment outside a Hospital Sterile Services Department.

Glutaraldehyde, peracetic acid and chlorine-releasing agents are all sporicidal disinfectants but contact times vary from a few minutes (peracetic acid, chlorine) to several hours (glutaraldehyde). Efficacy is dependent on thorough cleaning, the exclusion of trapped air and the concentration of the disinfectant used.

Many infection control practitioners do not refer to immersion in sporicidal disinfectants as a sterilization process because items have to be rinsed in sterile water afterwards to remove toxic residues. They are also difficult to dry and cannot be packaged to protect them from recontamination during storage.

A detailed account of the properties of disinfectants for instruments, equipment, environmental surfaces and the skin follows later in this chapter and is set out in Table 5.2.

Cycle parameters and the advantages and disadvantages of various sterilization options for use in the community are shown in Table 5.4.

Transmissible spongiform encephalopathies (TSEs)

The Advisory Committees on Dangerous Pathogens (ACDP) and Spongiform Encephalopathies

Table 5.4 Sterilization: recommended process options

Process	Cycle parameters	Advantages	Disadvantages
Heat-tolerant items			
Autoclave	121°C for 15 min 126°C for 10 min 134°C for 3 min	Highly effective Items may be wrapped (vacuum autoclave) No toxic chemical residues	Unsuitable for heat-sensitive items Moist process
Heat-sensitive items			
Sporicidal disinfectants, e.g. 2% glutaraldehyde*	Immersion 3–10 hr	Suitable for heat-sensitive items Point of use processing	Rinsing necessary to remove toxic residues Items cannot be wrapped
0.2–0.35% peracetic acid*†	Immersion 10 min	Inexpensive Sophisticated processing equipment required	Slow compared with heat Disinfectants often irritant,* corrosive and damaging
≥1000 ppm chlorine/chlorine dioxide*†	Immersion 10 min		Difficult to control process

*Exhaust ventilation and personal protective equipment required.
†Check instrument compatibility with manufacturer of medical device.

(SEAC) have jointly prepared guidelines (1998) on safe working practices and the prevention of infection from transmissible spongiform encephalopathy agents. These appear to be caused by infectious, self-replicating proteins or prions without detectable RNA or DNA. Prions are resistant to routine autoclaving, dry heat sterilization and immersion in most disinfectants at use concentrations. The advice currently given by ACDP, SEAC and the NHS Executive (HSC 1999/178) is that instruments that have been used on patients with known Creutzfeldt–Jakob disease or related disorders and 'at risk' patients where they have been exposed to the brain, spinal cord and eye tissue, must be disposed of by incineration. Instruments used on 'at risk' patients where there has been no involvement of the brain, spinal cord or eyes should be thoroughly cleaned, preferably using an automated system, and sterilized or disinfected using one of the following options:

- porous load steam sterilization at 134–137°C for a single cycle of 18 minutes (six times the length of the usual cycle)
- immersion in sodium hypochlorite, 20 000 ppm av. Cl, for 1 hour; or
- immersion in 2 mol l⁻¹ sodium hydroxide for 1 hour.

Very few instruments are likely to withstand these methods. Process compatibility should be verified with the instrument manufacturer before proceeding.

'At risk' patients identified in the guidelines are: recipients of human dura mater grafts, recipients of hormones derived from human pituitary glands, and people with a family history of CJD. Where a diagnosis of CJD is suspected, instruments used on such patients should be quarantined pending a confirmation of diagnosis. It would therefore seem prudent to use single use items wherever possible. This guidance has since been extended to instruments used for tonsillectomy as prions have been detected in laryngeal tissue.

Effective and thorough cleaning of surgical instruments to remove as much protein and organic debris as possible before sterilization or disinfection makes a major contribution to risk reduction. It is therefore essential that all existing decontamination procedures operate to the highest standards in line with expert guidance, HTM 2010, HTM 2030 and Health Service Circular 1999 (178). Traceability is also an important issue, particularly if instruments have to be quarantined and/or destroyed by incineration. A record should be kept of instrument identity, the decontamination procedure and the patient on which the instrument was ultimately used. This is rarely done in the community.

Although it is unlikely that prions will be encountered during the minor surgical procedures carried out in the community, the risk cannot be entirely ignored. Hospital Sterile Service Departments have instrument tracking systems and use properly validated, automated cleansing and sterilization procedures. This service is therefore preferred.

Incineration

Incineration by burning (800–1000°C) is a highly effective sterilization process which is carefully controlled to prevent toxic emissions and widely used for destroying infectious or sharp clinical waste.

PREPARATION OF INSTRUMENTS FOR REUSE

Handling dirty instruments

- Instruments may be soiled with potentially infectious material and should be handled with care. If instruments are to be transported they should be placed in a distinctive protective bag or container.
- Instruments should be cleaned as soon as possible, otherwise blood and other body secretions/excretions may dry onto surfaces, making subsequent removal difficult.
- Gloves, plastic apron and, if splashing is likely, a face mask or visor should be worn for protection during cleaning (Fig. 5.3).
- All single use (disposable) items, e.g. blades and needles, should be removed and safely contained. A yellow sharps bin or suitable clinical waste container should be used.

Cleaning: manual

Cleaning is an essential prerequisite to sterilization and disinfection (MDA 1993/96, Babb 1993a). Manual cleaning is as follows:

- Wearing appropriate protective clothing, rinse instruments under running water and then clean using warm water and detergent. A deep dedicated sink (not a wash hand basin) should be used.

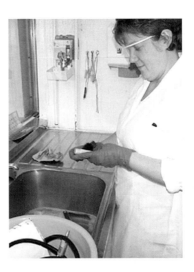

Figure 5.3 Nurse wearing suitable protective clothing for instrument cleaning, i.e. gloves, plastic apron and, if splashing is likely, a facemask or visor. Reproduced by kind permission of Hospital Infection Research Laboratory, City Hospital NHS Trust, Birmingham.

- Use a nylon cleaning brush to remove stubborn soil, taking care not to splash yourself or already cleaned items. Irrigate all lumened devices using a syringe or water jet. If cleaning is done below the water surface, splashing is less likely. After use all brushes and syringes must be cleaned and stored dry.

Cleaning: automated

This is preferred to manual cleaning since handling, and therefore infection risk, is reduced. Cleaning is also more efficient and thermal disinfection may be achieved during the process.

- Use an ultrasonic cleaner (Fig. 5.4) with a suitable detergent. Ensure items are totally immersed and all trapped air is expelled from lumens. Five to ten minutes ultrasonic cleaning should suffice; otherwise follow cleaner manufacturer's instructions. Check compatibility of the process with the instrument supplier. Some devices, e.g. endoscope telescopes, are damaged by ultrasonic cleansing.
- Ensure cleaning solution is changed regularly, e.g. after each sessional use. Clean and drain

the immersion tank after use. Store dry when not in use.

OR

- Use a washer disinfector (see Fig. 5.5) which meets the requirements of BS 2745 1993 (parts 1 and 3), i.e. initial low temperature wash, main hot water wash with detergent, disinfection rinse (items to reach 71°C for 3 minutes or 80°C for 1 minute or 90°C for 12 seconds).
- If drying does not form part of an automated cycle, dry with a non-linting cloth or in a dedicated drying area or cabinet.

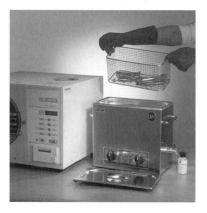

Figure 5.4 Benchtop ultrasonic machine for instrument cleansing. © Eschmann Holdings Limited. Reproduced by kind permission of Eschmann Holdings Ltd., Peter Road, Lancing BN15 8TJ, UK.

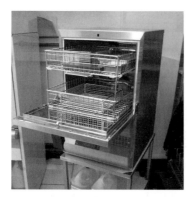

Figure 5.5 Small washer disinfector suitable for reusable heat-tolerant instruments and other items. © Dekomed Ltd. Reproduced by kind permission of Dekomed Ltd., 34 London Road, Hazel Grove, Stockport SK7 4AQ, UK.

Inspection

- After cleansing, check for residual soil in good light. A magnifying glass may help with small or complex items. Instruments must be free of tissue fragments, blood and other body fluids.
- Check that all components or parts of the instrument or set are present.
- Check movement of hinged joints, forceps, etc. These should be free to move but not over loose.
- Check alignment of forceps and that handle grips are firm.
- Check scissors are sharp and needles free from burrs.
- Check lumened devices are clean and free of obstruction. If this cannot be done visually, irrigate the lumens with water to check they are clear.
- All items must be dry.

Packaging

- Items should be packaged prior to steam sterilization only if a **vacuum-assisted** autoclave is used.
- Sterilization packaging, e.g. bags, sheets or pouches, should conform with BS/EN 868 Parts 1 and 2.
- For single instruments a bag or clear-fronted pouch is most suitable. This should contain an appropriate process indicator (see Fig. 5.6).
- Composite sets of instruments are best processed on trays. These should be wrapped in sterilization paper. A single sheet is applied

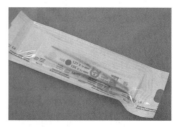

Figure 5.6 Pouch with process indicator suitable for single instruments which are to be sterilized in a vacuum steam sterilizer. Reproduced by kind permission of Hospital Infection Research Laboratory, City Hospital NHS Trust, Birmingham.

using one of two folding techniques (see Fig. 5.7). The wrapping is secured with process indicator tape and labelled for identification and traceability.

- Two types of sterilization paper bag are available with different closure methods, i.e. plain top and heat or 'self' seal. The packaging technique is the same.
- Items with sharp edges or points should be protected with covers or hoods to prevent them from penetrating the bag. Make sure items are placed in the bag with the handle nearest the closure.
- Label the bag with a description of the contents, date and sterilizer. This assists with instrument traceability, which is now an important issue.

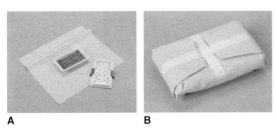

A   **B**

Figure 5.7 Folding technique for composite sets of instruments for steam sterilization. (A) Tray and wrap; (B) wrapped product.

Autoclaving

- Ensure there is sufficient water of a suitable quantity (i.e. distilled or water for irrigation) in the sterilizer chamber.
- Perform daily sterilizer performance tests as listed in Testing section, above.

Non-vacuum-assisted steam sterilizers

- Place clean dry instruments across tray ribs so that they do not touch and allow steam to circulate freely (see Fig. 5.8).
- Hinged instruments should be opened and gallipots inverted to facilitate sterilization.
- Place a process indicator on the tray. This will identify processed items on removal.

Vacuum-assisted steam sterilizers

- Packaged, narrow lumened and porous items must be sterilized in a vacuum-assisted steam sterilizer.
- Place packaged items on trays or within baskets to allow steam to circulate freely. Packages should be suitably labelled and exhibit a process indicator.

- Close door, select and initiate a cycle.
- Enter date, time, cycle details, etc. in the process log book.

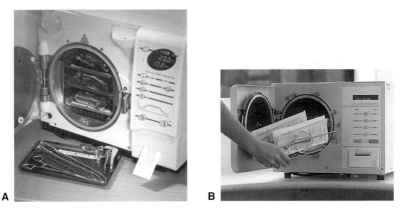

A   **B**

Figure 5.8 Loading non-vacuum- (A) and vacuum-assisted (B) steam sterilizers to allow steam circulation and penetration. © Eschmann Holdings Limited. Reproduced by kind permission of Eschmann Holdings Ltd., Peter Road, Lancing BN15 8TJ, UK.

Preparation for reuse

- On completion of a successful sterilization cycle, open sterilizer door when appropriate or when instructed to do so.
- Remove the load, processing tray or basket onto a clean dry surface. Take care not to damage packaging if present.
- Examine cycle print-out to confirm satisfactory cycle and keep record.
- Unpackaged items with process indicators should be kept clean and dry and preferably covered with a sterile field.
- Packaged items should be stored clean and dry.
- Packaging should be examined to ensure it is clean, dry and undamaged before opening. If it is not, items should be repacked and re-sterilized.
- The process indicator will identify processed items and the label will identify contents and processing data. This will assist with stock rotation and instrument traceability.
- Packaged instruments should be removed immediately prior to use. This will minimize handling and environmental contamination.

PROCESS OPTIONS FOR DISINFECTION

Most equipment-associated infection is due to inadequate cleaning and disinfection and not to a failure in sterilization practices (Ayliffe 1988). Thermal (heat) disinfection is preferred but, if the item is heat-sensitive, disinfectants may have to be used. It is important that the method chosen is effective against patient-associated organisms and also opportunistic pathogens present in the environment. The most effective stage of decontamination is thorough cleaning, and this should accompany or precede disinfection. Automated washer disinfectors (thermal and chemical) offer the safest, most reliable option providing they are suitably monitored and maintained. Cleaning and disinfection will ensure non-invasive items are free of infection risk and safe for handling or reuse (see Table 5.1).

Thermal (heat) disinfection

Exposure to hot water or steam is the most effective, and usually the least expensive, means of disinfection. Items normally processed in this way include instruments, respiratory equipment, human waste receptacles such as bedpans, linen and dishes/cutlery, etc. Process temperatures vary between 65°C and 100°C but, as a general rule, the higher the temperature the shorter the processing time. The method selected will depend on the thermal tolerance of the item, the time available for processing and whether or not disinfection is accompanied by mechanical cleaning.

In the UK, linen, which is fairly heat-sensitive, is cleaned and then disinfected at either 65°C for 10 minutes or 71°C for 3 minutes (NHS Executive 1995 HSG(95) 18). Other instruments and equipment are usually cleaned and disinfected at higher temperatures, that is, 80°C for 1 minute or 90°C for 12 seconds (BS2745 1993, NHS Estates HTM 2030 1995). Cleaning and thermal disinfection will render invasive devices (high risk), such as surgical instruments, safe to handle prior to sterilization and reuse, and non-invasive devices (intermediate risk) fit for immediate patient use. Examples of invasive and non-invasive heat-tolerant devices may be found in Table 5.1. Some guidelines (MDA 1993/96 and BMA 1989) identify immersion in boiling water (98–100°C) for at least 5 minutes as a suitable method of disinfection. However, cleaning does not accompany disinfection and hot/boiling water fixes protein. Washer disinfectors are therefore preferred.

Boilers

Boilers and pasteurizers are still used in some community establishments for disinfecting non-invasive, reusable, pre-cleaned instruments such as tongue depressors, vaginal specula and proctoscopes. Fortunately their use has been widely discouraged because of the difficulties in monitoring processing times and temperatures, the potential risk of scalding, removing items before they have reached disinfection temperatures, or because of the recontamination risk, particularly if instruments are left to soak in water at room temperature overnight or for longer periods. Consequently boilers are no longer recommended. There are now several ultrasonic cleaners, thermal washer disinfectors and benchtop autoclaves which are not prohibitively expensive and which rapidly and safely clean, disinfect and sterilize. These can be used for invasive and non-invasive items provided they tolerate processing temperatures. Alternatively, inexpensive single use items may be used.

Thermal washer disinfectors

Boiling water, or processing in a washer disinfector at temperatures between 65°C and 100°C, will destroy HIV, *Mycobacterium tuberculosis*, *Staphylococcus aureus*, salmonella and other non-sporing bacteria and viruses likely to pose an infection risk to patients or staff. Although some doubt has been cast about the thermal tolerance of Hepatitis B virus (HBV) at temperatures below 100°C, this and other non-sporing micro-organisms are unlikely to survive, providing thorough cleaning precedes thermal disinfection.

There are now several small cabinet type washer disinfectors (as shown in Figs 5.4 and 5.5) which are ideally suited to cleaning and disinfecting instruments, respiratory equipment, holloware such as bowls, kidney dishes and trays, and other items in community healthcare establishments. These cleanse items with rotating or fixed spray arms or using ultrasonic transducers. A typical cycle is as follows:

- An initial low-temperature wash (usually less than 35°C) to remove proteinaceous soil prior to the application of heat.
- Hot water wash (approx 55°C) with a suitable detergent to remove soil and oily residues.
- Thermal disinfection rinse. Items must reach >71°C for 3 minutes, 80°C for 1 minute or 90°C for 12 seconds (BS 2745 Part 1).
- Optional rinse and dry.

Useful advice on the selection, purchase, maintenance and monitoring of washer disinfectors can be found in British Standard 2745 Parts 1, 2 and 3 and Health Technical Memorandum (HTM) 2030 (1995) from NHS Estates.

The performance of thermal washer disinfectors can be established by monitoring the temperature of processed items and by checking soil removal and drying. Thermocouples and a recorder can be attached to processed items to ensure the specified time and temperature parameters are met. Water temperature indicators on the machines may not reflect the temperature of processed items, particularly if they are poor conductors of heat.

Although a range of test soils can be used to establish the efficiency of the cleaning processes a careful inspection of all processed items should reflect cleaning deficiencies. Usual reasons for failure are:

- initial wash temperature too high, i.e. above protein coagulation temperature
- blocked or misdirected jets
- excessive delays before processing
- badly placed instruments in processing trays
- failure to access soil, i.e. dismantle instruments and irrigate lumens
- incorrect use of detergents and rinse aids.

Tests have shown that cabinet and ultrasonic washer disinfectors (see Figs 5.4 and 5.5) are highly effective in removing soil and micro-organisms providing dirty instruments are not subjected to heat beforehand, for example autoclaving to make safe for handling before processing. If delays are likely before processing, instruments should be rinsed under running water in a dedicated sink or sluice, that is, not a wash hand basin.

Ultrasonic washers are more efficient in cleaning the external surfaces of intricate items, particularly where blood and body fluids have dried onto surfaces, but they are not recommended for some optical equipment. Always check process compatibility with instrument manufacturers before use. Lumened items will require irrigation manually if no provision is made for automated irrigation. This is particularly important prior to and following ultrasonic cleaning. Heat fixes protein and may block narrow lumens.

The reservoirs of ultrasonic washer disinfectors should be emptied, cleaned, and dried on a regular basis or organisms will proliferate in cleaning solutions and soil will be redeposited onto

Table 5.5 Disinfection: recommended process options

Process	Cycle parameters	Advantages	Disadvantages
Heat-tolerant items Washer disinfectors (linen, instruments,* bedpans, commode pans, urine bottles, holloware, dishes)	65°C for 10 min, 71°C for 3 min; 80°C for 1 min 90°C for 12 secs	Fully automated programmable cycles Cleaning a stage in the process Minimizes handling risks Performance easily monitored No toxic residues	Unsuitable for some complex lumened devices Equipment is expensive
Heat-sensitive items Disinfectants (environment, spillages, heat-sensitive instruments e.g. flexible endoscopes, equipment and skin)	Variable times at room temperature	Suitable for 'point of use' processing Rapid Inexpensive Often used with compatible detergent	Less effective than heat Often adversely affected by organic matter Some are irritant and sensitizing Items cannot be wrapped No process controls Items must be rinsed to remove toxic residues

*Invasive (surgical instruments), to make safe for handling prior to sterilization; non-invasive items, to make safe for reuse.

processed instruments. This may cause stiffness, friction and wear on hinged instruments. Tissue deposits left on reusable biopsy forceps and cytology brushes may become fixed during subsequent processing and lead to misdiagnosis. Cleaning is therefore essential to protect the quality of diagnostic samples and to ensure the effectiveness of subsequent disinfection and sterilization procedures.

Cleaned and disinfected items should be dried before packaging or subsequent storage as Gram-negative bacilli and other opportunistic pathogens, such as *Pseudomonas aeruginosa*, *Escherichia coli* and *S. aureus* acquired from the environment may proliferate. Drying may be carried out within the washer disinfector, in a separate drying cabinet, or by hand. A summary of disinfection options for heat-tolerant and heat-sensitive items can be seen in Table 5.5.

PROCESS OPTIONS FOR DISINFECTION: DISINFECTANTS

The only practical means of disinfecting most heat-sensitive instruments and equipment, environmental surfaces and the skin is to use disinfectants. A disinfectant is a chemical compound which destroys micro-organisms. Some are non-toxic and can safely be applied to the skin or living tissues: these are called antiseptics. Others are capable of destroying spores and are referred to as sterilants or cold sterilizing agents, although these do not have the same degree of assurance as that achieved by physical methods such as autoclaving. Items immersed in disinfectants cannot be packaged to prevent recontamination before use, and rinsing is often necessary to remove toxic residues. If the rinse water is not sterile this could result in recontamination.

Disinfectants may be used to destroy potentially pathogenic micro-organisms. Most are capable of destroying non-sporing bacteria, viruses and fungi. A detailed account of essential properties of disinfectants and their selection can be found earlier in this chapter and in Ayliffe, Coates and Hoffman (1993).

Disinfectants for instruments and equipment

Reusable heat-sensitive devices may be cleaned and disinfected using one of the following: alcohol, glutaraldehyde, peracetic acid, chlorine-releasing agents and other agents.

Alcohol

Ethanol 60–80% or isopropanol is widely used for disinfecting instruments in the community. It destroys most non-sporing bacteria, fungi and viruses in under 10 minutes on pre-cleaned surfaces. Its principal advantages are that it is rapidly effective and evaporates leaving surfaces dry. Rinsing to remove toxic residues is therefore unnecessary. Consequently it is useful for disinfecting items that are heat-sensitive and are required rapidly, such as thermometers, scissors, probes, handles, trolley tops, stethoscopes, forceps and dropped instruments. Items that are unsuitable for immersion, such as electrical equipment, may be wiped over with alcohol using a commercially-prepared and preferably packaged alcohol wipe. The principal problem associated with alcohol is its flammability. Great care should be taken if used close to a source of ignition.

Glutaraldehyde

Two per cent glutaraldehyde (for example Cidex, Asep, Totacide) is the most widely-used instrument disinfectant for flexible and other heat-labile endoscopes (Babb 1993b). Other aldehydes such as Gigasept (succine dialdehyde and formaldehyde) and Cidex OPA (0.55% orthopthalaldehyde) are also occasionally used. Glutaraldehyde has a wide spectrum of antimicrobial activity but is only slowly effective against mycobacteria such as TB and spores. It is non-corrosive and does not damage rubber, lens cements, polymer and other instrument components. Unfortunately the aldehydes are toxic, irritant and sensitizing and, as such, have become a principal target for risk management, assessment and hazard control, for example COSHH regulations (HSC 1998). Suitable gloves, such as nitrile, and fluid-proof protective clothing (apron) should always be worn and the disinfectant activated, used and discharged using enclosed exhaust-vented equipment (British Society of Gastroenterology 1993).

A wide range of washer disinfectors are now available which protect users from disinfectant exposure. A new Maximum Exposure Limit (MEL) of 0.05 ppm ($0.2\,\mathrm{mg\,m^{-3}}$) glutaraldehyde over a 15-minute and 8-hour Time Weighted Average (TWA) was published in 1999 (HSE 1999: 40/99). This MEL is approximately the odour threshold and must not be exceeded.

Immersion times vary depending on the instrument used, the nature of the clinical procedure undertaken and the microbial contamination expected. Most non-sporing bacteria and viruses are killed in 10 minutes but 20 minutes is required for *Mycobacterium tuberculosis*, for instance in bronchoscopes, and even longer periods to kill some bacterial spores. In the UK the disinfectant manufacturers, professional societies and the Department of Health have produced guidelines on the decontamination (cleaning and disinfection) of endoscopes which includes disinfectant suitability and contact times. Users are advised to follow these guidelines (see Table 5.6). Items should be thoroughly cleaned, disinfected and then rinsed in water of an appropriate microbiological quality, that is, sterile for invasive instruments or those entering sterile body cavities, to remove disinfectant residues without recontaminating the endoscope.

Peracetic acid

Formulations of 0.2–0.35%, such as Steris, NuCidex, Perasafe, Perascope and Gigasept PA, have recently been introduced as less irritant alternatives to glutaraldehyde. These are more rapidly effective than glutaraldehyde and destroy *Mycobacterium tuberculosis*, other bacteria and viruses in under 5 minutes and spores in 10 minutes, but they are more expensive, less stable and may cause superficial damage to some instruments and processors.

Peracetic acid appears to be less irritant than glutaraldehyde and is not identified as a sensitizer, but until it is more widely studied staff are advised to wear suitable protective clothing, that is, gloves, apron and goggles (if splashing is likely) and to enclose and use exhaust-vented processing facilities where practicable.

Chlorine-releasing agents

Chlorine dioxide (Tristel) has also recently been introduced as a glutaraldehyde alternative for

Table 5.6 Decontamination of endoscopes: national guidelines

Organization	Method	Contact time	Endoscope
British Soc. of Gastroenterology (Gut 1998, 42, 4, 585–593)	Automated cleaning with detergent followed by 2% glutaraldehyde or peracetic acid (0.2–0.35%) Rinse with potable water (bacteria-free for invasive procedures, e.g. Endoscopic Retrograde Cholangiopancreatography)	10 min* start of session and between patients 20 min* at end of session and for high level disinfection, i.e. AIDS patients, TB and immunosuppression 5 min[†] start and end of session and between patients	Flexible GI endoscopes, e.g. gastroscopes, sigmoidoscopes and colonoscopes
British Association of Urological Surgeons (British Journal of Urology 1993, 7, 5–9)	Preclean with detergent followed by 2% glutaraldehyde. Autoclave if heat-tolerant Rinse with bacteria-free or sterile water	10 min 1 hr for known or suspected mycobacterial infections	Cystoscopes: flexible (heat-sensitive), rigid (usually heat-tolerant)
British Thoracic Society (Thorax 2001, 56 (Suppl. I), i1–i21)	Wash with detergent followed by 2% glutaraldehyde. Rinse with bacteria-free or sterile water	20 min* between cases 1 hr* before immuno-compromised patients and after use on patients with TB or mycobacterial infection 5 min[†] all the above	Bronchoscopes
Medical Devices Agency (Device Bulletin DB 9607 1996)	Review of professional societies' and manufacturers' guidelines for endoscopes	Review of suitable agents and contact times	All endoscopes
Hospital Infection Society (J. of Hosp. Inf 2000, 45, 263–277 MAT Working Party Report)	Preclean with detergent followed by 2% glutaraldehyde or alternative[†] Rinse with bacteria-free or sterile water Autoclave if heat-tolerant (rigid)	>10 min*[†] 1 hr for known or suspected mycobacterial infections*	Arthroscopes, laparoscopes, other surgical endoscopes

*Glutaraldehyde.
[†]Peracetic acid.

endoscopes. This disinfectant is also highly effective, and its spectrum of activity is similar to peracetic acid. However, it is irritant to staff and damages some instruments and processing equipment. Its suitability for endoscopes is still under scrutiny.

Other agents

These include peroxygen compounds such as Virkon, and quaternary ammonium compounds like Dettol ED and Sactimed Sinald.

These are good cleansing agents and are more user-friendly. However, efficacy tests with spores, mycobacteria and enteroviruses have proved disappointing. These agents should be considered where non-damaging or more user- and environmentally-friendly products are required, and where the risk of infection with disinfectant-tolerant organisms is remote.

Compatibility

Under the Medical Devices Directive (93/42/EEC), the manufacturers of reusable instruments are required to state suitable methods of decontamination and this includes tolerances to heat, moisture, pressure and processing chemicals.

Before considering changing to a new disinfectant, users are advised to: inform their infection control practitioners, check disinfectant compatibility with instrument and processor manufacturers, carry out a COSHH assessment of the disinfectant, and implement suitable control measures, and also to cost the change bearing in mind the stability and use life of the agent. Many effective disinfectants are damaging, particularly if recommended contact times are exceeded. Use of an unsuitable disinfectant not authorized by the instrument or processor manufacturer may invalidate guarantees or service agreements.

Selection of disinfectants

A list of the properties of various instrument and environmental disinfectants can be seen in Table 5.2.

Endoscope washer disinfectors utilizing disinfectants

Endoscopic procedures are now carried out in several community-based healthcare establishments. Automated washer disinfectors are available which can be programmed to clean, disinfect and rinse the internal channels and external surfaces of flexible endoscopes and accessories (see Fig. 5.9). These provide a reliable standardized process, are convenient for the nurse and prevent staff contact with irritant processing chemicals. When purchasing such equipment it is important to establish that it is effective, non-damaging, safe, and sufficiently versatile to accommodate the various endoscopes used. It should also enable the user to select a suitable disinfectant contact time which will meet the requirements of national guidelines or local disinfection policies. To prevent instrument recontamination from the environment or patient-associated material the washer disinfector must have a 'self disinfect' facility and the rinse water must be of a high microbiological standard, that is, preferably sterile or passed through a bacteria-retaining filter (pore size 0.2 μm). Disinfection of the washer disinfector and associated rinse water pathways is recommended at the start of each session.

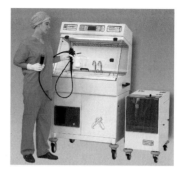

Figure 5.9 Enclosed, exhaust-ventilated washer disinfector with a water filtration facility for flexible endoscopes. © Labcaire Systems Limited. Reproduced by kind permission of Labcaire Systems Limited, 175 Kenn Road, Clevedon BS21 6LH, UK.

Reused disinfectants rapidly become diluted in automated systems due to carry-over of water or detergent. It is therefore important to establish when to change the disinfectant. If 2% glutaraldehyde is used, it is recommended that the concentration does not fall below 1.5% and that the post-activation life does not exceed that recommended by the disinfectant manufacturer, that is, 14 or 28 days for activated alkaline glutaraldehyde. Transfer of disinfectant to the rinse water also occurs if it is reused, increasing the risk of irritancy to the instrument user or patient. The rinse water should therefore be changed frequently, preferably after each cycle. Pumping air through the channels will express residual water but drying will only occur if hot air or alcohol is used. Storing a dry instrument will decrease the likelihood of microbial proliferation during storage, but all instruments should be disinfected before starting a new session.

The new generation of washer disinfectors have integral vapour handling systems which extract irritant fumes or recirculate vapour through a dedicated, absorbent charcoal filter. These are now considered essential when using glutaraldehyde to comply with the new Maximum Exposure Limit of 0.5 ppm ($0.2\,mg\,m^{-3}$) over a 15-minute and 8-hour TWA reference period (Health and Safety Executive EH40/99).

Advice on the selection, purchase, installation and performance of chemical washer disinfectors can be found in NHS Estates (1995) HTM 2030, from professional societies (see Table 5.6), the Medical Devices Agency (DoH) (1996) DB 9607, and Bradley and Babb (1995).

Disinfectants for the environment

Disinfectants are used to protect staff removing potentially hazardous material such as spilt blood, wound exudate, excretions and other infectious material from environmental surfaces (Ayliffe et al 1993, Babb 1996). They may also be used to disinfect surfaces in contact with instruments or the skin of patients if there is a known infection risk, for example following contact with the skin of an MRSA-colonized or infected patient. If spillages are not removed they become slippery, offensive or a source of bacterial proliferation.

Chlorine-releasing agents

The most widely-used agents for inanimate surfaces are the chlorine-releasing agents such as sodium hypochlorite (NaOCl) or sodium dichloro-isocyanurate (NaDCC). These are used for body fluid spills, work tops, patient supports, mattresses, infant feeding bottles, catering equipment and surfaces, sanitary ware (baths, WCs, wash hand basins), heat-sensitive linen, water treatment, and occasionally for heat-sensitive items such as respiratory equipment, dental impressions, tonometers and dialysers. NaDCC formulations are available as tablets, granules or powders. Some contain a compatible cleansing agent. The NaDCC formulations are often preferred to bleach (NaOCl) because they are easier to prepare and use and are slightly more efficacious and less damaging to surfaces. Chlorine-releasing agents are comparatively inexpensive and if used at a sufficiently high concentration are rapidly effective against a wide range of micro-organisms including the blood-borne viruses, mycobacteria and bacterial spores. They are inactivated by organic material, and high concentrations such as 10 000 ppm available Cl are recommended for direct application to blood, other body fluid spills and grossly contaminated surfaces (see Table 5.7). Chlorine-releasing

Table 5.7 Some uses of chlorine-releasing agents and solution strengths

Organic load	Task	Available Cl ppm
High	Blood and other spillages	10 000
Medium	Precleaned surfaces	1000
Low	Cleaned medical and catering equipment	200–500
Extremely low	Hydrotherapy pools, drinking water	4–6 0.5–1

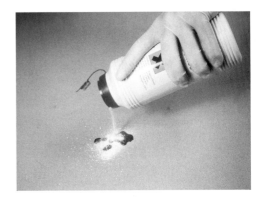

Figure 5.10 Removal of a small blood spill with NaDCC (chlorine-releasing) granules. Reproduced by kind permission of Peter Hoffman, Laboratory for Hospital Infection, Central Public Health Laboratory, London.

agents are corrosive to metals, and damage rubber and some other materials. This damage may be reduced if surfaces are cleaned first and a lower concentration used, for example 100–1000 ppm available Cl.

Chlorine-releasing agents should not be diluted in hot water or mixed with acids or inappropriate cleansing solutions, as a rapid release of chlorine may occur which could irritate the eyes and respiratory mucosa of the user.

Small spills of blood and other body fluids (less than 30 ml) are best removed by applying granules or powder directly to the spill (see Fig. 5.10). This can then be removed using one or more paper towels or wipes. This would however be impractical for larger spills, which should first be removed and a lower concentration of chlorine used, 1000 ppm av. Cl.

Tablets, powders and granules are all extremely stable, but once prepared at use concentration they should be used within 24 hours. Chlorine-releasing agents are also useful for disinfecting mops and other cleaning equipment if heat treatment is impractical.

The greatest risk when removing infectious spillage is from broken glass, needles and sharp instruments. These should carefully be removed with a suitable scoop and transferred to a sharps bin. This and all disposable cloths and cleaning materials should be disposed of in a yellow sealed bag or container as clinical waste. Suitable non-sterile gloves and a plastic apron should be worn when removing spillages or disinfecting environmental surfaces, as chlorine and other disinfectants are irritant to the skin.

Clear, soluble phenolics

Clear, soluble phenolics like Clearsol, Stericol and Hycolin are used for removing body fluid spills and disinfecting environmental surfaces. Some contain a compatible detergent, and cleaning may therefore be carried out at the same time as disinfection. Phenolics are now less widely used, as their virucidal activity is poor. They are not therefore recommended for blood spillages. They are, however, highly effective in destroying mycobacteria and other non-sporing bacteria, especially if present in faeces, sputum and other excretions. Phenolics are comparatively inexpensive, but are irritant, taint food and damage some plastics. They are therefore unsuitable for the skin, mattress covers and kitchen surfaces. Concentrations of 0.6–2% are usually advised, depending on the quantity of organic matter likely to be present.

Other environmental disinfectants

Other disinfectants suitable for the environment are the quaternary ammonium compounds such as Dettox, Trigene and the peroxygen compounds like Virkon. These are used for cleaning and disinfection in kitchens and other areas where the chlorine-releasing agents and phenolics are too irritant, taint food or damage surfaces. Their spectrum of activity, particularly against mycobacteria, spores and enteroviruses, is less good and they are not therefore advised for high or intermediate risk items (see Table 5.1). Most are however excellent cleansing agents and are more friendly to user and environment than the more effective chlorine-releasing agents. A review of the properties of environmental disinfectants can be seen in Table 5.2.

Control of substances hazardous to health (COSHH)

As an extension to the Heath and Safety at work Act, the COSHH regulations (HSC 1998) require all employers to assess the risk to health of using hazardous substances. This includes the pathogenic micro-organisms responsible for infection and the disinfectants used to destroy them. The most effective disinfectants, such as aldehydes, chlorine-releasing agents and phenolics, are irritant and sometimes sensitizing, and those that are safe tend to be less effective. Those responsible for formulating policy have therefore to achieve a balance in selecting effective agents which destroy the pathogens responsible for infection and yet are safe for the user and environment. If no safer alternative process is available, environmental controls and personal protective equipment will be necessary. The following course of action is advised:

- Consider the consequences of using or not using the agent.
- Eliminate or substitute a safer alternative, e.g. single use, heat processing or another disinfectant.
- Review the manufacturer's safety data sheet.
- If the disinfectant is irritant and/or sensitizing to the skin and eyes, make sure personal protective equipment is provided and used, i.e. gloves, waterproof aprons and if splashing could occur, eye protection.
- If the disinfectant is a respiratory irritant or sensitizer, contain and/or exhaust ventilate.

Risks can be further reduced if instruments are processed in a dedicated room with minimal occupancy, away from patient treatment areas.

A dated record must be kept of all relevant health and safety data, the risk assessment, policy for use including spillages, staff training and measurement for compliance with occupational exposure limits if necessary.

ENVIRONMENTAL CLEANING

The routine disinfection of floors, furniture, fittings, worktops and other surfaces remote from the patient is wasteful, unnecessary and may be damaging to the surface. Provided floors and other surfaces are cleaned without raising dust and adherent micro-organisms, they are unlikely to be carried to a susceptible site in sufficient numbers to cause infection. Regular and effective cleaning is, however, necessary to maintain the appearance of community healthcare establishments and to ensure the patient's confidence in the services they provide (Ayliffe, Babb and Taylor 1999).

Thorough cleaning and drying will control the microbial population and prevent unpleasant odours and the transfer of potentially infectious material. Cleaning alone may be sufficient for items and surfaces which are remote from the patient or in contact with normal healthy skin (see Table 5.1).

Cleaning procedures

Cleaning should remove and not redistribute soil and micro-organisms. Some environmental sites such as sink outlets, sluices, drains and lavatory pans, are heavily contaminated with Gram-negative bacilli and cleaning will only have a temporary influence on their numbers. Such areas are normally kept clean, but it is more sensible to regard them as grossly contaminated and take the necessary steps to prevent transmission, rather than to adopt expensive and often ineffective measures to keep them spotless, especially as the risk of infection from these sites is extremely low.

Two methods of environmental cleaning are used, dry and wet. If a dry method is used, dispersal of bacteria carrying particles such as *S. aureus* on skin squames into the air is the main risk, as these may be transferred to an open wound or the respiratory tract. Dry methods rely on mechanical action to dislodge and remove dust. Wet cleaning methods are more suitable for dirty hard surfaces and spillage. These do not raise dust but could lead to contamination of staff hands and other surfaces if poorly done.

Dry methods

Brooms redisperse bacteria-carrying particles into the air in large numbers. This method of cleaning should therefore be avoided in clinical areas. Dust attractant mops, sticky or static, gather and retain soil and micro-organisms and these are preferred. Their dust-holding properties may be extended to several days if the head is vacuumed after use or is washed and dried.

Vacuum cleaners are widely used on carpeted areas. A well-designed vacuum cleaner should not increase airborne bacterial counts, provided exhaust air is passed through a bacteria-retaining filter or bag and the exhaust is directed away from the floor. Dry dusting, particularly if high, may dislodge and disperse dirt and micro-organisms into the air. Damp dusting is preferable, although dry dusting with a vacuum head or dust attractant mop could also be used. If treatment rooms are not ventilated it is best to clean them at the end of the day or to keep wounds covered for at least 30 minutes after dusting has ceased. In addition to bacteria, many allergens such as dust mite faeces and feathers may be raised and inhaled if inappropriate dry cleaning methods are used.

Wet methods

Floors and other surfaces may be scrubbed or mopped with detergents and other cleaning agents. These techniques remove and suspend or dissolve soil and micro-organisms, which can then be disposed of down the sluice or drain. Dispersal of micro-organisms into the air during wet cleaning is unlikely. However, cleaning solutions soon become contaminated and bacteria grow in mop buckets and cleaning materials, particularly if they are soiled and kept moist for several hours, for instance overnight or a weekend. Cleaning solutions should be changed frequently and disposed of promptly when the task is complete. Moist surfaces encourage bacterial growth and should be regarded as a potential infection hazard. Surfaces used for clinical purposes, such as placing instruments or preparing food, should not be used until they are completely dry. If excessive amounts of water and detergent are used, as after cleaning a carpet, a wet vacuum machine may have to be used. This equipment must be kept clean, dry and properly maintained to prevent it becoming a source of bacterial aerosols.

Cloths, mops and other moist, soiled cleaning materials act as an ideal growth medium for micro-organisms. Bacteria normally reach their rapid or logarithmic phase of growth in three or four hours. If cleaning materials are left moist, dirty and warm, a few bacteria will become many millions overnight. If cleaning materials are reused the next day, or several hours later, they will effectively paint surfaces with a culture of potentially pathogenic micro-organisms. It is therefore important that disposable cleaning materials are used for a single task or for periods not exceeding two to three hours, and that reusable cleaning materials are cleaned, disinfected and dried before reuse. Disinfection can either be achieved by laundering in a washing machine or using an appropriate disinfectant such as a chlorine-releasing agent.

Outline policy for wet cleaning the environment

- Wearing suitable protective clothing, i.e. apron and gloves, prepare a fresh cleansing solution, e.g. detergent and warm water, in a clean dry container for each specific task.
- Apply the cleaning solution using a clean wipe, mop or brush.
- Do not put too much cleaning agent onto the surface as this may cause damage.
- Change the cleansing solution frequently to prevent a build-up of soil or micro-organisms which would recontaminate the surface.
- Rinse off the cleansing solution when it has had time to work.

- Dispose of the cleansing agent into a suitable sluice, sink (not wash hand basin) or drain.
- Dry the surface or allow it to dry.
- Remove the cleaning equipment to a suitable place. Make sure reusable equipment is cleaned, disinfected if appropriate, dried and stored in a designated and secure place.
- Dispose of single use cleaning materials.
- Remove gloves and protective clothing and wash hands before carrying out other duties.

If spillage of body fluids or other potentially infectious material occurs, or should the surface be in contact with the skin of an infected patient or one colonized with a multi-resistant strain of bacteria such as MRSA, a disinfectant may be required in addition to cleansing. For advice on the selection of a suitable agent and the method of spillage removal, see above.

DISINFECTION OF THE SKIN AND MUCOUS MEMBRANES

The purpose of skin disinfection is (Ayliffe et al 2000):

- To protect open wounds, damaged skin and other vulnerable sites from micro-organisms transferred on the hands of healthcare providers
- To protect the patient's tissues against his/her endogenous skin flora during surgery or an invasive procedure
- Occasionally to treat carriers and dispersers of multi-resistant strains such as methicillin-resistant *S. aureus* (MRSA).

The normal skin flora consists mainly of Gram-positive, coagulase-negative cocci such as *Staphylococcus epidermidis*, Micrococci, other staphylococci and aerobic and anaerobic diptheroids. These are known as residents, and rarely cause infection unless they are introduced during surgical or invasive procedures. The resident skin flora grow naturally on the skin and are extremely difficult to remove by normal skin cleansing procedures.

Many believe that the primary function of resident organisms is defensive, in that they protect the skin from invasion by more harmful micro-organisms. Reybrouck (1983) described the skin as self-disinfecting due to the arid conditions which are non-conducive to the survival of Gram-negative bacilli, the skin lipids which inhibit streptococci and the antimicrobial substances produced by the resident skin flora.

Micro-organisms, that is, bacteria and viruses acquired or deposited on the skin from other patients, health carers or the inanimate environment, are known as transients. These do not normally grow on the skin and are readily removed by thorough cleansing or disinfection. The transient flora includes most of the micro-organisms responsible for cross infection, such as *S. aureus*, *E. coli*, *P. aeruginosa*, salmonella spp. and rotaviruses.

Hand washing and disinfection

The hands are believed to be one of the principal routes of spread of infection (Garner and Favors 1985, Reybrouck 1986, Babb 1992, Infection Control Nurses Association 1998, Ayliffe et al 1999, 2000). Effective hand washing is, therefore, probably the most important infection control procedure. It is not unusual to find one third of healthcare providers carrying transient organisms on their hands at any one time and this increases during outbreaks, following contact with grossly contaminated surfaces and during lapses in compliance with hand washing and disinfection procedures. Numbers of transients on the hands can be as high as 10^{10}, for example after cleaning up an incontinent patient, although tens of thousands are more common (Ayliffe et al 1988).

The transient and resident flora can be removed or destroyed by the application of soap and water, antiseptic soaps and detergents or alcoholic hand rubs. Transients are superficial and are more easily removed or destroyed than the residents which colonize hair follicles, sebaceous glands and deeper layers and crevices of the skin. Table 5.8 indicates how, when and why the hands require cleaning and disinfection.

Social or routine hand washing

Thorough hand washing with unmedicated bar or liquid soap removes soil and most transient micro-organisms. This will normally suffice for tasks in community healthcare establishments, patients' homes and kitchens. It is essential to wash the hands after they have become soiled or contaminated with micro-organisms and before they make contact with a susceptible site on a patient or with food.

Table 5.8 Why, how and when to wash or disinfect hands. From a poster produced by J R Babb for *Professional Nurse* 1994.

	Social hand wash	Hygienic hand disinfection	Surgical scrub
Why	Use bar or liquid soap to render the hands socially clean and remove transient organisms	Use antiseptics to remove or destroy all/most transient micro-organisms	Use antiseptics to remove/destroy transient micro-organisms and substantially reduce detachable superficial resident micro-organisms. A prolonged effect is required
How	A thorough wash with a cosmetically acceptable bar or liquid soap	A thorough or defined wash for 15–30 sec. with an antiseptic soap or detergent, e.g. chlorhexidine, povidone-iodine or triclosan. Alternatively, apply an alcohol hand rub to disinfect clean hands	Scrape/brush nails if soiled and apply antiseptic soap or detergent e.g. chlorhexidine or povidone-iodine, to hands and forearms using a defined technique for approx 2 min. Dry hands on sterile towel. Alternatively, clean hands with soap and water and apply two or more applications of an alcohol hand rub
When	All routine tasks within healthcare establishments and catering areas	During outbreaks of infection, in high risk areas, when contact with infectious material is likely or at the discretion of those responsible for infection control	Prior to surgery or invasive procedures, and/or at the discretion of those responsible for infection control

Hygienic hand disinfection

Many antiseptic formulations are more effective in destroying transient micro-organisms than non-medicated soap. They are often preferred where the risks of hand transmission are particularly high, for example during outbreaks or if contact with infectious material is likely. Some aqueous formulations, like those containing chlorhexidine, povidone iodine or triclosan, have a residual or persistent effect which sustains antimicrobial activity so that the micro-organisms subsequently deposited on the skin are less likely to thrive. If a thorough technique is used, the more effective aqueous scrubs and alcoholic hand rubs may be 10 or 100 times more effective than soap alone. However, the possible detrimental effect that such agents may have on the resident skin flora, and the selection of antiseptic-resistant strains if these agents are routinely used, should be considered.

Surgical hand disinfection

During major surgical procedures a high proportion of surgical gloves are punctured or damaged by sharp instruments, needles and bone splinters. In one large study it has been shown that the clean wound post-operative infection rate increases threefold if gloves become damaged. It is therefore logical to use antiseptic formulations which are effective in removing or destroying both the transient and the superficial resident skin bacteria which would otherwise pass through the holes in the gloves, increasing infection risk. Effective antiseptic detergent scrubs such as those containing chlorhexidine and povidone-iodine, or alcoholic hand rubs, are therefore recommended prior to donning gloves for surgery. Products with a prolonged effect are preferred, to give lasting protection under the gloves. Sterile nail brushes or sticks may be used to clean nails prior to the first procedure of the session but are rarely required at other times. Frequent use of nail brushes damages the skin and may increase microbial proliferation. Hands should be dried, preferably on a sterile towel, before donning gloves.

Selection of soaps, detergents and alcoholic hand rubs

The efficacy of antiseptic soaps, detergents and hand rubs varies with the formulation and the nature of contamination. The efficacy of formulations for hygienic hand disinfection is assessed by a reduction in transient flora such as *E. coli* artificially applied to the hands or fingertips (Ayliffe et al 1988, Rotter and Ayliffe 1991). The most efficacious agents are those containing 60–80% isopropyl or ethyl alcohol, 4% chlorhexidine gluconate and 7.5% povidone-iodine, although unmedicated bar or liquid soap, if suitably applied, will remove 99% of the transient flora. Antiseptic formulations are more effective and alcoholic hand rubs, which are the most effective agents, will achieve reductions of 99.99% or more.

Surgical scrubs are usually assessed using a glove juice technique by measuring their immediate and prolonged effect (for example 3 hours) on the resident skin flora (Babb et al 1991). Although the rank order of effectiveness of antiseptics is similar to products for hygienic hand disinfection, the reductions in resident flora are less pronounced and no significant reduction occurs with unmedicated bar soap. The ranking order of effectiveness of antimicrobial soaps, detergents and hand rubs is: 1) 60–80% isopropyl alcohol, 2) 60–80% ethyl alcohol, 3) 4% chlorhexidine gluconate, 4) 7.5% povidone-iodine, 5) 2% trichlosan, 6) unmedicated soap (Ayliffe et al 1988, Babb et al 1991). The addition of aqueous antiseptics such as chlorhexidine, povidone-iodine and trichlosan to 60–80% alcohol does not improve the immediate effect but may enhance the prolonged or residual effect.

The application of alcohol as a solution or gel does not remove micro-organisms but rapidly destroys them on the skin surface. Alcoholic hand rubs are particularly valuable in areas devoid of wash hand basins or where access to a suitable clean hand wash facility is impractical. Alcoholic formulations do not contain the harsh detergents which are so often responsible for allergies and dermatitis. An emollient is necessary in detergent formulations and alcohol rubs to prevent the hands drying and chapping. Alcohol gels are particularly popular for community use as they are easily transported and used without leakage. Alcohol is flammable, and caution should be exercised when using it as a hand rub or skin disinfectant, particularly in the presence of a naked flame or diathermy equipment.

Studies using electronic counting equipment (Ayliffe et al 1988) have shown that hand washing frequency is much lower than that claimed. It is essential that soaps, detergents and alcoholic hand rubs used in healthcare establishments and those carried and used by community healthcare workers are cosmetically acceptable or they will not be used.

Hand washing technique

Studies have shown that certain areas of the hands are regularly missed during cleaning and disinfection, particularly if alcoholic hand rubs are used (Taylor 1978). Missed sites include tips of the fingers and thumbs, the surfaces most likely to pick up and transfer potentially infectious micro-organisms. A defined technique, which normally takes only 15–30 seconds, is shown in Figure 6.2 on page 81. This can be used for applying soaps and detergents and alcoholic hand rubs, ensuring all potentially contaminated surfaces are treated. The same procedure may be used for surgical scrubs, providing the forearms are included: 3–5 ml should suffice, but additional aliquots may be necessary for the more prolonged (2-minute) surgical scrub. **See Figure 6.2, page 81**.

When to wash or disinfect the hands

There is no set frequency for hand washing and disinfection. The need is determined by the tasks previously undertaken and those about to be performed. A social, routine or hygienic hand wash removes most transient organisms from hands. It is essential to wash or disinfect the hands after they become contaminated with potential pathogens and before these are conveyed to a susceptible patient site.

Frequent or over-diligent hand washing and disinfection may damage the skin and encourage the survival or proliferation of micro-organisms, but poor compliance with hand washing frequency

---

Box 5.4 Occasions when hands should be cleaned/disinfected (ICNA guidelines 1998, *Professional Nurse* poster, J R Babb 1994)

Before:
- commencing work
- preparing, handling or consuming food
- surgical procedures and injections
- administering medication
- dressing wounds
- inserting IV lines and catheters
- caring for immunocompromised patients
- donning gloves

After:
- contact with excretions and secretions
- using the lavatory, handling bedpans and urinals
- caring for isolated or barrier-nursed patients
- cleaning duties
- bedmaking and handling soiled or infectious linen
- removing soiled dressings
- handling clinical waste
- removing gloves

---

may result in infection transmission. The list of tasks in Box 5.4 gives some indication as to when the hands should be cleaned and/or disinfected.

Wash hand basins: design and location

Wash hand basins should be used exclusively for cleaning and disinfecting the hands and not for cleaning instruments or soaking clothing and equipment. One way of ensuring appropriate use is to install a hot/cold mixer tap and remove the plug.

The most suitably designed basins are those which deflect water away from the user. They should be located in examination and treatment rooms, lavatories, dirty sluice areas and kitchens. If they are not readily accessible they will not be used. A cosmetically acceptable liquid or bar soap and soft paper towels for hand drying should be readily available. Reusable (roller) towels soon become moist, contaminated and a potential source of infection. Hot-air dryers are available in some public lavatories but these are noisy, slow and should be avoided in clinical areas as they are likely to discourage hand washing.

Hand washing and disinfection compliance is likely to be poor if the wash hand basins are badly located or the hand wash formulations and paper towels are unpopular with staff. Alcoholic hand rubs may be issued if hand wash facilities are inadequate or not readily accessible, but the hands will still need to be cleaned. Liquid soaps should contain a bacteriostatic agent or preservative to prevent microbial proliferation during use. Containers and delivery systems should be disposable or readily accessible for cleaning prior to replenishment. Gram-negative bacilli are likely to grow on bar soap if stored moist or in a dish, but these are readily removed from the hands during rinsing.

Disinfection of the skin prior to surgery or an invasive procedure

Some minor surgical procedures are now carried out in community healthcare establishments, and a rapid reduction in skin flora (transients and residents) is required (Babb 1992, Ayliffe 1980). The most suitable agents are 60–80% isopropanol or ethanol. Provided the skin is clean, alcohol works rapidly and evaporates leaving the skin surface dry. The addition of other agents such as dyes, 0.5% chlorhexidine, or 10% povidone-iodine (now preferred to 1% iodine as it causes fewer skin reactions) may help to identify treated areas and prolong the antimicrobial effect, but they do not appear to enhance the immediate effect. Aqueous antiseptics such as 0.5% chlorhexidine and 10% povidone-iodine can be used on broken or damaged skin. Antiseptics should be applied with friction. This is most effectively done immediately prior to surgery and after shaving or clipping (Babb 1992).

Disinfection of the skin prior to injection

The need for disinfecting the skin prior to injection remains unclear, although the infection risk would appear minimal (Ayliffe et al 2000). Dann (1969) concluded that skin swabbing was unnecessary, but the study involved the use of healthy student volunteers and not elderly, compromised or MRSA patients. The British Diabetic Association also no longer advises skin disinfection prior to insulin injection. In spite of the lack of support for

skin disinfection, most infection control practitioners recommend it particularly for IV injections, sites close to discharging lesions or if faecal contamination of the skin is likely. Alcohol applied with a swab or wipe is by far the most effective agent, and rapidly evaporates leaving the skin dry.

Disinfection of mucous membranes

There is little evidence in support of the use of antiseptics for the disinfection of mucous membranes. Alcoholic formulations are usually too painful to apply, but have been used in the mouth prior to dental surgery. Antiseptics are soon diluted or inactivated by saliva, mucus and other body fluids and consequently have only a marginal effect. Chlorhexidine (0.2%) mouth washes are available for oral hygiene and these have been used for the treatment and prevention of gingivitis. The urethra normally has few commensal bacteria but is liable to become contaminated on passage of a catheter or instruments. A solution of 0.02% chlorhexidine instilled into the urethra, or applied with lignocaine, will disinfect the meatus prior to cystoscopy or catheterization. Cleaning with dilute Savlon or Savlodil (chlorhexidine 0.015% and cetrimide 0.15%) or a vaginal douche with 5% povidone-iodine followed by the use of 10% povidone-iodine gel, can be used for the vaginal mucosa. An obstetric cream containing 1% chlorhexidine gluconate may be used as an antiseptic lubricant during vaginal examinations.

Treatment of carriers of MRSA

Repeated applications of nasal creams containing antibiotics and antiseptics such as Bactroban (mupirocin) and Naseptin (neomycin and 0.1% chlorhexidine) have been successful in clearing multiresistant and/or highly communicable strains of *S. aureus* from the noses of patients and staff, but recolonization often occurs after treatment. Bathing or showering with an antiseptic soap or detergent has also been effective. Chlorhexidine, povidone-iodine, hexachlorophane and triclosan have all been used for this purpose with some beneficial effect (Ayliffe (chair) MRSA

Working Party Guidelines 1998). Each individual patient must be assessed fully before specific treatments are prescribed.

AUTHORISED PERSONS (STERILIZERS)

Professional advice on the selection, purchase, safe use, validation and periodic testing of benchtop steam sterilizers and washer disinfectors may be obtained from an Authorized Person (Sterilizers).

A list of such persons is available from the Institute of Healthcare Engineering and Estate Management, 2 Abingdon House, Cumberland Business Park, Northumberland Road, Portsmouth PO5 1DS. In addition to this, advice and support is also provided by the sterilizer manufacturers.

Summary of methods of decontamination of equipment or environment suitable for nursing homes and other community healthcare establishments

Equipment	Routine or preferred method *Acceptable alternative or additional recommendation*
Airways	Single patient use only (disposable).
Ambu bags	Clean, thermal disinfection in a washer/disinfector and dry. *Clean and disinfect by immersion in a chlorine-releasing agent (500 ppm av. Cl).*
Ambu lifts	Clean with detergent. *After known infected patient or MRSA carrier, clean and wipe with disinfectant,* *i.e. chlorine-releasing agent.*
Ampoules	Wipe neck with 70% alcohol, do not immerse.
Baths	Clean with detergent or cream cleanser and rinse. *After infected or MRSA patient clean and disinfect with a non-abrasive chlorine-releasing agent.*
Bedding	Laundering. *Preferably heat disinfect at 65°C for 10 min or 71°C for 3 min.*
Bedpans	Washer disinfector or use disposables. *Empty down WC, rinse and, if used on another patient, disinfect with a chlorine-releasing agent.*
Bowls (washing)	Each patient should preferably have their own bowl. Clean with detergent and dry. *Disinfect (heat or disinfectant) if known infection risk.*
Brushes: lavatory	Rinse in flushing water and store dry.
nail	Use only if essential, store dry. *A sterile or heat-processed brush should be used for surgical procedures.*
shaving	Single patient use only. *Autoclave if used for surgical procedures.*
tooth	Single patient use only.
Carpets	Vacuum at agreed frequencies. Periodic hot water/extract cleaning. *For infectious spillages disinfect with compatible agent if available, rinse and dry.*
Catheters	Single patient use only (disposable).
Combs	Single patient use only (disposable).
Commodes	Clean seat, pan and arm-rest after each use with detergent. *If contaminated, clean and wipe with disinfectant, i.e. chlorine-releasing agent* *or clear soluble phenolic.*
Crockery and cutlery	Machine wash, preferably above 80°C, and dry. *Hand wash with hot water and detergent, air dry.*
Curtains	Launder or dry clean six-monthly.
Drainage bags	Empty down WC or sluice (avoid splashing). Dispose of as clinical waste.
Dressing trolleys	Clean with detergent and dry. *Wipe clean surface with 70% alcohol.*
Duvets	Covers laundered (see Bedding). *Waterproof cover: clean with detergent and dry between patients. Disinfect* *with chlorine-releasing agent if contaminated with infectious material.*
Earphones/earpieces	Wipe with moist cloth and detergent and dry. *Wipe with 70% alcohol.*
Feeding cups	Machine wash, preferably above 80°C. *Hand wash with hot water and detergent, air dry.*
Feeds, bottles and teats	Clean and disinfect using hot water or steam. *Clean and disinfect by immersion in a chlorine-releasing agent (125 ppm av. Cl).*

Floors:
(dry cleaning) — Vacuum clean or use dust-attractant mops.
Do not use brooms in patient areas.

(wet cleaning) — Clean floor with detergent.
Disinfect infectious spillages with a chlorine-releasing agent.

Furniture and fittings — Damp dust with detergent.
Disinfect infectious spillages with a chlorine-releasing agent.

Lavatory seats, handles and rails — Clean with detergent.
Disinfect with a chlorine-releasing agent if contaminated.

Masks (O_2 ventilator) — Single patient use only (disposable).
Reusable masks: clean with detergent and dry or disinfect with 70% alcohol wipe.

Mattresses — Fit waterproof cover. Wipe with detergent and dry.
Apply disinfectant (chlorine-releasing agent) only if known infection risk.

Medicine glasses — Wash with detergent and dry.
Machine wash preferably at temperatures above 80°C.

Mops:
(dry, dust-attracting) — Vacuum head, wash or reprocess.
Do not overload.

(wet and buckets) — Rinse after use, wring and store dry, heat disinfect.
Rinse after use, soak in chlorine-releasing agent for 30 min and store dry.

Nebulizers — Single patient use only (disposable).
Clean with detergent between use on same patient, disinfect in accordance with manufacturer's instructions.

Pillows and supports — Covers laundered.
Waterproof cover: clean with detergent and dry between patients. Apply disinfectant (chlorine-releasing agent) only if known infection risk.

Plastic aprons — Single use (disposable).

Razors — Single patient use only (disposable).
Shared electric razors: remove head, clean and disinfect with 70% alcohol wipe after each patient use.

Rooms (terminal cleaning and disinfection) — Non-infected patients: clean surfaces with detergent and allow to dry.
Infected patients: clean and dry as above, disinfect surfaces close to patient with a chlorine-releasing agent, rinse and dry.

Sheepskins — Launder following manufacturer's instructions preferably at temperatures of 65°C for 10 min or 71°C for 3 min.

Sputum containers — Single use item (disposable).

Stethoscopes — Wipe with 70% alcohol.

Stoma bags — Single patient use, dispose of as clinical waste.

Suction equipment — Clean and dry, preferably thermal disinfection or sterilization.
Clean and soak in a chlorine-releasing agent.

Syringes — Single patient use, dispose of as clinical waste.

Thermometers — Single use (disposable) or clean with warm water and detergent, rinse and dry. Disinfect with 70% alcohol wipe.
Use disposable sleeve (oral/rectal), wipe with 70% alcohol.

Tooth mugs — Single patient use (disposable).
If reusable, thermally disinfect and dry.

Toys — Clean in detergent and dry.
If contaminated, launder or wipe with 70% alcohol or a chlorine-releasing agent.

Trolleys (food) — Clean with detergent and dry.

Urine bag holders — Clean with detergent and dry.

Urine bags — Single patient use, dispose of as clinical waste.

Urine bottles — Washer disinfector or use disposables.
Empty down WC or sluice and, if used on another patient, disinfect with a chlorine-releasing agent.

Ventilators — Damp dust with detergent and water. Change filters at appropriate intervals.
tubing — Disposable or *thermal disinfection.*
humidifiers — Disposable or *thermal disinfection.*

Vomit bowls and receivers — Washer disinfector or use disposables.
Empty down WC or sluice, clean with detergent, disinfect with a chlorine-releasing agent, rinse and dry.

Wash basins and showers — Clean with detergent or cream cleanser. Disinfectant not normally required.
Disinfect with a non-abrasive chlorine-releasing agent.

Waterbeds — Clean with detergent and dry.

Unless otherwise stated, the chlorine-releasing agents should be used at a concentration of 1000 ppm av. Cl.

REFERENCES

Advisory Committee on Dangerous Pathogens (ACDP) and the Spongiform Encephalopathy Advisory Group (SEAC) 1998 Guidance on Transmissible Encephalopathy Agents: Safe Working and the Prevention of Infection. HMSO, London

Ayliffe G A J 1980 Review article: The effect of antibacterial agents on the flora of the skin. Journal of Hospital Infection 1: 111–124

Ayliffe G A J 1988 Equipment related infection risks. Journal of Hospital Infection 11 (Suppl. A): 279–284

Ayliffe G A J (Chairman) 1998 Revised guidelines for the control of methicillin-resistant *S. aureus* infection in hospitals. Report of a combined working party of the BSAC, HIS and ICNA. Journal of Hospital Infection 39: 253–290

Ayliffe G A J, Babb J R, Quoraishi A H 1978 A test for 'hygienic' hand disinfection. Journal of Clinical Pathology 31: 923–928

Ayliffe G A J, Babb J R, Taylor L S 1999 Hospital Acquired Infection: Principles and Prevention, 3rd edn. Butterworth-Heinemann, Oxford

Ayliffe G A J, Coates D, Hoffman P N 1993 Chemical Disinfection in Hospitals. Public Health Laboratory Services, London

Ayliffe G A J, Fraise A P, Geddes A M, Mitchell K 2000 Control of Hospital Infection: a Practical Handbook, 4th edn. Arnold, London

Ayliffe G A J, Babb J R, Davies J G, Lilly H A 1988 Hand disinfection: a comparison of various agents in laboratory and ward studies. Journal of Hospital Infection 11: 226–243

Babb J R 1992 The action of disinfectants and antiseptics and their role in surgical practice. Chapter 6. In: Taylor E W (ed.) Infection in Surgical Practice. Oxford Medical Publications, Oxford

Babb J R 1993a Methods of cleaning and disinfection. Central sterilization, central service. Official publication of the European Society for Hospital Sterile Supply. ESHSS, Weisbaden-Nordenstadt, 227–237

Babb J R 1993b Disinfection and sterilization of endoscopes. Current Opinion in Infectious Diseases 6: 532–537

Babb J R 1994 Handwashing and disinfection: why, how and when. From a poster for Professional Nurse, Austin Cornish Publishers, London

Babb J R 1996 Application of disinfectants in hospitals and other healthcare establishments. Infection Control Journal of South Africa 1: 4–12

Babb J R, Davies J G, Ayliffe G A J 1991 Test procedure for evaluating surgical hand disinfection. Journal of Hospital Infection 18 (Suppl. B): 41–49

Bradley C R, Babb J R 1995 Endoscope decontamination, automated vs. manual. Journal of Hospital Infection 30 (Suppl.): 537–542

British Association of Urological Surgeons 1993 Decontamination of urological equipment: interim report of a Working Group of the Standing Committee on Urological Instruments of the BAUS. British Journal of Urology 7: 5–9

British Dental Association 2000 Advice sheet A12 Infection control in dentistry. British Dental Association, London

British Medical Association 1989 A code of practice for sterilization of instruments and control of cross infection. British Medical Association, London

British Society of Gastroenterology Working Party 1993 Aldehyde disinfectants and health in endoscopy units. Special report. Gut 34: 1641–1645

British Society of Gastroenterology 1998 Cleaning and disinfection of equipment for gastrointestinal flexible endoscopy. Working party report. Gut 42: 583–593

British Standards Institution 1993 British Standard 2745 Parts 1–3. Washer disinfectors for medical purposes. British Standards Institution, London

British Standards Institution (European Standard) 1997 BSEN 868 Packaging materials for sterilization of wrapped goods. Parts 1, 2, 3, 4, 5, 6. London

British/European Standard 1994 BSEN 554: Sterilization of medical devices – validation and routine control of sterilization by moist heat

British Thoracic Society 2001 Guidance on diagnostic flexible bronchoscopy. Thorax 56 (Suppl. 1): i1–i21

Dann T C 1969 Routine skin preparation before injection. An unnecessary procedure. Lancet 1: 96–98

Farrow S C, Kaul S, Littlepage B C 1988 Disinfection methods in general practice and health authority clinics: a telephone survey. Journal of the Royal College of General Practitioners 38: 447–449

Garner J S, Favors M S 1985 Guidelines for handwashing and environmental control. American Journal of Infection Control 14: 110–129

Health and Safety Commission 1998 Control of Substances Hazardous to Health Regulations. HSE Books, London

Health and Safety Executive 1999 EH 40/99 Occupational Exposure Limits. HMSO, London

Health Service Circular (HSC) 178 1999 Variant Creutzfeldt–Jakob Disease (vCJD): Minimising the risk of transmission. NHS Executive, London

Hoffman P N, Cooke E M, Larkin D P et al 1988 Control of infection in general practice: a survey and recommendations. British Medical Journal 297: 34–36

Hospital Infection Society Working Party Report 2000 Decontamination of minimally invasive surgical endoscopes and accessories. Journal of Hospital Infection 45: 263–277

Infection Control Nurses Association 1998 Guidelines for Hand Hygiene. ICNA, Bathgate

Institute of Sterile Services Management (ISSM) 1998a Quality standards and recommended practices for sterile service departments. ISSM c/o Fitwise, Bathgate

Institute of Sterile Services Management 1998b Sterile Services Resource Manual. ISSM c/o Fitwise, Bathgate

Medical Devices Agency 1993/96 Sterilization, Disinfection and Cleaning of Medical Equipment: Guidance on Decontamination, Part 1 Principles; Part 2 Protocols; Part 3 Procedures (in preparation). Microbiology Advisory Committee to the Department of Health. HMSO, London

Medical Devices Agency 1996 Decontamination of endoscopes. Device Bulletin MDA DB 9607. Department of Health, London

Medical Devices Agency 1997 The purchase, operation and maintenance of benchtop steam sterilizers. Device Bulletin MDA DB 9605. Department of Health, London

Medical Devices Agency 1998a Medical device and equipment management for hospital and community-based organisations. Device Bulletin MDA DB 9801. Department of Health, London

Medical Devices Agency 1998b The validation and periodic testing of benchtop vacuum steam sterilizers. Device Bulletin MDA DB 9804. Department of Health, London

Medical Devices Agency 2000a Guidance on the purchase, operation and maintenance of vacuum benchtop steam sterilizers. Device Bulletin MDA DB 2000(05). Department of Health, London

Medical Devices Agency 2000b Single use medical devices: implications and consequences of reuse. Device Bulletin MDA DB 2000(04). Department of Health, London

Medical Devices Directive 93/42/EEC 1998 Council Directive 14 June 1993 concerning medical devices. Official Journal of the European Committee L169 36 12.7.93

Morgan D R, Lamont T J, Dawson J D, Booth C 1990 Decontamination of instruments and control of cross infection in general practice. British Medical Journal 300: 1379–1380

NHS Estates 1994/95 Sterilization. Health Technical Memorandum 2010. HMSO, London

NHS Estates 1995 Washer disinfectors. Health Technical Memorandum 2030. HMSO, London

NHS Executive 1995 Hospital laundry arrangements for used and infected linen (HSG (95) 18). Health Publications Unit, Heywood, Lancs

NHS Management Executive Health Service Guidelines HSG (93) 26 1993 Decontamination of equipment prior to inspection, service or repair

Reybrouck G 1983 Role of the hands in the spread of nosocomial infections. Journal of Hospital Infection 4: 103–110

Reybrouck G 1986 Review article: Handwashing and hand disinfection. Journal of Hospital Infection 8: 5–23

Rotter M L, Ayliffe G A J 1991 Practical guide on rationale and testing procedures for disinfection of hands. World Health Organization, Geneva

Safety Action Bulletin SAB(94)22 1994 Instruments and appliances used in the vagina and cervix: recommended methods of decontamination. Department of Health, London

Sneddon J, Ahmed S, Duncan E 1997 Control of infection: a survey of general medical practices. Journal of Public Health Medicine 19: 313–319

Taylor L J 1978 An evaluation of handwashing techniques (parts 1 and 2). Nursing Times 74: 54–55, 108–110

White R R, Smith J M P 1995 Infection control in general practice: results of a questionnaire survey. Journal of Public Health Medicine 17: 146–149

6

Home nursing

J. Lawrence

INTRODUCTION

Historically, many publications and guidelines have concentrated on the issue of hospital-acquired infection and means of prevention. Healthcare over the last few years has seen many changes. These changes have arisen from a reactive, fragmented service to a needs-led service for all.

At the time of writing, changes are taking place in re-shaping services within communities. Primary Care Trusts will have a leading role in these changes to cover the whole spectrum of hospital, community and primary services. Health authorities will be replaced by fewer and smaller strategic health authorities with responsibility for strategy and performance management (Department of Health 2002a).

A second publication, 'Getting Ahead of the Curve' (Department of Health (Chief Medical Officer) 2002b), outlines a strategy for combating infectious disease and other aspects of health protection. Within this strategy infection control measures are highlighted as being essential to reduce illness and death from tuberculosis, healthcare-associated infection, antibiotic-resistant organisms, blood-borne and sexually transmitted infections.

Health Trusts are required to have satisfactory arrangements in place for infection control, and these are currently guided by Controls Assurance Standards (Department of Health 1999a). Part of the requirements are to ensure:

- an Infection Control Committee is in place
- there is a functioning Infection Control team

- day-to-day working practice and responsibility are clearly illustrated
- there are clear responsibilities of the Trust concerned
- there is an annual infection control programme
- there are written policies and procedures available for prevention and control of infection.

There are many staff involved in the process of infection control in the community and these can include:

- Consultant in Communicable Disease Control
- Community Infection Control Nurse
- Environmental Health Officer
- Public Health Laboratory Personnel
- Medical Microbiologist
- District Nurses and Health Visitors
- School Nurses and Doctors
- Social Services/Home Care
- General Practitioners and Practice Nurses
- Occupational Health staff
- Residential/Nursing Home owners and managers.

The infection control nurse is normally the only full-time member of the infection control team and is a source of advice and information for all community issues related to infection control.

Amongst much technological advance and changing disease patterns, the need to provide healthcare closer to, and in, the home environment has become apparent. It is also essential that collaborative approaches to care in the community are undertaken. Nurses must adapt their practice in order to deliver healthcare that is relevant and evidence-based. This practice must be constantly reviewed and exercised within the professional code of practice. Due to changes in the systems of process and service, nurses have a vast area of collaborative working to achieve effective client outcomes for those in their care. Amidst all these changes, problems associated with infection remain ever present. In 1999 the then Chief Nurse stated that 'Communicable disease control will always be a fundamental element of all healthcare' (Moores 1999). For many years infection control was heavily concentrated towards the hospital

environment, but it is important to remember that those patients in hospital are part of the community prior to any admission and after discharge.

There is now a very rapid turnover of patients being admitted and discharged, with acute surgery ranging from minor to major. Patients also undergo various treatments that take place at the local General Practice or within the home itself. Indeed, it is no longer unusual for patients to be treated at home with various types of invasive devices.

Patterns and the way care is delivered have also altered, for example Social Services providing home care with responsibilities for basic hygienic needs of patients. Figure 6.1 shows the possible number of services that can be involved in care-giving for patients in the community.

The community nurse is concerned with the total healthcare of the individual and his/her family. This includes helping to prevent and control infection (Griffiths 1981). In 1993, however, Castledine pointed out that 'hygiene itself does not appear to have a dramatic and stimulating appeal' in comparison to other subjects. Further to this the House of Lords Select Committee (1998) stated that 'infection control and basic hygiene should be at the heart of good management and clinical practice'. It is essential to remember that the basic principles of hygiene lie at the heart of good health. The nurse, therefore, has an essential role to play in the prevention and control of infection within the community home setting.

Services are changing in regard to care taking place in the home. An example of this is the introduction of intermediate care teams. These are designed to prevent avoidable admissions to acute care, and facilitate the transition from hospital to home (Department of Health 2000). Such initiatives demonstrate that much more care will take place in the home. In order to achieve a service of high quality, it is also important to include the patient in all decision-making processes (Department of Health 1998).

PHYSICAL ENVIRONMENT

Social, cultural and environmental conditions vary widely, depending on the community

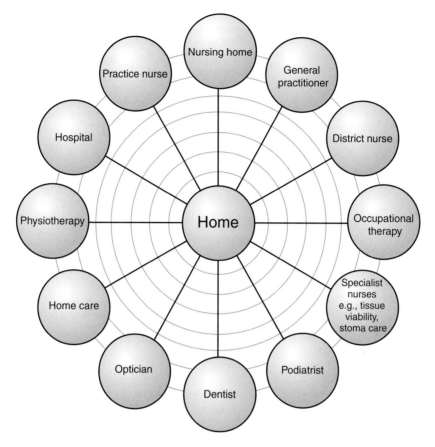

Figure 6.1 The healthcare services web.

concerned. For example, rural farming communities differ vastly from large inner cities.

The patient being cared for in the home is a form of 'isolation nursing' as the numbers of staff involved in the care process can be considerably smaller than in a hospital ward. The nurse does not have the same amount of control over the environment as in the hospital setting (Lawrence 1994). Indeed, the nurse is a guest in the patient's home and it is important to tailor care in agreement with the patient or the carer. The following checklist may be useful when setting up care in the home and its relationship to infection control.

- Was the patient recently discharged from hospital?
- History of known infections/antibiotic treatment

- Any infections whilst in hospital?
- What other staff/services are involved in the care process?
- What procedures need to be carried out?
- Where will procedures be carried out?
- Can hands be washed in the home?
- Will large amounts of clinical waste be generated?
- Will a sharps box be required and safely stored in the home?
- Is there adequate space to store necessary equipment?
- Are there any other family members ill or immunocompromised?

The information received from the hospital by a district nurse is extremely important. Ideally, discharges should be planned to 'anticipate a patient's community needs' (Newman 1991). This allows the district nurse to plan and make suitable arrangements to allow for continuity of care. It is not always possible to know when a discharge will take place, but it should have at least 48 hours notice. Due to the increasing amount of day surgery and early discharges this timescale can be difficult to achieve, but every effort must be made to meet the needs of the patient when being discharged home.

Conditions in patients' homes may vary considerably and it is necessary to plan care in consultation with the patient and their carers. The district nurse has no control over the environment and must always try to adhere to the wishes of the patient.

Whatever the conditions, 'practice should always be in the interest of the patient and be competent, safe, evidence-based and continually evaluated against agreed standards' (Joint Committee of Professional Nursing, Midwifery and Health Visiting Associations England 1997).

STANDARD INFECTION CONTROL PRECAUTIONS

As a routine measure, standard infection control precautions (SICP) are applied in the delivery of healthcare to all patients at all times. The purpose of the precautions is to minimize the risk of transferring micro-organisms to others.

The term 'Universal Precautions' was originally applied to all body fluids and was described by the Centers for Disease Control in the USA (CDC 1987). This was in response to hazards associated with blood-borne viruses. Not all body fluids contain blood-borne viruses, and the guidance was altered to exclude body fluids that did not contain blood (CDC 1988). The term SICP will be used throughout the chapter. They will be discussed under the following headings as related to the home environment:

- Hand decontamination
- Protective clothing
- Safe handling and disposal of sharps
- Safe disposal of clinical waste
- Safe handling of contaminated linen

- Dealing safely with spillages of blood and body fluids
- Decontamination of reusable devices and equipment.

Hand decontamination

Hand washing today remains one of the most important measures in the prevention and control of infection. Micro-organisms are invisible to the naked eye, which makes it difficult for healthcare staff to recognize their importance. Hands are frequently implicated as the route of transmission in outbreaks of infection (Wilson 2001). Skin itself supports the growth of a wide range of microbes which are known as normal flora or resident skin flora. The transient microbes are those that are acquired on the hands from contact with objects, other people and the environment. Transient micro-organisms can be easily removed with hand washing (Fig. 6.2), thus reducing the risk of spreading infection (ICNA 1997).

Studies on hand washing in the community are not in abundance as most are centred around the hospital and clinical environment. In a literature review by Ward (2000), it was noted that the Health and Safety Regulations require that both hot and cold running water should be available in areas where employees are expected to wash their hands. This obviously applies to hospital and where clinical services are based, and cannot be enforced in the homes of patients (Fig. 6.3). Carlisle (1998) pointed out that there is a lack of understanding in the acute sector in terms of what is manageable in the community. It requires skill on the part of the nurse to overcome the problems associated with the environment in which they need to carry out care.

It is the responsibility of the nurse to ensure that hand decontamination is carried out before each and every episode of care and after any activity or contact that potentially results in hands becoming contaminated (*epic* Project 2001). In order to ensure that hand decontamination is carried out in a patient's home, the following practice options are suggested:

1. Where running water and soap are available and access to the sink is clear, the nurse

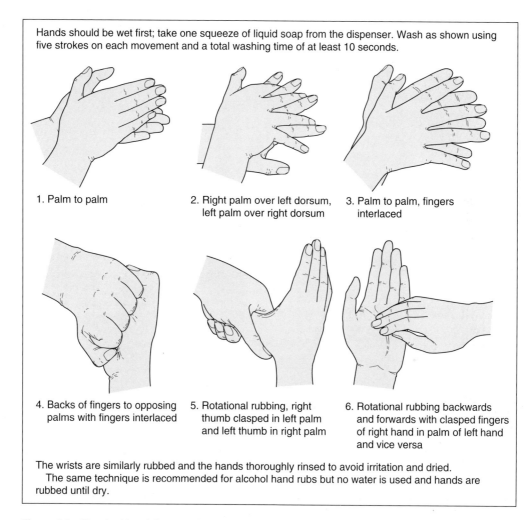

Hands should be wet first; take one squeeze of liquid soap from the dispenser. Wash as shown using five strokes on each movement and a total washing time of at least 10 seconds.

1. Palm to palm

2. Right palm over left dorsum, left palm over right dorsum

3. Palm to palm, fingers interlaced

4. Backs of fingers to opposing palms with fingers interlaced

5. Rotational rubbing, right thumb clasped in left palm and left thumb in right palm

6. Rotational rubbing backwards and forwards with clasped fingers of right hand in palm of left hand and vice versa

The wrists are similarly rubbed and the hands thoroughly rinsed to avoid irritation and dried.
The same technique is recommended for alcohol hand rubs but no water is used and hands are rubbed until dry.

Figure 6.2 Standard hand decontamination technique. Based on that of Ayliffe, Babb and Quoraishi (1978).

can carry paper hand towels to use in the client's home.

2. When soap is not available, the nurse can carry her own supply of liquid soap/hand towels as recommended by the employer/infection control team.

3. If access is difficult or facilities limited, the nurse can employ an alcohol hand rub.

It must be remembered that alcohol is not a cleansing agent and is not recommended in the presence of physical dirt (Larson 1995 in ICNA 1997). The hand rub must come into contact with all surfaces of the hand. Hands must be rubbed together vigorously, paying particular attention to the tips of the fingers, the thumbs and the areas between the fingers, and until the solution has evaporated and the hands are dry (*epic* Project 2001).

Protective clothing

The purpose of protective clothing is to prevent potentially pathogenic micro-organisms being transmitted from the nurse's clothing to another patient. Its use also prevents contamination of the nurse's own clothing or uniform. Employers have a responsibility to ensure the provision of protective clothing for safe working practices (Health and Safety Executive 1992).

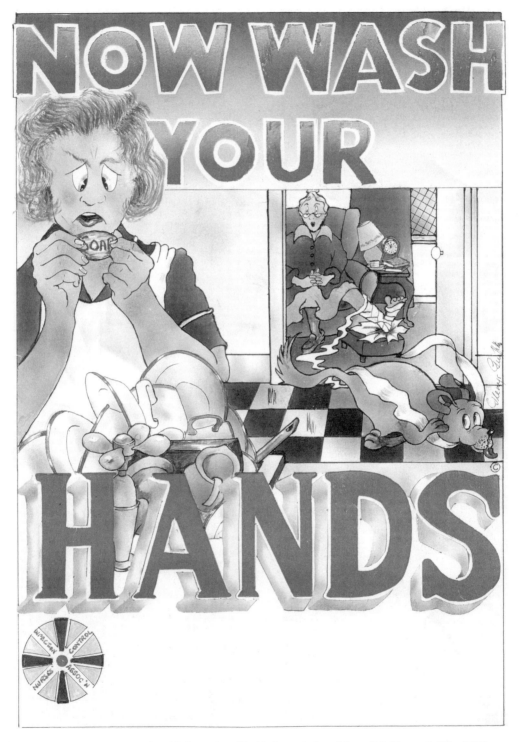

Figure 6.3 'Now wash your hands'. Reproduced by kind permission of the artist, Glenys Griffiths RGN.

Table 6.1   Level, type of contact and recommended protective clothing. Reproduced with kind permission of Nursing Times, where this first appeared (July 14, Volume 95, No. 28, 1999)

Example procedure	Anticipated level of contact	Recommended protective clothing
Cleaning of large blood spillage. Dealing with haemorrhaging patient. Minor invasive procedures where spraying of blood is possible, for example, angiogram, insertion of central venous device, endotracheal/tracheal suctioning	Contact with blood and risk of splashing. Risk of respiratory secretions to the face	Gloves (sterile or non-sterile as appropriate), apron, face protection
Insertion and removal of urinary catheter. Emptying and removal of wound drain/urinary drainage bag. Removing and replacing wound dressing. Cleaning patient who has had an episode of incontinence	Contact with body substance. Possible risk of splashing	Gloves and apron. Face protection based on individual assessment of splash risk
Rectal examination. Insertion of enema, suppositories, pessaries. Vaginal examination. Oral toilet	Contact with mucous membrane and body secretions. Clothing exposure	Gloves and apron
Blanket bath. Lifting and handling patients. For example, positioning for X-ray. Physiotherapy where contact with uniform is anticipated	Close contact with patient and bedding. Contamination of uniform/clothing is probable	Plastic apron. Wash hands after removal of apron

The main items of protective clothing involved in home care include: disposable latex or non-latex powder-free gloves, disposable plastic aprons, protective eye wear and masks for the protection of mucous membranes. Protective clothing recommended for various patient contact situations is given in Table 6.1.

Gloves

When direct contact with blood or body fluids is anticipated, staff should wear seamless, non-sterile disposable gloves (for example latex or non-latex and powder-free). The gloves **must** be discarded after each procedure and hands must be washed. Disposable gloves are single use items and must be discarded after each use or procedure (ICNA 2002).

Washing gloves is not recommended as the soap solution can cause glove damage. If punctured unknowingly, this may cause body fluid to remain in direct contact with skin for prolonged periods (Adams et al 1992).

Aprons

When direct contact with blood or body fluids is anticipated, staff should wear a plastic disposable apron. Nurses' uniforms can become contaminated, and organisms can be disseminated from uniforms to patients, but the correct use of plastic aprons can prevent this redispersal (Curran 1991).

Face protection

Face protection involves the use of protective eyewear and/or mask. This will only be necessary when splashing of blood or body fluids to the face/mucous membranes is anticipated.

Sharps management

Nursing staff are exposed daily to many hazards during the course of care giving. One of these hazards is the potential risk from needlestick injury. It will not always be possible to determine who may be infected by bacteria or viruses, therefore safe practice must be adhered to at all times.

Employers must have detailed local guidelines and policies on procedures for dealing with sharps and any consequent inoculation injury. Inoculation injury also applies to contamination of abrasions with blood or body fluids, scratching involving broken skin, and splashes of blood or body fluids into the eyes or mouth. 'Sharps' include needles, scalpels, broken glass or other items that may cause a laceration or puncture (Wilson 2001).

Needlestick injuries are the most common type of occupational injury among nurses (Russell 1997). The circular MDA SN2001 (19) from the Medical Devices Agency, Department of Health highlights the dangers to staff and advises safe practice.

Safe practices for prevention of injury include the following:

- Needles which have been used must *never* be re-sheathed broken or bent.
- Sharps must not be passed directly from hand to hand and handling must be kept to a minimum.
- Dispose of a syringe and needle as one complete unit directly into a sharps container as soon as possible after use.
- Never leave sharps lying around. It is the responsibility of the user to ensure safe disposal.
- Sharps containers should only be three quarters full prior to sealing and disposal.
- Always label the sharps box with the source and the date.
- Ensure secure closure and locking when the container is three-quarters full.
- Ensure the sharps container conforms to BS 7320 (MDA 2001a).
- Always locate containers in a secure position out of reach of others.
- Carry used sharps containers by the handle.
- Do not dispose of sharps with other clinical waste.

Any exposure to blood and body fluids through a sharp object, bite or splashing into the eyes or mouth must be followed up immediately to prevent the risk of infection from blood-borne viruses. Cuts and abrasions on exposed skin must always be covered with a secure waterproof dressing. Disposable gloves may be required if hands are extensively affected (UK Health Departments 1998). Actions to be taken are shown in Figure 6.4. It is the responsibility of individual staff to ensure that the correct procedure is followed to prevent the risk of infection.

Whilst working in a community setting it is not always as easy to reach the local occupational health and accident and emergency departments. It is therefore advisable to check on local policy and guidance to ensure the correct procedure is being followed. The community employer has

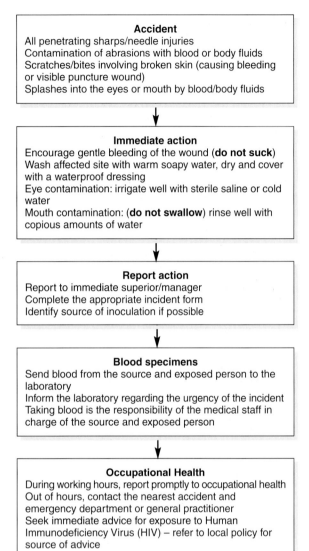

Figure 6.4 Action following accidental inoculations with blood/body fluids.

a responsibility to secure arrangements for staff working in the community setting. These arrangements can normally be set up through the local infection control committee in conjunction with occupational health and the acute hospitals.

Sharps containers

All sharps containers must conform to the British Standard Specification 7320/UN3291 and be available for use when required.

Discarded syringe needles, cartridges, broken glass and any other contaminated disposable sharp instrument or item is classed under Group B in the categorization of clinical waste (Health and Safety Commission 1999). In the community setting staff will be required to carry containers to dispose of sharp instruments. The containers may be sited in a patient's home but only following a risk assessment regarding how safe this practice will be. No specific guidance is available regarding the carrying of a sharps container in a car by a healthcare worker or carrying it manually. The following practice is suggested in order to eliminate risks to others.

- The sharps container must be of a type approved under the requirements of the Carriage of Dangerous Goods Regulations (1996).
- A sharps container can be carried in the healthcare worker's car providing it is sited safely and the employer accepts this practice as agreed by the infection control committee.
- The sharps container must have a suitable mechanism that allows the contents of the container to be retained safely prior to its being locked.
- When storing the container in a car boot, ensure it is positioned in a secure manner to prevent any spillage of the contents.
- The car must be securely locked when left unoccupied at any time.
- Small containers are available for use (for instance, pocket/bag size). These must be positioned in a bag to avoid spillage and the mechanism for containing prior to final locking must be secure.
- Always label the container with the date and source prior to disposal.
- Lock the sharps container securely when three-quarters full and place in the dedicated area prior to collection for final disposal.

Clinical waste management

Managing clinical waste in the home setting has never been addressed fully, as much of the information and guidance relates to the hospital and/or other clinical settings. Guidance was published in 1999 by the Health Services Advisory Committee (HSAC) of the Health and Safety Executive, but this assumed that clinical waste generated in the home environment consisted of 'small amounts' and it was only handled by the patient or their immediate family. There still remains no clear advice on management in the home. The following information and guidance is to assist the staff who are responsible for ensuring safe practice when dealing with clinical waste arising from home care.

Definitions

Clinical waste is defined (HMSO 1992) as 'any waste which consists wholly or partly of human or animal tissue, blood or other body fluids, excretions, drugs or other pharmaceutical products, swabs or dressings, syringes, needles and other sharp instruments' which unless rendered safe may prove hazardous to any person coming into contact with it. This also includes other waste arising from medical, nursing, dental, veterinary, pharmaceutical or similar practice, investigation, treatment, care, teaching or research, or the collection of blood for transfusion, being waste which may cause infection to any person coming into contact with it.

Clinical waste is disposed of by placing into a plastic bag, which is yellow in colour and usually printed with the words 'clinical waste, incineration only'. The local council disposes of all domestic waste into black plastic bags or a 'wheelie bin' system for collection. A yellow bag with black stripes is for non-infectious waste such as waste from the Group E category (see Table 6.2).

Clinical waste is further defined into categories as shown.

Safe practice

It is essential that employers have clear written guidance for staff dealing with clinical waste in the home setting. The 1999 COSHH regulations require that employers who generate clinical waste must ensure that the risks from it are properly controlled. This involves assessing the risk, developing policies, putting arrangements into place to manage the risks and monitoring the way these arrangements work (Lawrence and Fuller 2000). The Controls Assurance standard for waste

Table 6.2 Safe disposal of clinical waste (Health Services Advisory Committee 1999)

Group	Waste for disposal
A	Identifiable human tissue, blood, animal carcases and tissue from veterinary centres, hospitals or laboratories Soiled surgical dressings, swabs and other similar soiled waste Other waste materials, for example from infectious disease cases, excluding any in groups B–E
B	Discarded syringe needles, cartridges, broken glass and any other contaminated disposable sharp instruments or items
C	Microbiological cultures and potentially infected waste from pathology departments and other clinical or research laboratories
D	Drugs or other pharmaceutical products
E	Items used to dispose of urine, faeces, and other bodily secretions which do not fall within group A. This includes used disposable bed pans or bed pan liners, incontinence pads, stoma bags and urine containers

Box 6.1 Example of collaborative working (for clinical waste disposal)

- Discuss with infection control, district nursing, public health and the local council
- Agree what constitutes 'clinical waste' according to the guidance and legislation
- Design a form to request services to remove clinical waste from a patient's home (see Fig. 6.5)
- Supply district nurses with the form for use
- Evaluate at periodic intervals
- Ensure contact details of a named person are available at the local council to enable rapid communications when problems arise

management is concerned with the safe segregation, handling, transport and disposal of clinical waste (DoH 2001). This standard contains the criteria necessary to ensure safe systems are in place.

Disposal of clinical waste from the home environment

Guidance on the disposal of clinical waste has placed much focus on the hospital setting. The publication of the 'Safe Disposal of Clinical Waste' (HSAC 1999) did make reference to producers of clinical waste other than hospitals, but failed to give specific guidance for community nursing on a national basis.

The increase in treatments carried out in the home raises the amounts of waste that will require to be disposed of. The guidance only stated that 'employers have a duty to ensure that clinical waste generated is disposed of safely'. In some parts of the United Kingdom many problems are encountered by healthcare workers dealing with clinical waste when guidance is confusing or not always easy to interpret or follow. At the time of writing a review is taking place aiming to rationalize the approach to the disposal of waste in the community.

Legislation is an essential element in the safe handling, segregation and disposal of clinical waste (Lawrence and Fuller 2000). A collaborative approach is advised in order to comply with legislation and guidance and to ensure that safe, effective and sensible systems are in place for clinical waste to be collected and disposed of in the correct manner (Box 6.1).

Waste from human hygiene (Sanpro waste) may carry micro-organisms, and it has been shown that domestic waste contains more organisms than that found routinely in clinical waste (Phillips 1999). Examples of waste in this category include (HSAC 1999):

- sanitary towels
- tampons
- nappies
- stoma bags
- incontinence pads
- other similar wastes, provided they do not contain sharps.

Other items which may contain micro-organisms and are placed in domestic waste include pregnancy testing kits, condoms and blood cholesterol testing devices.

All of the above items may be put into the domestic waste provided it is adequately wrapped and free of excess liquid (HSAC 1999). Deciding which type of disposal is required for patients' waste should be assessed by the nurse on the first visit when agreeing their programme of care.

CLINICAL OR CHEMICAL TOILET WASTE COLLECTION		
Request for Service/Cancellation of Service* ***(Please delete as appropriate)**		
To be completed by nurse or medical professional. Please tick and date		
SERVICE REQUESTED	**Request commenced**	**Cancelled**
Clinical Waste Group A – Soiled surgical dressings, swabs and other soiled waste from treatment areas – to be incinerated. (Weekly)		
Clinical Waste Group E – Items used to dispose of urine, faeces and other bodily secretions/excretions, not falling in Group A, including disposable bed pans, bed pan liners, incontinence pads, stoma bags and urine containers – to go to landfill. (Weekly)		
Chemical Toilet Waste Collection. (Weekly)		

PATIENT DETAILS

Name:	
Address:	
District:	Full Postcode:
Tel No:	
House Type	e.g. flat, semi etc.

ORIGINATOR DETAILS

Signed:		Print Name:
Base:		Contact Tel No:

Any comments: _____

_____

Designation

_____

Send completed form to:

Mr/Ms _____   Telephone: _____

Refuse Collection Agency _____

Street _____

Figure 6.5 Clinical or chemical toilet waste collection: request/cancellation form. Reproduced by courtesy of Leeds Community and Mental Health Services NHS Trust.

Linen

Linen used by patients in their own home is normally laundered using a domestic washing machine. Current guidance on laundering is dedicated to acute settings and residential care, and does not address the home environment. Thorough washing and rinsing at low temperatures (40–50°C) will remove most organisms and should be sufficient in most circumstances, particularly in domestic washers (Ayliffe et al 2000).

Items being laundered include personal clothing and household linens, such as bedclothes.

The task can be carried out by the patient, home care worker, relatives or friends. Advice includes the following:

- Employ a plastic bag to contain the items ready for laundering.
- Do not soak any items in solutions.
- Household gloves (dedicated for the purpose) should be used for handling the soiled linen.
- Gross faecal soiling on items should be carefully sluiced down the toilet before placing in the machine.
- A hand wash can be carried out using household gloves when a washing machine is not available (suitable for personal clothing).
- Hands must be thoroughly washed following handling of soiled items.

It may be necessary to use an outside laundry agency for those patients with no assistance, or access to a washing machine, or those with significant continence problems. These arrangements will need to be put in place through Social Services in collaboration with the patient and the district nurse. Further information and advice can be sought from the infection control nurse/team.

Linen which is heavily contaminated with blood can be cleaned using (UK Health Departments 1998):

- the hot wash cycle of a domestic washing machine to a temperature of at least 80°C
- dry cleaning at elevated temperatures, or dry cleaned cold followed by steam pressing.

Incineration may be necessary for gross soiling.

Blood and body fluid spillage

All spillage must be dealt with as soon as possible to prevent contamination to others and prevent damage to surfaces in the home environment (see Box 6.2).

Should any abrasions, cuts or eczematous lesions become contaminated with blood or body fluids, it must be reported as an accidental inoculation and the local policy must be followed.

Box 6.2 Spillage procedure in the home

- Wear a disposable plastic apron and disposable latex or non-latex gloves.
- Soak up as much spillage as possible using disposable kitchen towel roll or paper towels.
- Use detergent and water to clean the area using a disposable cloth or a cloth that can be disposed of.
- *Do not* use hypochlorite on a carpet as this will bleach the carpet.
- Discard cloth, gloves, apron and paper towels into a yellow clinical waste bag. Where no clinical waste collection service is in use, wrap all items to be disposed of in double wrapping and place in the domestic waste system. When blood spillage is a frequent occurrence, it is advisable to make arrangements for a collection service.
- Wash hands thoroughly on completion of the procedure.

PRACTICES

Home care

The home care division of social services provides a service of personal hygiene and household duties to patients in their own home. The district nurse works in collaboration with this service, ensuring that care being given is delivered in a safe and effective manner. When direct care, such as bathing or emptying urine drainage bags, is to be carried out, home care staff require education and training in infection control to minimize the risks of infection to the patient and themselves. This also fulfils the requirements of health and safety.

Training should include the following:

- Standard infection control precautions
- Specific infections such as wound infection, chest infections, urinary tract infections, scabies

- Wound care
- Catheter care
- Antibiotic resistance and its implications
- Care of equipment.

Aseptic techniques

The purpose of aseptic techniques is to prevent microbial contamination of tissue, fluid or sterile equipment, and contamination of susceptible sites. (The key principles are described in Chapter 8, Residential and nursing homes.)

When carrying out aseptic procedures such as dressings in a patient's home, the nurse does not have specific equipment as in acute settings, for example a dressing trolley; therefore adaptation and creativity are often required. In some areas district nurses use a portable tray/trolley that can be used as a working field.

Urinary catheter care

Catheter care, when carried out in the home setting, is usually for patients with long-term or permanent catheters. Care should be aimed at preventing the introduction of new uropathogens (Fig. 6.6) and minimizing other health-related problems. Urinary catheters not only affect the patient's psychological and social well-being; they may also cause significant health problems, including urinary tract infection, stricture formation, urethral perforation, encrustation, bladder calculi and neoplastic changes (Lothian 1998).

Bacteria can enter the bladder via the following routes:

- Introduced during the insertion of the catheter
- Along the side of the catheter
- Along the lumen of the catheter.

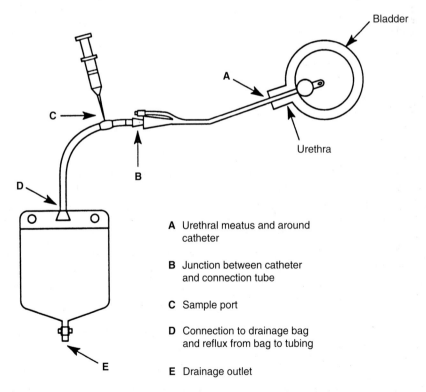

A Urethral meatus and around catheter

B Junction between catheter and connection tube

C Sample port

D Connection to drainage bag and reflux from bag to tubing

E Drainage outlet

Figure 6.6 Potential points of entry of micro-organisms into the bladder of a catheterized patient. Reproduced by kind permission from Wilson J 2001 *Infection Control in Clinical Practice*, 2nd edn. Baillière Tindall, Edinburgh.

Box 6.3 Catheter insertion: guidelines for practice (adapted from Wilson 2001)

- Select the appropriate catheter for insertion
- Use sterile equipment
- Prepare the patient and position comfortably
- Clean the perineum and urethral meatus using soap and water, water or saline
- Wash hands thoroughly and wear sterile gloves
- Instil anaesthetic lubricating gel into the urethra
- Insert the catheter directly into the urethra
- Inflate the balloon with the correct amount of sterile water
- Connect to the chosen drainage system
- Document the type, size and material of the catheter and the date of insertion.

Catheter insertion

Insertion of a catheter must be carried out using an aseptic technique, as set out in Box 6.3.

Figure 6.7 illustrates an example catheter liaison record which can be used for accurate documentation. The selection of a catheter must be carefully assessed in regard to the size, balloon size and material. Appropriate selection is essential to minimize trauma to the delicate mucosa of the bladder and urethra (Pomfret 1996).

Shorter-length urinary catheters are available for use on female patients, which allow less kinking and movement of the catheter. Selecting the type of material is dependent on the expected duration of use (see Chapter 8). The urinary catheter should not be changed unless the lumen is blocked or encrustation has occurred (Bryan and Reynolds 1984).

Cleansing of the perineal area can be carried out as part of the routine daily shower or bath. Cleaning should also take place after faecal contamination following bowel movements, to prevent bacteria from the bowel flora entering at the urethral meatus.

Drainage system management

The key elements for managing the drainage system are:

- Maintenance of a closed drainage system, which is central to the prevention of catheter-associated infection (*epic* Project 2001)

- Use of a sampling port for urine specimens
- Avoidance of unnecessary disconnections of the closed system
- Use of an aseptic technique for drainage bag changes
- Advice to patients to ensure that the drainage bag is lower than the bladder but not on the floor (Ayliffe et al 2000)
- Advice to the patient and/or others involved to empty the drainage bag when full
- Use of disposable plastic apron and disposable latex/non-latex gloves when emptying the drainage bag: there is an anticipated risk of contact with a body substance and possible risk of splashing (McDougall 1999)
- Decontamination of hands before and after all procedures.

Leg bags

Patients who are ambulant may find the use of a leg bag combined with an overnight drainage bag beneficial (Fig. 6.8). They also promote a degree of privacy and dignity for the patient. Leg bags are designed with a connection to prevent the closed system being broken.

Although opinion differs anecdotally, the overnight drainage bag should be emptied down the toilet and the bag ideally disposed of as clinical waste. Drainage bags must not be washed or reused. They are manufactured and intended for single use (Medical Devices Agency 2000).

Bladder installations

Bladder irrigation is carried out to instil a therapeutic agent designed to act intravesically on bladder tissue or to irrigate the bladder and/or an indwelling catheter by fluids which act by physical or chemical forces at the bladder and/or catheter surface (Getliffe 1996).

Gates (2000) examined research findings relating to catheter care and why and how urinary catheter encrustation occurs. This was to allow nurses to assess the evidence before deciding whether to irrigate catheters. The evidence concluded that catheter maintenance solutions

CATHETER LIAISON RECORD

Patient name: _____ Ward _____

G.P. contact number: _____

District nurse contact number: _____

Hospital insertion: ( )

Community insertion: ( )

Date of insertion: _____

Name and contact number of health professional inserting: _____

_____

Type of catheter: Urethral ( )   Suprapubic ( )

Reason for catheterization: _____

_____

_____

Long-term ( )   Short-term ( )

Size (ch) _____ Material _____

Length: Long ( )   Short ( )

Drainage systems

Leg bag: Short tube ( )   Long tube ( )   Make/brand _____

Catheter valve: Yes ( )   No ( )

Support straps: ( )   Support sleeve: ( )

Overnight drainage system required: Yes ( )   No ( )

Management plan for transfer to community

Information given and understood by the patient: Yes ( )   No ( )

Site of next change: Catheter clinic ( )   Home/District Nurse ( )

Approximate date of change: _____

Equipment provided on discharge: _____

_____

Patient information leaflets given: (list) _____

_____

General comments _____

_____

Signature/position/contact number:

Print name: _____

Signature: _____

Contact number: _____

Figure 6.7   Catheter liaison record. Adapted by kind permission from Guidelines for the Urinary Catheterization of Male/Female Patients in Primary and Secondary Care (Adults and Children), Leeds Teaching Hospitals Trust.

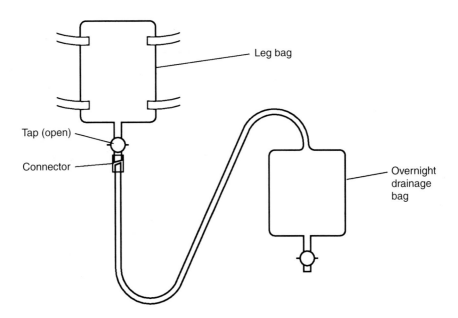

Figure 6.8 Overnight drainage system for a leg drainage bag. Reproduced by kind permission from Wilson J 2001 *Infection Control in Clinical Practice*, 2nd edn. Baillière Tindall, Edinburgh.

should be used with reservation, and as a considered management tactic rather than as a first line treatment. Consideration must also be given to individual variations between patients. There is no evidence to demonstrate that bladder instillations prevent urinary tract infection, therefore careful risk assessment should take place before carrying out the procedure.

Urinary sampling

The integrity of the closed drainage system must be maintained and the principles of asepsis adhered to. Guidelines appear in Box 6.4.

Catheter removal

The catheter is removed as soon as the patient condition allows. The procedure includes the following:

- Use disposable procedure gloves and a plastic disposable apron to contain splashing from body fluids
- Deflate the catheter balloon in accordance with the manufacturer's instructions and document the amount of fluid removed

Box 6.4 Urinary sampling: guidelines for practice

- Sampling of urine must only take place via the sampling port
- A sterile syringe and small bore needle should be used, although some systems may have a needle-free sampling port. This needle-free port avoids the risk of inoculation injury
- The urine sample should be transferred to a specimen container, avoiding contamination
- The specimen should be labelled and the request form completed and placed in the plastic specimen bag
- The specimen will normally be transported via the general practice of the patient concerned

- Dispose of items preferably as clinical waste
- Decontaminate hands before and after the procedure
- Normal urination should occur within six hours
- Document and monitor urinary output.

For some patients in the community it may be necessary for this procedure and/or change of catheter to be carried out in a hospital day unit to allow the appropriate monitoring to take place.

Catheter valves

These valves are designed to attach directly to the catheter as an alternative to a leg drainage bag. The valve will maintain the normal empty-ing and filling cycle of the bladder and needs to be released regularly. A thorough assessment is required to determine that the patient has the mobility and manual dexterity to operate the valves and that full bladder sensation is present. It is advisable to work in collaboration with the continence adviser when considering use and the assessment process.

The valves are normally changed every 5–7 days. However, it is important to follow the manufacturer's instructions for their use and management.

Intravenous therapy

Intravenous (IV) therapy in the home setting is normally considered for patients who require long-term venous access for a variety of therapies. Before being discharged, early assessment of any patient being considered for home intravenous therapy is important to decide if the treat-ment and patient are suitable for management in the community (Kayley 1995). Many patients in the community manage their own therapy, for example in cystic fibrosis, renal conditions and human immunodeficiency virus (HIV). Another type of self-management is patient-controlled analgesia using an infusion device. This device is of particular value for pain relief which allows analgesia to be self-administered when required.

Most patients receiving IV therapy at home will be those requiring long-term access to the central venous system such as chemotherapy, total parenteral nutrition and haemodialysis.

Intravenous therapy is associated with compli-cations, of which infection is one. These infec-tions include (ICNA 2001):

- entry site infection
- tunnel infection
- bloodstream infection
- endocarditis.

(Other types of complications are listed in Chapter 8, Residential and Nursing Homes.)

Every year, almost 6000 patients in the UK acquire a catheter-related bloodstream infection (*epic* Project 2001). Figure 6.9(A) illustrates extrinsic and intrinsic sources of infection, and 6.9(B) routes of access of contamination and related factors.

Catheter types

A variety of IV catheters are listed in Table 6.3.

Patients needing long-term therapy require a tunnelled catheter such as Hickman, Groshong. These allow for vascular access and stability. The other type is a totally implantable intravascular device, such as Port-A-Cath, which is tunnelled under the skin but has a subcutaneous port with a self-sealing septum accessible by needle punc-ture. Evidence does not support routine use of these catheters (Van Der Pijl and Frissen 1992, reprinted in ICNA 2001).

Peripherally-inserted central catheters can be used at home. A study (Flynn 1999) reported the use of this system for orthopaedic patients self-administering IV antibiotics at home, which prevented patients being hospitalized for weeks or months.

A patient in their own home may have a lower risk of acquiring infection as risks of cross-infection from other patients are lower (Wilson 2001).

An important factor when caring for patients with IV devices at home is the training and educa-tion of staff. Nurses must be able to demonstrate that they have undertaken appropriate training and acquired skills to enable them to provide this care safely (Kayley 1995).

Catheter insertion

Devices for long-term vascular access are usually inserted in the hospital setting in the operating theatre or a designated clean area.

Catheter insertion site

Daily inspection of the site is required to ensure that infection is not present and that the device is secure. Infection may be present without local signs as the patient may have a pyrexia 'which cannot be attributed to another cause' (ICNA 2001). Local signs of infection will include pain, inflammation and swelling.

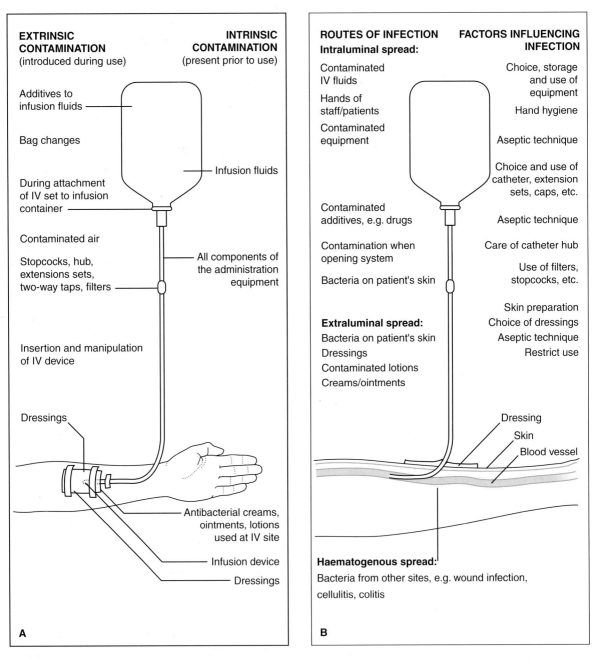

Figure 6.9 (A) Extrinsic and intrinsic sources of infection. (B) Routes of access of contamination and factors which influence development of IV infection. Reproduced by kind permission from Infection Control Nurses Association 2001.

Catheter site dressings

Considerable controversy exists about which type of dressing is most effective (Wilson 2001). The types in use are sterile gauze and transparent film dressings to cover the insertion site. Transparent film dressings allow good visibility of the insertion site and have good stability. Changes are also less frequent than with other dressing types. Some studies (Fitchie 1992, Conly et al 1989, Fox 2000) suggest that film dressings can cause moisture to

Table 6.3 Intravascular catheters (reproduced by kind permission from Infection Control Nurses Association 2001)

Type of device	Common site	Usage	Main complications	Replacement
Peripheral venous catheter (PVC)	Forearm/hand/ lower limb	Drugs/fluid administration	Phlebitis/BSI	48–72 hours
Peripheral arterial catheter	Radial/femoral artery	Blood sampling/ BP monitoring	Site infection/BSI	Unresolved
Peripherally-inserted central venous catheter (PICC)	Antecubital fossa	Drug/fluid administration	Site infection/BSI	Unresolved
Central venous catheter (CVC)	Subclavian/jugular veins	Drug/fluid adminstration, haemodynamic monitoring	BSI/thrombus/ pheumothorax	Signs of site infection/ BSI/mechanical failure
Pulmonary artery catheter (PAC)	Subclavian/jugular veins	Cardiac/haemodynamic monitoring	BSI/thrombus/balloon failure/pulmonary artery occlusion	3–4 days
Tunnelled CVC	Subclavian vein	Drug/nutrition administration, haemodialysis	BSI/tunnel infection (low rate)	Signs of site infection/ BSI/mechanical failure
Totally implanted catheter (TIC)	Central veins	Drug administration	BSI (low rate)	Signs of site infection/ BSI/mechanical failure

become trapped resulting in an increase in the incidence of catheter-related infection by as much as 50%. Guidelines should be available at a local level to guide staff on the type of dressing and the manufacturer's instructions for application and use. The insertion site dressing should always be changed when it becomes loose, soiled or damp and if the site is not visible. Topical antimicrobial agents are not recommended and should not be used routinely (Maki and Mermel 1998).

Aseptic techniques must be applied to minimize the risk of introducing infection when dressings are being changed.

Stopcocks and caps

Stopcocks allow an increase in the number of entry ports for adding drugs and fluids and for blood sampling. After each use they must be flushed thoroughly using normal saline for peripheral vascular catheters and routine flushing using a heparin solution for central venous catheters (ICNA 2001, *epic* Project 2001).

Caps must be replaced with a new sterile one after they have been removed from the circuit.

Administration sets

Intravenous tubing and stopcocks should be replaced at 72-hour intervals unless otherwise

clinically indicated and replaced following administration of blood, blood products, or lipid emulsions (*epic* Project 2001).

Infusion devices for ambulatory use

These devices are indicated when administration of continuous or intermittent infusion is required and can be managed in the home setting. This includes chemotherapy, analgesia and/or total parenteral nutrition.

The patient-controlled analgesia (PCA) devices consist of a pump and a timing device. This allows the patient to press a button and deliver a prescribed dose of analgesia via the IV route. In most cases this self-administration can boost the confidence of the patient as they are in control, are more comfortable, and have freedom and flexibility. It must be noted however that some patients may not welcome the independence and autonomy offered by PCA (Cowan 1997). This should be addressed when considering this method. Patients who will be using ambulatory devices must be fully educated in their use and management. As well as PCAs, infusion pumps are used for administering other prescribed medication such as antibiotics and chemotherapy.

The choice of type of device for use will be determined by the therapy and use proposed, and local guidance. At all times follow the advice and instructions given by the manufacturer of the product in use.

Enteral feeding

Enteral tube feeding has become an increasingly common method of nutritional support. There are however hazards associated with enteral feeding which can make it a source for the growth of micro-organisms. Liquid nutrients provide an ideal medium for bacteria and can cause cross contamination to the feeding system during setting up and handling the equipment.

Selection of equipment

Various types of feeding systems are available for use alongside numerous items of equipment required for a fully functioning system suited to the patient, such as extension sets, syringes and other connections. It is important to select a system which has a hazard-reducing design, that is, no parts easily touched during assembly that come into contact with the feed. Choose a delivery system that requires a minimum number of connections (Anderton 1994).

Feed preparation

Pre-packaged sterile ready-to-use feeds should be used in preference to feeds requiring reconstitution, dilution or additions (Aidoo and Anderton 1990). This also reduces the handling during preparation. Decanting is sometimes necessary as patients may be unable to tolerate other types of feed. When this type of feed or powdered modular feeds are required, the following points should be noted:

- Decontaminate hands thoroughly using soap and water before and after all handling of equipment and the preparation process. In the absence of soap and water in the home, an alcohol rub preparation can be used.
- Decant in a clean environment such as an area of a patient's kitchen designated for the purpose and set up with all the necessary equipment.
- Limit the feed hangtime to 12 hours (Payne-James 1991).

- Once a feed is opened but not connected to a sterile giving set it should be treated as a non-sterile feed, and the hangtime limited to 4 hours.
- Always use utensils for powdered modular feeds which have been thoroughly washed and dried and designated for this use only.
- Sterile water is the preferred option for mixing feeds and is essential for immunocompromised patients (Anderton 1995). Alternatively, cool boiled water may be used and can be stored, covered, in the refrigerator to be used within 24 hours.
- Clean the outside surface of all bottles, cans and cartons using an impregnated wipe (70% isopropyl alcohol) (Anderton 1995).
- Use full-strength formula and avoid adding water, medication, or other substances directly into the container.

Administration of feeds

The following key points are for all types of feeding:

- All persons involved in the handling and administration of enteral feeding must be suitably trained/educated to carry out the process in a safe manner.
- Hands must be thoroughly decontaminated prior to administration.
- Inner surfaces of the equipment must not be touched.
- A no-touch technique should be adopted when preparing the feed during priming and connecting to the administration set/feeding tube.
- Protective clothing is not required unless splashing of body fluids is anticipated.
- Feed must be labelled with the patient's name, date and time of feed and documented in the nursing notes.

Table 6.4 outlines problems encountered in enteral feeding, and possible causes, and Figure 6.10 shows sources of contamination.

Drug administration

Medication may be required to be given to patients who are receiving nutritional support.

Table 6.4 Enteral feeding: problems and possible causes

Problem	Possible causes
Contaminated feed	During manufacture, reconstitution or decanting
Preparation of feed and equipment have become contaminated	Touch contamination of feed/equipment. Poor hand decontamination. Excessive manipulation of the system. Poor no-touch technique during preparation
Storage of feed	Failure to refrigerate where appropriate and storing in contaminated areas
Poorly-designed equipment	Prone to touch contamination during assembly/use
Misuse of equipment	Prolonged use of administration sets/syringes
Contaminated additive	Medication or flush solutions
Site problems	Percutaneous site (PEG)* colonization or infection
Cross infection	Failure to adequately decontaminate equipment

*PEG = Percutaneous endoscopic gastrostomy

It is preferable to use aqueous solutions to elixirs and crushed tablets as they may adhere to the wall of the tube and can result in blockage, which will encourage bacterial growth. Where it is necessary to use elixirs they can be diluted with the same amount of cool boiled water. The tube must be flushed before and after administration of medication. When more than one drug is required, 5–10 ml of water should be flushed through in between each drug bolus. The amount will be dependent on adult or paediatric medication.

Gastrostomy site care

The site must be kept clean and dry using soap and water. It is useful, where possible, to teach the patient to do this at least once daily and advise on the need for good hand hygiene. A dressing is not required unless there is a discharge from the site that can be covered using a loose, absorbent key-hole dressing.

Local or percutaneous infections around the site of the skin entry may result in induration, swelling, soreness, pain and even ulceration of the skin. Early recognition is important to permit early

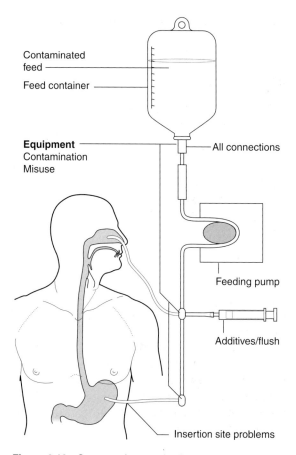

Figure 6.10 Sources of contamination.

treatment. In addition to treatment it is essential to question why this happened. A change in procedure may be required to prevent any recurrence. Any infection must be carefully documented in the patient care plan and reported to the general practitioner. Advice can be sought from the infection control nurse when infection is persistent despite treatment, for example colonization of the site with methicillin-resistant *Staphylococcus aureus* (MRSA).

Enteral feeding equipment and decontamination

The equipment to be used for enteral feeding will be agreed following an assessment of the patient's needs and the most suitable type of feeding. Collaboration with nursing staff in the acute

Table 6.5 Decontamination methods for enteral feeding equipment

Item	Method
Canned feeds	Clean top using an alcohol wipe (70% isopropyl alcohol) or swab. Do not dry using a cloth.
Connectors	Thoroughly wash in detergent and hot water. Rinse and air dry. Store in a clean container with a lid. Change every 7 days or follow manufacturer's instructions. Where packaging states the item is single use only, then discard after each use (MDA 2000).
Extension sets:	
a) single patient use	Thoroughly wash in detergent and hot water. Rinse and air dry. Store in a clean container with a lid. Change every 7 days or follow manufacturer's instructions. Some extension sets are not removed following feeding, therefore thorough flushing following a feed is required.
b) single use	Discard after single use.
Giving sets	Use a new set every 24 hours. In the case of intermittent feeds a new feed bag can be attached to the same giving set **immediately** and stored in the refrigerator. Remove and return to room temperature before feeding.
Pumps	Wipe over daily using a damp cloth to keep dust-free. Any spillage on the pump must be cleaned immediately.
Syringes used for flushing, checking and medication	If the syringe is designed for single use it should be discarded after each use. Some enteral feeding syringes are designed to be re-used, and these can be washed thoroughly in detergent and hot water, rinsed and air dried and stored in a covered container. Change every 7 days or follow manufacturer's instructions.
Bolus feeding sets:	
a) single patient use	Thoroughly wash in detergent and hot water. Rinse and air dry and store in a clean container with a lid to keep dust-free, or follow the manufacturer's instructions.
b) single use	Discard after single use.

setting is useful to ensure that the system will be managed safely in the home setting. To prevent transmission of infection it is essential that decontamination of equipment is carried out in between use and before returning to a central store.

Table 6.5 gives a summary of the common items of equipment used and method of decontamination. For further details on Cleaning, disinfection and sterilization please refer to Chapter 5.

EQUIPMENT FOR HOME CARE

Cleaning and decontamination of equipment used in the home

Amidst the changes in healthcare and technology, medical devices play an important role in treatment and subsequent care. In the process of caring for a patient in the home setting there are numerous medical devices in use. Medical devices are described as any instrument, apparatus, appliance material or healthcare product, excluding drugs, used for or by a patient or service user (MDA 2001b).

All devices in use require decontaminating during and after use by the patient. To ensure

- DO NOT REUSE
  Synonyms for this are:
  - Single-use
  - Use only once

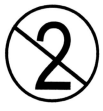

Figure 6.11 Packaging symbol for single-use medical devices (MDA Device Bulletin DB 2000(04)).

safe systems of work and to prevent the transmission of infection, it is essential that decontamination of equipment is carried out. This is in accordance with the requirements of Controls Assurance documents on the decontamination of medical devices and reusable medical devices (DoH 1999b).

Contamination is defined as the soiling of objects or living material with harmful, potentially infectious or other unwanted material (MAC 1996, 2000). (Classification of equipment in relation to risk is described in Chapter 5, Cleaning, disinfection and sterilization, Table 5.1.)

Within a local setting, it is advisable to seek out the policy for decontamination to ensure that practice is safe and prevent the spread of infection.

All equipment designated for single use must not be re-processed (MDA 2000 (04)). The device is designed and intended to be used during a single procedure, then discarded. *At all times follow the instructions from the manufacturer.* A symbol is used on the packaging of devices indicating it is for single use only: this symbol appears as Figure 6.11.

Table 6.6 is a list (not exhaustive) that may be used by nurses and home care staff in the home

Table 6.6 Decontamination of equipment in the home

Item	Method of decontamination
Bandages	Not to be washed and reused, particularly when exudates/strikethrough are present. Follow manufacturer's instructions for use with specialized bandaging for venous and arterial ulcers.
Bathing aids	Clean with detergent. Keep as dry as possible to prevent build-up of mildew especially on the underside of seating equipment. Manufacturers also give guidance on the maintenance of slings and bathing accessories. Slings can usually be laundered on a regular basis.
Bowls (patient wash type)	Clean with detergent and store dry.
Bedding	Launder in the washing machine on the hottest wash. Items can be sent to outside services as local arrangements.
Bedpans	Empty down the toilet and rinse and dry thoroughly. Store covered to keep dust-free.
Brushes (lavatory)	Rinse in the flushing water of the toilet and store dry.
Chairs (special)	Clean with detergent.
Commodes	Clean with detergent.
Commode pots	Empty, rinse thoroughly and dry, replace in the commode.
Cushions (pressure-relieving)	Clean with detergent. Follow manufacturer's instructions.
Feeding cups	Hand hot wash and air dry.
Hoists	Clean with detergent. Follow manufacturer's instructions for the care and maintenance of the hoist and associated equipment.
Masks (oxygen)	Single patient use. If reusing, wash in detergent, rinse and air dry. Wipe over using alcohol (70% wipe). Change equipment every 7 days.
Mattresses	Clean with detergent. Allow drying before turning or placing patient on. Make sure the cover is intact. A chlorine-releasing agent may be used for contaminated areas following blood or body fluid spills. Only use the agent if necessary, as prolonged use may damage the mattress (Ayliffe et al 2000). Many different types of mattresses/pressure relieving beds are in use, therefore follow the instructions of the manufacturer for maintenance and care.
Nebulizers	Single patient use only. Clean with detergent in between use. Disinfect according to the manufacturer's instructions. Change mask and tubing weekly. Discard after treatment is complete.
Stethoscopes	Wipe with 70% alcohol (wipes).
Suction equipment: a) catheter	Single use only.
b) tubing	Single patient use. Flush through after each use. Change every 7 days unless copious amount of secretions are present, then change daily.
c) bottle	Empty down the toilet and clean with detergent and dry. Follow the manufacturer's instructions for care and maintenance, depending on the type of machine. Clean the machine prior to returning to a loan store.
d) filters	Change when discoloured and at least every 3 months (Wilson 2001).
Urinary equipment: a) catheters	Single use.
b) drainage bags	Single patient use. Do not wash out and reuse. Change every 7 days. Overnight drainage bags connected to leg bags to be discarded after use.
c) urine bottles	Empty down the toilet and rinse thoroughly. Clean with detergent before returning to a loan store.

setting. It identifies the suggested methods of decontamination. For full details, including types of disinfectant and their use, please refer to Chapter 5 on Cleaning, Disinfection and Sterilization.

When new items of equipment are introduced, the method for decontamination must be adhered to alongside the daily use and maintenance.

REFERENCES

Adams D, Bagg J, Limaye M et al 1992 A clinical evaluation of glove washing and re-use in dental practice. Journal of Hospital Infection 20: 153–162

Aidoo K E, Anderton A 1990 Decanting – a source of contamination of enteral feeds? Clinical Nutrition 9: 157–162

Anderton A 1994 What is the HACCP (hazard analysis critical control point) approach and how can it be applied to enteral tube feeding? Journal of Human Nutritional Diet 7: 53–60

Anderton A 1995 Reducing bacterial contamination in enteral tube feeds. British Journal of Nursing 4: 368–377

Ayliffe G A J, Babb J R, Quoraishi A H 1978 A test for 'hygienic' hand disinfection. Journal of Clinical Pathology 31: 923–928

Ayliffe G A J, Fraise A P, Geddes A M, Mitchell K 2000 Control of Hospital Infection: a Practical Handbook, 4th edn. Arnold, London

Bryan C S, Reynolds K L 1984 Hospital-acquired bacteremic urinary tract infection. Epidemiology and outcome. Journal of Urology 132: 494–498

Carlisle D 1998 Intravenous therapy at home. Nursing Times 94(23) June 10

Castledine G 1993 Hygiene Standards. British Journal of Nursing 2(12)

Centers for Disease Control 1987 Recommendations for the prevention of HIV transmission in healthcare settings. Morbidity and Mortality Weekly Report August 21 36 (2S)

Centers for Disease Control 1988 Update: universal precautions for prevention of transmission of HIV, Hepatitis B virus and other blood borne pathogens in healthcare settings. Morbidity and Mortality Weekly Report June 24 37: 24

Conly J M et al 1989 A prospective randomised study comparing transparent and dry gauze dressings for central venous catheters. Journal of Infection and Disinfection 159: 310–319

Cowan T 1997 Patient-controlled analgesia devices. Professional Nurse 13(2)

Curran E 1991 Protecting with plastic aprons. Nursing Times 87: 38, 64–68

Department of Health 1998 A First Class Service: Quality in the New NHS. NHS Publications, London

Department of Health 1999a Health Services Circular HSC 1999/123 Governance in the new NHS. Department of Health, London

Department of Health 1999b Health Services Circular HSC 1999/179. Controls Assurance in Infection Control: Decontamination of Medical Devices. Department of Health, London

Department of Health 2000 Shaping the Future NHS: Long term Planning for Hospitals and Related Services (Consultation document). NHS Executive, London

Department of Health 2001 Controls Assurance Standards – waste management. Department of Health, London

Department of Health 2002a Shifting the Balance of Power: the Next Steps. DoH Publications, London

Department of Health 2002b Getting Ahead of the Curve. A report by the Chief Medical Officer. DoH Publications, London

epic Project 2001 Developing national evidence-based guidelines for preventing healthcare associated infections. Journal of Hospital Infection 47 (Suppl.) January

Fitchie C 1992 Central venous catheter related infection and dressing type. Intensive and Critical Care Nursing 8: 199–202

Flynn S 1999 Administering intravenous antibiotics at home. Professional Nurse 14(6)

Fox N 2000 Managing the risks posed by intravenous therapy. Nursing Times 96(30): 37–39

Gates A 2000 The benefits of irrigation in catheter care. Professional Nurse 16(1): 835–838

Getliffe K A 1996 Bladder instillations and bladder washouts in the management of catheterized patients. Journal of Advanced Nursing 23: 548–554

Griffiths G 1981 Infection in Institutions and in the Community. Medical Education (International) Ltd, 1270–1271

Health and Safety Commission Health Services Advisory Committee 1999 Safe Disposal of Clinical Waste. HSE Books, Sudbury

Health and Safety Executive 1992 Personal Protective Equipment at Work Regulations (EEC Directive). HMSO, London

Health and Safety Executive 1999 Control of Substances Hazardous to Health Regulations. HSE Books, Sudbury

House of Lords Select Committee on Science and Technology 1998 Government response to Antibiotic Resistance. HMSO, London

HMSO 1992 The Controlled Waste Regulations SI 1992/588. HMSO, London

HMSO 1996 The Carriage of Dangerous Goods (Classification, Packaging and Labelling) and use of Transportable Pressure Receptacles Regulations SI 2092. HMSO, London

Infection Control Nurses Association (ICNA) 1997 Guidelines for Hand Hygiene. ICNA, Bathgate

Infection Control Nurses Association (ICNA) 2001 Guidelines for Preventing Intravascular Catheter-related Infection. Infection Control Nurses Association, Bathgate

Infection Control Nurses Association (ICNA) 2002 Glove Usage Guidelines. ICNA, Bathgate

Joint Committee of Professional Nursing, Midwifery and Health Visiting Associations (England) 1997 A Celebration of Nursing and Health Visiting: Essential Ingredients of Healthcare. London

Kayley J 1995 Home Intravenous Therapy. Primary Health Care 5(8): 39–46

Larson E 1995 APIC guidelines for handwashing and hand antisepsis in healthcare settings. American Journal of Infection Control 23(4): 251–269. Quoted in ICNA 1997 Guidelines for Hand Hygiene. ICNA, Bathgate

Lawrence J 1994 Infection control for district nursing. In: Worsley M A et al (eds) Infection Control: A Community Perspective. Infection Control Nurses Association, Cambridge, Chapter 3

Lawrence J, Fuller A 2000 Safe Disposal of Clinical Waste in the Community. Educational Supplement. CDNA Issue 2 Vol 1, Community and District Nursing Association

Lothian P 1998 The dangers of long-term catheter drainage. British Journal of Nursing 7(7): 366–379

Maki D G, Mermel L A 1998 Infections due to infusion therapy. In: Bennett J V, Brachman P S (eds) Hospital Infections, 4th edn. Lippincott-Raven, Philadelphia, 659–725

McDougall C 1999 A Clean Sheet: Nursing Times Infection Control Supplement 95(28), July 14

Medical Devices Agency 1995 MDASN9516 Decontamination of Medical Devices and Equipment prior to investigation, inspection, service or repair. MDA, London

Medical Devices Agency 2000 Single-use Medical Devices: Implications and Consequences of Reuse. MDA DB2000 (04). MDA, London

Medical Devices Agency 2001a Safe use and disposal of sharps. MDA SN2001 (19). MDA, London

Medical Devices Agency 2001b Devices in Practice: a guide for health and social care professionals. MDA, London

Microbiology Advisory Committee (MAC) Part 1 (1996), Part 2 (2000) Sterilisation, Disinfection and Cleaning of Medical Equipment: Guidance on decontamination from the Microbiology Advisory Committee to the Department of Health. MDA ISBN 1 85839 518 6. Medical Devices Agency, London

Moores Y 1999 Message. British Journal of Infection Control, 1: Issue 1

Newman C 1991 Receiving Patients from Hospital. In: S K Armitage, Continuity of Nursing Care. Scutari Press, London

Payne-James J J 1991 Enteral nutrition and the critically ill: infection risk minimisation. British Journal of Intensive Care Sept/Oct: 135–141

Phillips G 1999 Microbiological aspects of clinical waste. Journal of Hospital Infection 41: 1–6

Pomfret I J 1996 Continence clinic catheters: design, selection and management. British Journal of Nursing 5: 245–51

Russell P 1997 Reducing the incidence of needlestick injuries. Professional Nurse 12(4)

UK Health Departments 1998 Guidance for Clinical Health Care Workers: Protection Against Infection with Blood-borne Viruses. Recommendations of the Expert Advisory Group on AIDS and the Advisory Group on Hepatitis. Department of Health, London

Van der Pijl H, Frissen P H 1992 Experience with a totally implanted venous access device (Port-A-Cath) in patients with AIDS. AIDS 6(7): 709–713. Reprinted in ICNA 2001 Guidelines for Preventing Intravascular Catheter-related Infection. ICNA, Bathgate

Ward D 2000 Handwashing facilities in the clinical area: a literature review. British Journal of Nursing 9(2)

Wilson J 2001 Infection Control in Clinical Practice, 2nd edn. Baillière Tindall, London

7

Nurseries and schools

S. Ross

INTRODUCTION

This chapter aims to provide the reader with an insight into the importance of preventing and controlling infection in day care facilities for children. Its aim is to discuss the variety of facilities currently available within the United Kingdom and the factors which may influence the spread of infection, and to provide suggestions to prevent and control infection.

Day care facilities for children are believed to have been available since the early 1800s (Osterholm 1987). The various types of child care available and the number of children attending demonstrate their immense popularity. It has been suggested by Baker (1987) that the growth in demand for child care provision has many influences, including social and economic factors such as: the increased proportion of single-parent families; a growth in the divorce rate; more mothers establishing or continuing professional careers; and a greater awareness of equal opportunities.

The principal types of day care provided in England in 1998 highlight the diversity of the facilities available, and the increasing demands for such provision (Department for Education and Employment 1999). Day care for children can be provided in a number of different ways and in different settings. The Children Act of 1989 was a landmark in child care legislation as it comprehensively looked at the needs of children, including the regulation of day care services (DoH 1990).

The types of care currently provided include day nurseries and child minders, playgroups, out-of-school clubs, family centres, and facilities within schools.

Day nurseries

Day care nurseries are facilities that care for children for the length of the adult working day. Children may attend full or part time, depending on individual requirements. They may be run by Social Services Departments, Education Departments, voluntary organizations, private companies, individuals as a business, or community groups.

Since 1988, the number of day nurseries has more than trebled, with 91% of places being provided by registered nurseries. These facilities currently provide an estimated 223 000 places within 6700 day nursery premises (DfEE 1999).

Child minders

Child minders look after children aged under five and school-age children outside school hours and in the holidays. Provision of this service is usually on domestic premises, most commonly in the child minder's own home. The parents and child minder negotiate the terms and conditions. The Children Act 1989 extended registration to those places provided by child minders. In 1998, there were 94 700 registered child minders providing 370 700 places (DfEE 1999).

Playgroups

Playgroups provide sessional care for children, usually aged between three and five. They aim to provide learning experiences through structured play opportunities in groups and with involvement of the parents/guardians. The number of playgroups is estimated at 15 700 providing 383 600 places for children. This figure has fallen since the peak of 1991 when there were 18 000 playgroups established (DfEE 1999).

Provision for school-age children

There has been a substantial rise in the number of out-of-school clubs providing sessional care to children before and after school. In all, some 92 300 places were provided in 1998 from 3100 clubs.

Holiday schemes are a relatively new concept, and provide care for children all day during school holidays. In the year ending 31 March 1998, there was a total of 6200 holiday schemes (17% more than in 1997) and 256 500 places (a rise of nearly 23%).

Family centres

A family centre is a place used or attended by children of any age with or without their parent/guardian. They provide a range of services and facilities for children, adults and whole families. At 31 March 1998, approximately 490 centres were provided for children aged under five, 20 for children five and over, and 320 catered for children of all ages and their families.

Schools

All children are required by law to start school at the beginning of the term after their fifth birthday, and to maintain their attendance until they are approaching sixteen years of age. The Government provides education for children via the Local Education Authority (LEA) in the form of primary and secondary schools.

In England in 1998, 4 460 646 children attended LEA primary schools and 3 072 822 attended LEA secondary schools for their educational needs. In addition to this, LEA's also cater for pupils of primary and secondary school age with emotional/behavioural difficulties and moderate or severe learning difficulties. 98 427 children attended such schools, whilst 4955 children attended similar establishments which were maintained by voluntary bodies. This statistical information was provided by the Department for Education and Employment (DfEE 1998).

FACTORS INFLUENCING THE SPREAD OF INFECTION

The phenomenal growth of child care provision can create a huge challenge for personnel working within the field of infection control. Infections are very common in childhood and are responsible for much of the illness in the under-fives. Susceptibility to infection in this group is increased because immune defences are not fully developed, and because young children may lack prior exposure or complete immunization to many infectious agents.

It is essential that quality care is provided to the children receiving day care. Their welfare and development are paramount and all their needs, including social, cultural, developmental, physical and emotional requirements, should be met.

This section will provide the reader with an explanation of the factors which may contribute to the spread of infection within schools and other child care establishments.

Factors relating to the child

There are a number of factors which may influence the transmission of infectious agents within such establishments. Russell (1987) suggests that the major factor is the prevalence of the infectious agent in the population represented, as well as the number of susceptible children present. Black et al (1981) highlight that the age of the children and the hygienic practices of staff are also important factors.

Younger children who attend nursery or similar day care provision are particularly susceptible to infectious diseases, for several reasons. These were identified by Berg (1988) as being:

- young age and consequent immature immune system
- the degree of close contact between the children
- lack of hygienic practices. This may be due to age or lack of understanding
- sharing of a number of facilities and types of equipment
- lack of prior encounters with the infectious agent
- ability and desire to be extremely mobile
- decreasing maternally-acquired antibodies
- behavioural characteristics of children, that is, their natural curiosity and intimacy with others
- presence of bites and abrasions
- incomplete immunizations. By the age of two all children should have received three doses of diphtheria, tetanus, whooping cough, *Haemophilus influenzae* type B, meningitis C and polio immunizations. They should also have received at least one dose of measles, mumps and rubella immunization (MMR), unless there are contraindications. By the age of five, children should, in addition, have received a booster vaccination of diphtheria, tetanus and polio and a

second dose of MMR (Department of Health 1999).

In addition to these factors, some children may have medical conditions that make them particularly vulnerable to infections which would be considered minor in most children. Such children include those being treated for leukaemia or other cancers, children on high doses of oral steroids, and children with conditions which may seriously reduce their immunity and ability to combat infection. These risk factors can relate to all children, whether attending nurseries or schools.

It is worth noting that children with an infection may subsequently transmit the agent to others at the nursery or the school, as well as other contacts within their private home and the community at large.

Evans (1992) suggests that day nurseries and hospitals share many of the same factors which can predispose to infection, and reminds people of the importance of sound infection control practices in order to prevent outbreaks of infection.

Staff-related factors

There is no doubt that the practices and knowledge of staff caring for children can influence the prevention and/or control of infection. It is extremely important that staff working with children are suitably qualified or working towards an appropriate qualification, or are supervised by appropriately-trained personnel. The Children Act of 1989 details these considerations and suggests that half of the staff should hold a child care qualification. This should be either a qualification endorsed by the Nursery Nurses Examination Board, nursing or teaching. In addition, guidance is provided on staffing ratios to ensure adequate supervision of the children. For day nurseries, the Secretaries of State suggest minimum acceptable ratios of 1:3 for under 2-year-olds, 1:5 for 2–5-year-olds. In nursery schools, the Children Act advises a minimum of one qualified teacher to 26 children, with an overall adult to child ratio of 1:13. The second member of staff should have a recognized qualification in nursery work.

The level of staff knowledge and awareness of infection control can influence the potential risk of infection spreading. Staff education is an essential component in preventing disease. A study in 1988, exploring infection control practices in 12 day care centres, showed that 70% of employers did not provide their staff with in-service education relating to infection control (Lopez et al 1988).

Environmental factors

Environments in which children are cared for should always be warm, light, welcoming and comply with current legislation. The Health and Safety at Work Act (1974) and Control of Substances Hazardous to Health Regulations 1999 (COSHH), are both key pieces of current legislation which require the assessment and control of hazards, including exposure to infectious agents.

A number of studies have identified the important role that the environment can have in reducing the risk of cross infection (Jewkes and O'Connor 1990, Kaltenthaler et al 1995, Early et al 1998). The provision of appropriate and adequate facilities can also play an important role in maintaining good infection control practices. Kaltenthaler et al (1995) surveyed 20 primary schools in Leeds and assessed the presence of faecal bacteria on the hands of children and environmental surfaces, as well as the level of children's knowledge towards basic hygiene. The researchers found that those children with good hygiene knowledge had less faecal contamination on their hands. Schools whose children had higher bacterial counts on their hands were also more likely to have reported outbreaks of gastrointestinal illness in the past. This study also revealed that classroom carpets were the most heavily contaminated areas sampled from the environment. This is cause for concern as the children frequently touch the carpeted areas when sitting down to listen to the reading of a story.

A study by Jewkes and O'Connor in 1990 surveyed the sanitation facilities in schools in one health district. Their findings were quite alarming, and evidence of inadequate resources was found. Locked toilets and poor standards of cleaning in some schools were also found to be important factors. An earlier American study (Koopman 1978) found that the provision of soap, toilet paper and clean towels had a greater influence on the number of cases of diarrhoea in the school than did the number of toilets per school.

Laborde et al (1993) examined the effects and likelihood of faecal contamination on the level of diarrhoeal illness in children attending nursery. They found that there was a higher level of contamination in the room used by the children aged 18 months and less in the rooms used by children aged 9 months to 3 years. This study also identified that the classroom sinks were a source of contamination and that toys had a higher level of faecal organisms than any other equipment sampled. This highlights the importance of recognizing the role of inanimate objects in the spread of infection. Children, whether attending day nurseries or schools, will share the majority of available equipment including toys and high chairs as well as the actual environment.

In a study undertaken in 1990 by Holaday et al, the environment, and the hands of children and staff, were sampled to detect micro-organisms over a six-month period. They found that those facilities with formal hand washing procedures had lower levels of contamination than those without. The researchers swabbed a number of objects, including:

- bathrooms
- toilet seats
- floors
- wash hand basins
- nappy changing surfaces
- handles
- table tops
- toys
- drinking fountain.

The study found widespread contamination in the classroom (on the floor, table tops and taps), and in the kitchen floor and work surfaces. The study concluded that the contaminated hands of children and staff members probably played an important role in disseminating faecal bacteria to these areas.

THE WAY IN WHICH INFECTION SPREADS

Micro-organisms use a range of different routes to find new hosts and transmit infection. They may spread through direct contact with the body fluids of an infected individual, for example, glandular fever is transmitted by kissing and rubella transmitted from mother to baby in utero (Wilson 2001).

Alternatively, some micro-organisms depend on people, animals or inanimate objects to transmit themselves from one thing to another. This route of transmission is referred to as indirect contact.

The routes of microbial transmission as described by Wilson (2001) are as follows:

- **Inhalation**: small particles of dust or droplets of water carry microbes into the respiratory tract via the mouth or nose. Examples include influenza, measles and tuberculosis.
- **Inoculation**: micro-organisms may be introduced via the skin and mucous membranes by accidental injury, injection, bites or during surgical incision. Examples include Hepatitis B, malaria and *Clostridium tetani*.
- **Transplacental**: micro-organisms may cross the placenta from the maternal to the foetal circulation to cause congenital infection. Examples of this route include rubella and syphilis.
- **Ingestion**: micro-organisms enter the gastro-intestinal tract with contaminated food or water. Examples include salmonella, polio and many viruses which cause gastrointestinal upset, including Norwalk virus and rota-virus.
- **Sexual intercourse**: microbes may be transferred from the genital tract of one partner to the other during sexual intercourse. Examples include herpes simplex type 2 and gonorrhoea.

THE PREVENTION AND CONTROL OF INFECTION

Many facilities caring for children employ good measures to reduce the risk of infection. The overall aim is to ensure a healthy environment for the development of children, but consideration has to be given to employ measures to minimize the spread of infection. This section will suggest some ideas that may help to prevent and control episodes of infection in establishments which care for children.

The environment

Environmental factors can play a major role in the spread of micro-organisms (Holaday et al 1990) and it is very important that interventions are employed to minimize these risks. In nursery facilities for children under two years of age, separate rooms must be provided for babies and toddlers to rest, sleep and play and be equipped with appropriate furnishings to promote restfulness. There must be at least 18 inches (half metre) between cots/beds for reasons of health and safety. The Children Act (1989) provides guidance regarding the appropriate standards of space for children. The Act emphasizes the importance of providing a warm, welcoming environment. The space recommendations are detailed in Table 7.1.

In addition, there should be sufficient toilets (1 per 10 children), of child sizes with an individual flushing mechanism and toilet lids (Fig. 7.1). A dedicated nappy changing area with easily cleansable, impervious surfaces should be available (Chorba et al 1987). Adequate and appropriate facilities are a crucial factor in the promotion of infection prevention. The number, location and type of hand washing facilities is a prime consideration. A survey undertaken in 1990 following an outbreak of viral gastro-enteritis in a school identified a number of problems (Jewkes and O'Connor 1990). The research team found that toilets were kept locked from children; there was an inadequate number of toilets and wash hand basins; there was a lack of hot water; toilet paper was not always available and toilet areas were not always adequately cleaned. These findings are very concerning, as these principles are fundamental in maintaining a good infection prevention strategy. Attempts to promote and teach good basic hygiene, including hand washing, will be undermined by inadequate facilities.

In a more recent American study, Early et al (1998) explored the effect of several interventions

Table 7.1 The recommended standards of space provided when caring for children (The Children Act 1989)

Age of child	Square feet	Square metres
Up to 12 months	40	3.7
Between 1 and 2 years	30	2.8
Between 2 and 5 years	25	2.3

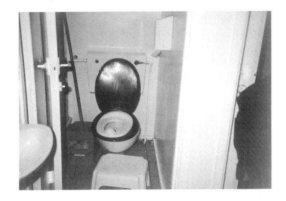

Figure 7.1 Correct type of toilet in nursery facilities.

on the frequency of hand washing. Some environmental problems discovered during this study included the inaccessibility of toilets, lack of time and opportunity in the school day to reinforce hand washing behaviour, and difficulties in keeping the resources stocked up. They identified that 66% of soap dispensers were non-functional, 78% of areas used bar soap and one third of hand air dryers were mechanically inoperable.

The furniture and fixtures provided within these environments should create a warm, cheerful and stimulating environment. Consideration must be given prior to their purchase of whether such resources can be easily cleansed without damage to their durability and function. Written cleaning schedules should be available and monitored to ensure that they are being appropriately and adequately followed. Such schedules should provide the following information:

- when something is cleaned
- what equipment is used
- whose responsibility it is to perform this task
- which agents are used.

It is important that such practices and schedules are monitored, evaluated and revised as necessary. Normal cleaning methods should be employed. It is not necessary for baths, toilets, etc., to be cleaned with any special disinfectants. Hot water and detergent is usually sufficient. Inadequate routine cleaning of the environment has been identified as a potential source for the transmission of enteric disease. A study undertaken in 1995, investigating 20 primary schools in Leeds, found that schools where children had a higher bacterial count on their hands were more likely to have reported outbreaks of gastro-enteritis in the past. This study found that classroom carpets were the most contaminated areas sampled from the environment. The authors recommended that carpeted areas in schools should be shampooed weekly (Kaltenthaler et al 1995).

Staff

There are a number of factors to consider relating to the staff member when addressing the prevention and control of infection in child care provision. These include:

- staff knowledge and education
- experience and qualifications of staff
- staffing levels
- staff health
- practices of staff
- adequate supervision of children.

Education and knowledge

All staff providing care for children are acting 'in loco parentis' and, therefore, have enormous responsibilities to ensure safety of the children. A key factor in promoting this philosophy is the level of staff knowledge surrounding infection risks and control measures. Staff should have a recognized certificate, experience of, or be working towards, an appropriate qualification. If this is not the case, such personnel must be appropriately supervised. It is also important, although not compulsory, for staff to receive educational input about the subject of communicable disease

control. Such subjects may include:

- common childhood diseases
- transmission modes
- possible sources of contamination
- infection control practices.

In the study by Lopez et al (1988) it was found that staff did not understand how diseases were transmitted. The authors concluded that, in their opinion, the level of education did not correlate with the knowledge needed to prevent, recognize, control or report the infectious diseases common to nurseries.

Gillis et al (1989) developed a model health educational programme using a video and a resource book to provide education to staff working in nurseries. The authors claim the programme resulted in significant reductions in respiratory illness and improvements in staff knowledge and practice.

Another important consideration is the number of staff available to allow adequate supervision of children during their daily activities. Table 7.2 shows the minimum staff/child ratios suggested by the Children Act (1989).

These ratios are the minimum acceptable level. The person in charge on site becomes supernumery when more than 12 children are received. The given ratios must be maintained at all times in each room where children are cared for, and when looked after outside or off site. This includes meal times, rest times and during staff breaks. In calculating the staff:child ratio, students on placement must not be included, nor must they have sole care of children. Some facilities may be required to have staffing levels greater than those above. Examples of this may include:

- where children have special needs
- where groups leave premises

Table 7.2 Minimum staff/child ratio (The Children Act 1989)

Age of children	Minimum ratio
0–2 years	1 adult to 3 children (1:3)
2–5 years	1 adult to 5 children (1:5)
5 years+	1 adult to 8 children (1:8)

- where premises may present particular difficulties, e.g. not ground floor.

RIDDOR

Under the Reporting of Injuries, Diseases and Dangerous Occurrences Regulations (1995) (RIDDOR), employers are required to notify the appropriate enforcing authority (either the Local Authority or the Health and Safety Executive) where an employee is found to be suffering from a work-related disease. Adult staff may be susceptible to childhood infections due to the decline of childhood antibodies, non-contact with a particular disease or an incomplete vaccination programme. An ill adult may also pose a communicable disease risk to the children. Guidelines should be available providing advice to staff regarding restriction of work practices or exclusion from work. These guidelines must be brought to the attention of all staff prior to their employment. Further advice may be sought from local infection control personnel, the Infection Control Nurse and Consultant in Communicable Disease Control.

Immunization

All staff should ensure via their GP that the routine immunization for polio, tuberculosis, diphtheria, tetanus, measles, mumps and rubella have been received. Female workers of childbearing age should be sure that they are immune to rubella (german measles), as they will be at risk of exposure to infection. A simple blood test will determine the possible need for vaccination before starting work.

Practices

In nurseries it may be useful to assign each child to a particular staff member for the duration of the day. Dividing children into small groups may help reduce disease transmission. The practices of staff have a vital role to play in minimizing the spread of infection. They should ensure adequate supervision of children, particularly during meal times and toileting. Hand washing is the single

most effective method for preventing infection. In a classic study by Black et al (1981), the introduction of a hand washing programme for staff and children in nurseries decreased the incidence of diarrhoea by 50%. Children should be encouraged to wash and should be supervised when washing their hands, as set out in the next section.

Good hygiene practices

Effective hygienic practices apply to everyone every day and, therefore, should be universally adopted, in order to protect against the wide range of potential infections. It is not always possible to identify staff and/or children suffering with, or incubating, an infection. Many carriers of infections will be unaware of their condition and the only sensible approach to infection prevention and its control is to take adequate precautions in all cases. This is known as adopting universal or standard infection control precautions.

Hand washing

Staff must be aware of the correct hand washing technique and when it is appropriate for themselves and the children to wash their hands.

Personal hygiene is one of the most basic yet most important health promotion issues. It is vital as a measure of infection control and also for social acceptance (May 1998). Hand washing is the single most effective means of reducing cross infection. The purpose of hand washing is to remove or destroy any micro-organisms that have been picked up on the hands, thereby preventing their transmission to others and protecting oneself. The earlier in life people start learning about hand washing, the better.

Poor hand hygiene among children can promote the spread of infection. Children must be encouraged and supervised to wash their hands:

- after visiting the toilet
- before eating, including snacks
- before drinking
- after playing outside

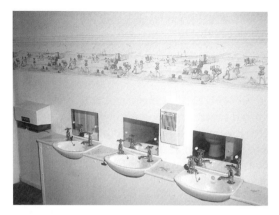

Figure 7.2 Appropriate facilities for hand washing are crucial.

- after playing with sand or water
- after touching animals.

Figure 7.2 is an example of a children's hand washing area.

Staff must wash their hands:

- before preparing or serving food
- before feeding children
- before eating or drinking
- after going to the toilet
- after assisting children at the toilet
- after changing nappies
- after dealing with any body fluids
- after any cleaning procedure
- after caring for sick children
- after handling soiled clothing or items
- after dealing with waste
- after removing disposable gloves and/or aprons.

In Chapter 6, Home Nursing, Figure 6.2 illustrates hand washing technique, which can be used as an aid to teach children.

- Hands must be wet under warm running water. (Hot water from the taps used by children should be regulated to deliver at a maximum 43°C to avoid scalding.)
- Hands should be washed vigorously for 30 seconds.
- Particular attention should be paid to thumbs, fingertips and in between fingers.

- Hands should be thoroughly rinsed under running water.
- Hands should be dried thoroughly after washing. To reduce the risk of cross infection, clean individual hand towels should be provided, preferably disposable paper towels. Alternatively, hot air dryers may be used.

A number of studies have been undertaken to explore the effects of hand washing on the level of reported infection, and interventions which may affect the levels of hand washing. Lopez, DiLiberto and McGuckin (1988) looked at infection control practices over a six-month period in six nurseries. A questionnaire was formulated to establish practices, some of which involved hand washing. Ninety-six per cent of the respondents identified that they taught children how to wash their hands. However, the self-reported mechanisms used may not reflect true practice.

May (1998) used health belief theoretical frameworks to promote hygiene issues in an infants' school. The programme involved the author and a school nurse, teaching, advising and instructing staff and pupils in hand washing techniques as well as acting as an information resource. Older pupils were appointed as monitors of toilet and hand washing areas and requested to inform the caretaker if areas needed cleaning or stocks replenishing. Hand washing times were set during the day – before entry into class, after breaks and toileting times. The children were taught to identify factors which might transmit diseases from person to person such as poor hand hygiene, sneezing and coughing.

As previously mentioned, in their study, Holaday et al (1990) identified that centres with formal hand washing procedures had a lower level of bacteria on their hands than those without formal procedures.

Also previously mentioned, Kaltenthaler et al (1995) investigated the presence of faecal indicator bacteria on hands and environmental surfaces. (Faecal streptococci were used as the indicator organism.) They also assessed and scored hand washing knowledge for each child. Those children with good hygiene knowledge had less faecal contamination on their hands. Those schools with higher hand counts were more likely to have reported an outbreak of gastro-enteritis in the past. The study also showed that those schools in high deprivation areas had higher bacterial hand counts.

An American study aimed to improve hand washing in school children by introducing a number of controlled interventions (Early et al 1998). These included:

- peer educational programme
- use of hand-wipes impregnated with alcohol, emollient and lemon fragrance.

The study identified that education alone was not effective at increasing and sustaining the frequency of hand washing. The introduction of both interventions had the greatest level of success. They concluded that education and accessible, convenient hand hygiene products may result in a sustainable increase in the frequency of hand washing.

Evans (1992) sampled 62 staff and 118 children's hands on arrival at a nursery, before meals, after toileting and before leaving for home for a two-week period. In week one, the largest number of isolates were found on arrival at the nursery, with a gradual decrease being noted throughout the day. The author suggests the improvements may be due to an increase in staff awareness and the effects of an observer being present during such practices. During the second week, a significant reduction was seen on the staff hands on arrival at the nursery, suggesting that staff anticipated that their hands would be sampled on arrival. During the same period, the number of isolates on children's hands were highest on arrival at the nursery but reduced sharply with hand washing after toileting. The author concluded that the results suggested that staff and children came from home with their hands contaminated with bacteria and that this level can be reduced by hand washing throughout the day.

All staff should always ensure that cuts and abrasions are covered with a waterproof dressing to provide protection for themselves and others. This brief review of the literature **clearly provides the evidence** of the extreme importance of hand washing for both staff and children in nurseries and schools.

Use of protective clothing

It is recognized that basic protective clothing is required when dealing with incidents where contact with body fluid is anticipated. It is recommended that single-use, disposable latex or vinyl gloves should be worn for tasks where there is a risk of exposure to blood or other body fluids, whether through direct contact with children or contact with contaminated clothing, toys or equipment (for example, nappy changing, cleaning potties, etc.).

Disposable plastic aprons should also be worn for tasks where there is a risk of splashing blood or other body fluids onto clothing. This applies whether a child is known to have an infection or not (Wilson and Breedon 1990). Disposable gloves and aprons must be disposed of after each task and never used for more than one child. After use they should be disposed of into an appropriate waste bag. Under Health and Safety Legislation, employers are required to ensure the adequate provision of protective clothing for staff.

General cleaning

Normal cleaning methods using a detergent solution (for example, washing up liquid) and hot water and thorough drying will be adequate for most surfaces, furniture and fixtures. It is important that a regular programme of cleaning is agreed and followed by relevant staff. No special disinfectants are necessary for toilets or sinks. However, it is advisable to use separate disposable cloths for different areas. An easy system to follow is to have a different coloured cloth for different areas. Evans (1992) demonstrated the importance of ensuring good environmental cleanliness.

Changing mats/nappy changing

A common infection problem seen in children under five years is diarrhoea. Hygienic practices involving toileting and/or nappy changing are vitally important. Changing mats should always be used, and covered with disposable paper towels which should be discarded after each child. If soiling occurs, the mat should be washed with hot water and detergent and thoroughly dried. The changing mats should be checked on a regular basis and discarded if the cover is torn or cracked.

A designated area should be set aside for nappy changing. Tables and surfaces used for play or preparing/serving food must not be used for nappy changing. Bonner and Dale (1986), when examining the incidence of giardiasis in children from day centres, identified that diarrhoea was more likely to occur when the same people who change nappies also prepare or serve food. With this in mind, it is helpful, if possible, to designate separate staff to these duties.

Furniture

Table tops must be cleaned using hot water and detergent immediately prior to the service of food. Evans (1992) highlighted a problem with the nursery she studied, when children were allowed to climb on the top of tables and were permitted to eat food from unwiped tables and chairs.

Toilet areas

Toilet areas must be cleaned frequently during the day and immediately if soiled. Particular attention should be paid to toilet handles, door handles, toilet seats and hand wash basins, especially taps. In an outbreak situation, infection control personnel may advise the use of disinfectants.

Waste and laundry

Purchase and use of disposable nappies should be recommended, as they are much easier to deal with when soiled. Following their use, they should be placed in an impervious bag, tied securely and discarded into an appropriate waste bag. Plastic bin liners must not be accessible to children. Non-disposable-type nappies should be soaked in a bucket of hot soapy water for a short period of time, before being washed in a washing machine. It is preferable for child care facilities not to launder soiled clothing but to place it into a sealed plastic bag and send it home for washing. However, if laundry equipment is used it should be located away from the kitchen area to reduce the risk of introducing faecal pathogens from soiled clothing. Such washing machines should have a cold pre-wash cycle, followed by a hot wash. It is advisable to purchase an industrial-type machine. Although initially expensive, they are cost-effective in the long term. The use of potties should be avoided if at all possible but, if used, the contents of potties should be carefully emptied into the toilet, the potty washed with detergent and hot water, rinsed and dried thoroughly after each use.

Female hygiene

Menstrual sanitary pads need safe disposal, preferably by incineration. Girls must be given privacy and adequate facilities to wash their hands following changing of sanitary protection.

Spillages

Spillages of vomit, urine and excreta should be cleaned away immediately using hot water, detergent and disposable paper towels or cloths. It is important to wear disposable gloves and apron, disposing of all materials into an impervious bag. People cleaning up spillages of blood or any body fluid which contains visible blood should follow the procedure given in Box 7.1.

Disinfectants may damage furnishings and carpets and should, therefore, not be used on these surfaces. Spillages of blood or other body fluids on such surfaces should be cleaned with detergent and water. It is advisable that carpeted areas are shampooed as soon as possible after contamination.

Note

Disinfectants are hazardous substances and employers are legally required to carry out a risk

---

Box 7.1 Instructions for dealing with a blood spillage

- Put on gloves and apron.
- Treat the injured/ill person.
- Cover the spill with paper towels and pour over undiluted household bleach **OR** cover the spillage with hypochlorite (bleach) granules.
- After five to ten minutes, mop up the spillage with additional paper towels/disposable cloths.
- Wash the area thoroughly with detergent and water.
- Discard *all* waste into a plastic bag, seal and dispose off into an appropriate waste bag.
- Wash hands.
- Soiled clothing should be placed into a plastic bag and sealed. They can be safely cleaned by a standard washing machine cycle. A cold pre-wash cycle will help to dispel any blood, followed by a hot wash.

---

assessment on their use in order to comply with the Control of Substances Hazardous to Health Regulations 1999 (COSHH). The manufacturer's guidance given on the product label must always be followed.

Any splashes of blood on the skin, eyes or in the mouth from another person should be washed off immediately with copious amounts of water (and soap if on the skin). Any bites and scratches that result in bleeding should be allowed to bleed freely, washed and covered with a waterproof plaster. It is very important to report the incident to the manager/employer to ensure it is properly documented.

In outbreaks of diarrhoea and/or vomiting, hypochlorite 1000 ppm may be recommended for environmental disinfection.

The child

An individual child may present a risk to other children and staff if suffering from an infectious disease. Prior to the enrolment of a child, parents should be asked to complete a health record which gives details on a child's general well-being, history of childhood infections and their immunization record. (Missed immunizations may be noted and parents reminded.)

Exclusion

Children's lack of prior exposure to infection and their lack of hygienic practices enhance the potential for infection to spread. An ill child is also at risk of spreading an infection to anyone he or she has contact with. It is the responsibility of the parent or guardian to inform staff at the child facility if the child is unwell. A major source of conflict between parents and staff arises over ill children. Parents criticize staff for excluding children, believing their child has become ill because of exposure to a disease at the nursery or school, whilst staff may be critical of parents who attempt to bring sick children to the nursery/school. One study (Landis et al 1988) compared the opinions of day care staff, working mothers and paediatricians regarding the exclusion of sick children. The results showed that day care staff were more conservative than mothers and paediatricians. All parties in the study agreed that unwell children, those with a temperature and other specific signs and symptoms such as diarrhoea, should be excluded from the child care facility. Children who have been in contact with infections but who themselves remain well, should not be a cause for concern.

It is very important to have written policies regarding the exclusion of a sick child. Head teachers can exclude children and staff from school if they have a communicable disease. This should reflect medical advice, and such advice can be gained from the local Consultant in Communicable Disease Control (CCDC). Local infection control nurses can also advise as necessary.

A trend is emerging in parts of America to provide day care for ill children. This is being approached in several ways:

- A 'sick wing' – cohorting children with similar illness together
- Staff from the nursery caring for the ill child in its own home
- Day care centres specifically designed to care for ill children.

Play and equipment

Equipment and toys should be chosen to enable the children to develop their social, emotional, cognitive and physical skills. Toys often have porous surfaces and crevices in which organisms can thrive, and because some children have a tendency to put things into their mouths, the risk of their acquiring an infection from such objects is increased (Laborde et al 1993). Where a British Standard exists, equipment purchased must conform to it, and consideration should be given as to the ease of decontamination. A study of toys in a paediatric ward highlighted the need for frequent and regular cleaning of toys (Suviste 1996). The author recommended toys to be thoroughly washed with detergent and dried. She also suggested that toys used by children with infectious diseases should be decontaminated with hypochlorite solution (1000 ppm – one thousand parts per million dilution). It is wise to avoid soft toys which cannot be machine washed.

Other equipment which could present a potential problem includes towels, toothbrushes and hairbrushes. Such toiletry items should not be shared, and systems must be put into place to control this (Fig. 7.3).

Feeding bottles/teething aids

Where facilities provide child care for young children who are being bottle fed, provisions to ensure their adequate decontamination must be made. If the child is less than one year old or susceptible to infection, feeding bottles and teething aids should be cleaned in detergent and water prior to being disinfected. Methods of disinfection may include the use of a 'Milton' cold sterilizing unit, using 1:80 dilution of hypochlorite solution changed daily, or a steam sterilizer.

Sand/water/playdough

Children are often involved in play activities (Fig. 7.4) involving sand, playdough, water and baking. Such equipment may be an ideal vehicle to transmit infections, and good standards of hygiene must prevail during such activities. Children should always wash their hands prior to and following these activities. During an outbreak of diarrhoea and vomiting, these activities should cease. It is advisable to have a system in place where the play tanks are drained, the water/sand discarded, the tank washed with neutral detergent and thoroughly dried and the sand/water replenished. Consensus opinion suggests this should occur on a monthly basis and more frequently if contamination occurs in between these times. Children suffering from enteric illnesses and runny noses should be discouraged from taking part in baking sessions.

Sensory equipment

Many child care facilities now utilize leisure equipment initially used for people who have a

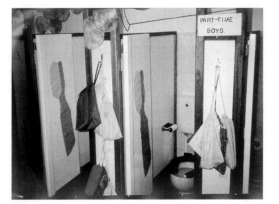

Figure 7.3 Storage for personal items.

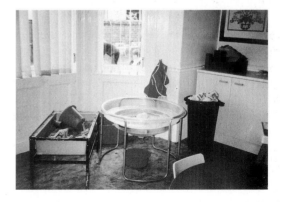

Figure 7.4 Play equipment: an ideal vehicle to transmit infections.

sensory impairment. This varied equipment provides stimulation and in some cases offers a therapeutic intervention. Examples include optical displays, bubble tubes, linelites, water beds, ballpools and soft foam wedges/bean bags. It is important to have a written cleaning schedule, detailing when equipment is cleaned and the cleaning products used. Most equipment can be cleaned using neutral detergent and water. Abrasive cleaners should be avoided as they may damage the product. It is extremely important to ensure all crevices are thoroughly cleaned.

Food hygiene

The hygienic preparation of food, combined with effective cleaning of food preparation areas and equipment and a high standard of personal hygiene, is extremely important in ensuring the safe delivery of food to children. Ideally, those staff involved in toileting children or nappy changing **should not** be involved in food handling.

Policies and procedures in relation to the preparation, storage and serving of food should be familiar to all staff within the child care setting and should be adhered to. In larger facilities it is advisable to have an industrial-type dishwasher. Kitchen sinks should not be used for any other purpose but for cleaning of kitchen equipment, and a separate wash hand basin is **legally required**. Bars of soap and cloth hand towels may harbour micro-organisms, and it is preferable to use liquid soap dispensers which cannot be re-filled and disposable paper towels.

In the study by Lopez et al (1988), 94% of child care facilities had a specially designated food preparation area but 45% used the same sink for food preparation and for other utility purposes. Food handlers should be aware of their statutory obligations under the Food Safety (General Food Hygiene) Regulations 1995. In line with this current legislation, all staff who handle food (Fig. 7.5) must receive food hygiene training which is commensurate with their food handling duties.

Staff must not handle food if suffering from:

- skin infections
- infected wounds

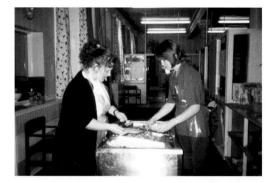

Figure 7.5 Staff handling food must receive appropriate training. Reproduced with permission.

- sores
- diarrhoea and/or vomiting.

They must notify the local Environmental Health Department if they suffer from any communicable disease. Meal times must be adequately supervised to ensure the children follow good hygienic practices.

Policies

It is extremely important that all facilities which provide care for children have written infection control policies and procedures. These should provide information and advice on all the subject matter discussed within this chapter. Such policies should be:

- concise, yet as specific as possible (for example, cleaning policies should indicate the cleaning agent and frequency of cleaning)
- written so that both staff and parents can understand them
- given to parents to read prior to a child's enrolment to the facility.

It is also useful if staff place information boards displaying advice or other educational material relating to infectious diseases and/or infection prevention (Fig. 7.6).

Animals

If pets are kept within the child care facility, there should be a named individual who is responsible

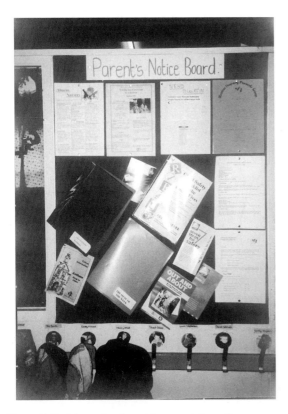

Figure 7.6 Information board for parents/guardians.

for their care. If an animal is brought onto the premises the individual organizing the specific event should agree hygiene and safety matters with the pet's owner. Pets should never be allowed in kitchen areas and any animal faeces must be cleaned up immediately. Litter boxes should not be accessible to children. It is advisable to exercise such animals away from areas where children may play. Animals' living areas must be kept clean and young children should not play with animals unsupervised. Children must wash their hands after handling animals, their bedding, or cleaning cages, etc. Particular care should be taken with reptiles and exotic pets as they can transmit or be carrying bacteria such as salmonella (Payne 2000).

Visits to farms or zoos

The individual(s) responsible for an outing to a farm or zoo must familiarize themselves with the infection risks from such visits. It is helpful to visit the area prior to the actual outing. Factors to be considered are set out in the following checklists.

Prior to visits, staff must check that:

- the area appears well run and maintained
- public areas appear reasonably clean, including toilets
- outdoor picnic areas are secured from animals
- suitable hand washing facilities are available, including hot and cold running water, soap (preferably liquid), and either disposable paper towels or a hot air hand dryer
- these facilities are accessible for the age of the children visiting
- first aid facilities are available
- slurry pits, manure stacks and sick animals are secured from access
- drinking water taps are designated in clean areas.

During the visit, there are additional considerations. These include:

- that appropriate footwear and impervious outdoor clothing is worn in wet, muddy areas or any area where there may have been animal faeces
- ensuring that children are adequately supervised by an appropriate number of adults
- advising the children not to place their faces against the animals
- reiterating the importance of hand washing to the children:
  - after touching the animals or their bedding
  - after feeding the animals
  - before eating
  - before drinking
  - after any contact with the animals
  - after contact with any equipment used on the animals.
- reminding the children that they must not eat or drink anything whilst visiting the farm/zoo due to the risk of infection from hand-to-mouth contact. This includes chewing gum, sweets, crisps, etc.

- supervising the children during hand washing
- consumption of food in an area well away from where the animals are kept
- warning children not to consume the following:
  — unpasteurized products such as milk, cheese, yoghurt
  — anything which may have fallen on the ground
  — any products for animal consumption
- ensuring children avoid contact with manure or slurry
- that at the end of the visit, children should thoroughly wash and dry their hands before departure. Any contaminated footwear should be cleaned as much as possible to remove faecal matter.

COMMUNICABLE DISEASES

A child with an infectious disease usually shows general signs of illness before a rash or other indicative symptoms develop. The child may complain of feeling unwell, shivering attacks or feeling cold, headache, vomiting or sore throat. Such symptoms should make staff suspicious. In such circumstances, it is recommended to contact the parent/guardian so that their child can be collected with a view to consulting their GP if necessary.

Exclusion policy

Despite the disruption to the family, an exclusion policy must be available to prevent and control infection. The purpose of exclusion is to separate a child or member of staff with a potentially infectious disease from others, to reduce the risk of the infection spreading. (Refer also to the exclusion section and communicable diseases in this chapter.)

Vulnerable children

Some children may have a medical condition which may make them particularly vulnerable to infections that would rarely be a problem to most children. This includes:

- children being treated for leukaemia or other cancers

- children taking high doses of oral steroids
- children with any illnesses affecting the immune system.

The following alphabetical list provides details of some communicable diseases, the recommended minimum period of exclusion and any additional relevant information.

Specific communicable diseases

AIDS (Acquired Immune Deficiency Syndrome)

AIDS is caused by the Human Immunodeficiency Virus (HIV). The virus gradually destroys the immune system so that the individual is susceptible to infections of all kinds.

Children with AIDS or HIV infection may have acquired it via contaminated blood products, such as those used to treat haemophilia, or (increasingly) by being born to HIV-infected mothers. Individuals may have acquired it sexually or by needle-sharing drug use. The essential points for schools are:

- The child with HIV/AIDS is vulnerable to infection *from* others; he/she is not a major source of infection *to* others.
- However, the blood of such a child is infective and should be dealt with as previously described. (These are routine measures for all blood spills.)
- The condition is lifelong, and schooling and other activities should be as normal as possible.

Exclusion None.

Athlete's foot

A fungal infection which causes irritation and discomfort, mainly between the toes. The skin becomes inflamed and cracked, and may bleed. Treatment is simple and effective and is always advisable.

Exclusion None.

Chickenpox

An acute but mild viral illness with a slight fever and itchy skin rash. The rash begins as small, raised blotches, which turn to blisters filled with clear fluid. Later, these turn yellow, break and become crusted and scabby. The rash may involve the whole body, including the scalp, inside the mouth and on the eyes. Some children have a few spots, whilst others are covered.

Spread is from person to person by direct contact, droplets or airborne deposits from the respiratory system. Incubation period is 2–3 weeks. Infectivity is usually 1–2 days before the rash appears but does not last more than five days after the blisters first appear.

Exclusion For five days after the blisters appear. See also Shingles.

Special information

- Vulnerable children are especially susceptible to chickenpox. If they are exposed to this, parents/carers must be notified promptly so they can seek further medical advice if necessary.
- Chickenpox can also pose a risk in pregnancy if the woman has not previously had the disease. If a pregnant woman is exposed in early pregnancy (the first 20 weeks) or very late in pregnancy (the last three weeks before birth) she should promptly inform her GP and whoever is providing ante-natal care. This will allow a blood test to be taken to check her immune status (DoH 1999).
- Hands should be washed after touching or treating spots of an infected person.

Conjunctivitis

The first signs of infection are excessive watering and irritation of the eye, followed by a swelling and possible discharge of pus from the eye – 'sticky eye'. It is spread by direct contact with discharge from the eye of the infected person. It can also be spread by contact with contaminated fingers, tissues and other items. Treatment is with a course of antibiotic eye drops or ointment.

Exclusion Whilst the child is ill or the sticky eye persists.

Special information

- Thorough hand washing after touching the affected eye.
- Never share eye ointments/drops, tissues or towels.

Diphtheria

A bacterial infection of the tonsils, throat and nose. First there is a sore throat and later a greyish/white membrane develops. Deaths occur as a result of the poisons produced by the bacteria or the obstruction of the air passages. Most infection in England has come from abroad, Eastern Europe and the Indian sub-continent being the greatest risk.

Report this dangerous disease immediately to the CCDC.

Incubation period is usually 2–5 days. Infectivity is usually two weeks or less. Diphtheria can be prevented by immunization, so children who have not been immunized are at unnecessary risk.

Exclusion Immediate.

Diarrhoea and vomiting

Diarrhoea and vomiting can be caused by a number of different germs including viruses (such as rotavirus), parasites (such as amoeba or giardia) and bacteria (such as salmonella, campylobacter, shigella and *E.coli*).

Different germs may cause different symptoms. The most common cause is by eating contaminated food or drinking contaminated water. It can also be spread from person to person (via unwashed hands), especially in children.

Exclusion In general, people should stay away from the child care facility until they have been free from symptoms for 48 hours and feel well.

Special information

- Personal hygiene must be very strict.
- Toilets, seats and handles must be cleaned daily and additionally if soiled.
- Discontinue water play, playdough, sand play and cooking activities during an outbreak.

Fifth disease or slapped cheek (parvovirus)

This is a viral infection which often affects red blood cells. It is caused by a human parvovirus. Anyone can acquire this infection but the disease seems to occur more often in schoolchildren. It is spread by exposure to secretions from the nose and throat of infected people. Initial symptoms include a slight fever and tiredness; later a red rash appears on the cheeks, giving a slapped face appearance. The rash may then extend over the body and tends to fade and re-appear. People with fifth disease appear to be contagious during the week prior to the appearance of the rash.

Exclusion   Is ineffective, as nearly all transmission takes place before the child becomes unwell.

Special information

- Some studies have shown that there is an increased risk of miscarriage within the first 18–20 weeks of pregnancy.
- In people with chronic red blood cell disorders (e.g. sickle cell disease), infection may result in severe anaemia.
- During outbreaks, pregnant staff or people with red blood cell disorders should consult their doctor as soon as possible.
- Strict hand washing should be performed following contact with secretions.

German measles (rubella)

A viral disease which produces a blotchy rash and slight fever. It is a mild disease, but is important if a pregnant woman becomes infected as it may seriously harm her baby.

Rubella spreads by contact with droplets from the respiratory system or direct contact with infected individuals. The incubation period is 14–23 days and the child is infectious for one week before the rash appears until one week after its onset.

Exclusion   Whilst the child is ill, until at least 5 days after the appearance of the rash.

Special information

- If a woman who is not immune to rubella is exposed to this infection in early pregnancy, her baby can be affected. Female staff should have a blood test to check their immunity to rubella, and if appropriate, offer immunization. Any pregnant woman who comes into contact with the infection should notify her GP promptly.

Hand, foot and mouth disease

This virus of humans has nothing to do with the foot and mouth disease of animals. It is more common in children than adults and outbreaks usually occur in hot summer weather. The person initially suffers from a sore throat and fever-like symptoms; blisters and grey ulcers then appear on the palate, inside the mouth and on the palms and soles of the feet. The rash can also affect the back of the hands and fingers, particularly the nail folds and the armpits. In small children the nappy area may be involved. It is caused by the Coxsackie Virus.

Spread is mainly by direct contact with nose and throat secretions, faeces and fluid from the blisters of the infected person. The disease is mild, and children usually recover in a few days; adults may take longer. There is no specific treatment or vaccine. Incubation period is 3–5 days.

Exclusion   No need to exclude from school unless the child is obviously unwell or feverish.

Special information

- Prompt and thorough hand washing when handling discharges or faeces.
- Prompt washing of soiled articles.
- Toilets including seats and handles must be cleaned daily or when soiled.

Hepatitis (jaundice)

Hepatitis A is a virus spread by mouth. There is fever, tiredness, loss of appetite, abdominal pain or discomfort possibly followed by jaundice within a few days. (Many young children never become jaundiced.) Spread is encouraged by poor hygiene, particularly lack of hand washing after visiting the toilet. Close contacts may be protected from infection by immunization. The incubation period is usually four weeks. Infectivity is highest in the later half of the incubation period before the symptoms occur, and continuing for a few days after the onset of jaundice.

Exclusion   Exclude from school for one week after the onset of jaundice. Report it promptly because it spreads easily.

Special information

- Ensure strict personal hygiene.
- Toilets including seats and handles must be cleaned at least daily or when soiled.

- No sharing of towels or flannels.
- During an outbreak, discontinue water play, playdough, sand play and cooking activities.

Hepatitis B is rare in schoolchildren. Symptoms are similar to Hepatitis A, and progress to jaundice. Spread is usually by blood but other body fluids also contain this virus. A small number of individuals become carriers. They feel well but their blood is infectious. You will not know who is a carrier, so it is important to deal with all blood spills carefully. The condition should be reported promptly.

Exclusion Only if unwell.

Special information

- Cover cuts and broken skin with a waterproof plaster.
- Wear disposable gloves when dealing with blood and body fluids.
- A vaccine is available for families and sexual partners of people with Hepatitis B.

Other Hepatitis viruses such as C, D, E, F and G are known to exist but are still rare. The measures against Hepatitis A and B above will help prevent them.

Impetigo

A localized patch or patches of infected skin caused by a bacterium which may also cause food poisoning if transferred from the skin to food. The affected area becomes red, swollen, weeping and crusted. It commonly affects the face but can occur anywhere on the body. Antibiotic treatment by mouth may speed healing.

Exclusion Until the lesions have dried up or can be covered. Recovery is usually 24 hours after treatment.

Special information

- *People with impetigo must not handle food.*
- Thorough hand washing is essential after contact with lesion or contaminated items.
- No sharing of clothing, bedding, towels, etc.

Lice (pediculosis, nits)

Tiny insects, smaller than a match head, which live on the skin and hair of the human body (see Fig. 13.1). The commonest variety are head lice. Louse eggs (nits) (Fig. 13.2) are tiny cream dots attached firmly near the scalp to single hairs. They are hard to dislodge. Empty eggshells are whiter and easier to see, and are further away from the scalp (at least 1 cm). Tiny black specks of louse droppings may be seen on the pillow. Lice spread by direct head-to-head contact with an infected person (child or adult). They cannot jump, swim or fly.

Exclusion None.

Special information

- Treatment is only required if live lice are seen in the hair (not nits).
- The best way of controlling head lice is for parents/carers to check hair every week.

Advice and information on head inspection and the treatment for lice can be obtained from the school nurse and local chemists.

Measles

An acute, highly infectious disease. It may start like a bad cold with fever, runny nose, red eyes and cough. The red blotchy rash usually starts on the face about 3–7 days after the onset of fever and spreads all over the body. The incubation period is about 10 days from exposure to onset of fever. It is spread by direct contact with secretions from the nose or throat of an infected person. Immunization prevents the infection.

Exclusion Until fully recovered from the symptoms, usually five days from onset of the rash.

Special information

- If a vulnerable child is exposed to measles, the parent/carers should be informed promptly so that they can seek further medical advice as necessary.

Meningitis

An infection of the brain linings by either a virus (usually mild) or bacterium (much more serious). The commonest bacteria are Hib, meningococcus and pneumococcus. Symptoms include headache, flu-like illness, stiff neck, vomiting, drowsiness and even coma. The individual may become ill very quickly. The same bacteria can invade the bloodstream (septicaemia) without affecting the brain linings. Headache and neck stiffness may not occur but there may be a purple rash. Typically the rash is non-blanching: if a drinking glass is pressed firmly against the rash, and the rash remains visible under pressure, then this is indicative of meningococcal infection. Meningitis is spread by direct close contact with the nose or throat discharges of an infected person. Close contacts (household and kissing partners) are treated with antibiotics as advised by the CCDC. There is usually no need to treat contacts at school or nursery.

Hib meningitis can be prevented by immunization. There is no vaccine against the commonest British strain of meningococcus, type B. There is a vaccine now available against meningitis C.

Exclusion Until fully recovered.
Special information

- *Report cases promptly: contacts, however, are no cause for concern by schools.*
- It is not necessary to exclude siblings and other contacts.

Mumps

Mumps results in a fever with swelling and tenderness of the salivary glands, usually those in front of the earlobes. Mumps is most infectious in the 48 hours before symptoms start. The incubation period is about 18 days. Immunization prevents it. Mumps is spread by direct contact with saliva and discharges from the nose and throat of infected individuals.

Exclusion Until fully recovered.

Poliomyelitis

Polio has been almost eradicated by immunization but might still be acquired abroad. It is an acute illness which damages the nervous system, resulting in weakness, paralysis or even death. It is usually spread by close association with the infected person but it may be spread by the faecal–oral route if sanitation is poor. Immunization prevents

it, so unimmunized children and adults are at unnecessary risk.

Report this dangerous disease immediately to the CCDC.

Ringworm

This condition is NOT caused by a worm. It is a skin infection caused by a type of fungi. It is spread by direct skin-to-skin contact with an infected person or animal, or indirectly by contact with contaminated items such as combs, hairbrushes, clothing, or shower room floors, etc. Ringworm of the body appears as a flat, spreading ring-shaped area. The edge is reddish and may be crusted.

Exclusion None.
Special information

- Hand washing after contact.
- Towels, clothing, pillows, etc. should not be shared.
- Good standards of cleanliness should be maintained in showers, baths and communal areas.

Scabies

An infestation by a tiny mite, about 1/3 mm long, which burrows into the skin and causes great irritation, leading to scratching. The burrows are typically seen in the webs between the fingers, but may be elsewhere on the body. Spread requires close contact. It is important that all households/close contacts of a person with scabies observe carefully for a rash developing.

Exclusion The child may return once treatment is complete, usually next day.
Special information

- Itching may persist for 1–2 weeks following treatment and does not necessarily indicate a failure of the treatment.

Shingles or herpes zoster

A recurrence of the chickenpox virus usually occurring in adults, and seldom in children. The rash appears over the area supplied by a single sensory nerve. Commonly, this will be a strip of skin round one side of the chest, less often one side of the head and face. There will be pain and illness. The rash can spread chickenpox (not shingles) to anyone who is not already immune.

Exclusion Until all the spots have dried and crusted over, usually 5–7 days.

Tuberculosis (TB)

TB usually affects the lungs (pulmonary TB). The symptoms may be vague illness, weight loss and a cough. The cough can spread infection to others, for example in the classroom. However, only a minority of TB cases are ever infectious and even those will stop being infectious after a couple of weeks of treatment. Immunization by BCG gives a high degree of protection.

Report cases of TB promptly to the CCDC.

Exclusion Will be decided by the hospital specialist.

Verruca

A wart on the sole of the foot. It is usually painless and will disappear given time. However, if it rubs against the shoe or is on a weight-bearing part of the foot, it may be painful. If so, or if it is spreading on the foot, it may require treatment.

Exclusion None.
Special information

- Verrucae should be covered before swimming.

Whooping cough (pertussis)

This starts insidiously with catarrh and an irritating cough which gradually gets worse and occurs in paroxysms. The incubation period is usually 7–10 days but may be much longer. The cough, with its characteristic 'whoop', may last for 8 weeks. The child becomes exhausted with the effort of coughing and may be left with damage to the lungs. It is most infectious at the catarrhal stage before the whooping begins. Treatment may reduce the period of communicability but does not help the individual much. Immunization largely prevents it.

Exclusion Until at least 21 days from the start of the paroxysmal cough or 7 days after the start of antibiotic treatment.

Worms

Many varieties of worms can inhabit the human body but in Britain the commonest ones are threadworms and roundworms. These are acquired when eggs from the parasites are conveyed to the mouth. After hatching, the worms live in the gut and pregnant female worms deposit their eggs in the faeces or outside the anus. Poor hygiene, scratching of the anus and inadequate hand washing enable eggs caught under the nails to be transferred to objects, food or mouths.

Threadworms (pinworms) are very common, and may not cause symptoms. If troublesome, they may cause disturbed sleep due to itching round the anus, irritability, scratching, and often soreness. Diagnosis may be made by seeing the worms like threads, on the anus, especially at night before bathing or going to the toilet. They may also be seen in the faeces. Threadworms of animals are not transmissible to people. The person is infectious as long as eggs are being laid on the skin. Eggs remain infective for at last 2 weeks. Treatment is effective and all family members should be investigated and, if necessary, treated at the same time. Good personal and domestic hygiene is essential.

Exclusion No reason to keep children away from school as long as good personal hygiene is followed and treatment is being carried out.
Special information

- Thorough hand washing after going to the toilet and before eating or preparing food is always essential in preventing the spread of infection.
- Keep nails short and clean.

CASE STUDIES

Case study one (Nursery)

Jon is a four-year-old who arrives at nursery with a rash on his upper body. The rash has formed a band on his trunk and he is complaining that it is very sore.

Jon had chickenpox when he was eighteen months old and it appears that Jon now has shingles.

1. Is Jon infectious to the other children and staff at the nursery?
2. What advice should be given to staff and parents?
3. Is it necessary to exclude Jon from nursery and, if so, for how long?

Points to consider

- Shingles only occurs in people who have had chickenpox in the past.
- Shingles is not spread from person to person. However, the spots are infectious while they are 'weepy' and contact with an infected individual may cause chickenpox in someone who has not had it before.

- It is unusual for children to get shingles and consideration should be given to the child's immune state and whether Jon has any other medical conditions.
- Staff and parents should be given information as above.
- Shingles can present a risk to children who have a medical condition which may make them vulnerable: for example, children with cancer or receiving treatment for cancer.
- Shingles may also pose a danger to pregnant women who have not previously had chickenpox. If a woman is exposed in early pregnancy (the first 20 weeks) or very late in pregnancy (the last 3 weeks before birth) she should promptly inform her GP and whoever is providing ante-natal care. A blood test can reveal whether an individual has immunity to chickenpox.
- Affected individuals should be excluded from nursery for 5 days from the onset of the rash, although they are infectious just before the rash actually develops.

Case study two (School)

The headmaster of a local special school providing education for children with both physical and learning difficulties seeks your advice. During a rehearsal for a school concert, a child vomited whilst on the stage. Over the following two days, many of the children who were on the stage at the time have become ill with symptoms of vomiting and subsequent diarrhoea. Twenty-three pupils and three staff have reported symptoms.

1. What action should be taken?
2. What information would you want to know?
3. What might be happening here?
4. What advice should be given?
5. Whom should you inform and what actions are likely to occur?

Points to consider

- The headmaster should inform the CCDC (Consultant in Communicable Disease Control) in the Public Health Department. It is very helpful if the school can draw up lists by class/year group, showing who is well or ill and the date the illness was reported to them.
- Following discussion, an initial assessment of the potential size and scale of the problem will be made. Information which would be required includes:
  — percentage of those on stage who are ill
  — percentage of the rest of the school ill now and recently. Remember, the illness could be coincidental.

(continued)

- It is likely that the CCDC will convene an Outbreak Control Group to
  — investigate the cause
  — formulate a plan of action to control the problem
  — draw general lessons from the experience.
- Key personnel involved will include:
  — the CCDC
  — Infection Control Nurse(s)
  — Environmental Health Officers (EHOs)
  — the headmaster and teachers
  — representative from the local education authority
  — school nurse.
- What might be happening?
  — probably spread of viral gastro-enteritis from person to person
  — it is unlikely to be food poisoning, but it must be considered
  — it is unlikely to be water supply, environmental poisons, etc.

Suggested action

A visit to the school from the CCDC, Infection Control Nurse and Environmental Health Officer to establish the current practices within the school and the environment, in collaboration with the school staff.

1. Factors which they will wish to explore include:
   — how spillages are cleaned up
   — the standard of cleanliness
   — facilities for hand washing and drying
   — process followed at meal times
   — processes undertaken when dealing with incontinent pupils
   — supervision of toileting and hand washing of pupils
   — how equipment is decontaminated
   — how play equipment is decontaminated.
2. Advice and support they will provide:
   — hygiene and decontamination in the school
   — the importance of good hand hygiene to pupils, staff and families
   — requesting parents to keep children at home until they are symptom-free for 48 hours,

and same advice for staff to ensure that a 'relapse'/recurrence does not develop
   — advice on cleaning procedures and for attention to be paid to door handles, taps and flushing mechanisms.
3. Liaison with EHOs to obtain food histories and stool samples from those with symptoms.
4. Provide written information for parents and children – a meeting may also be held in school to give verbal advice and information.
5. Media management – the outbreak may attract publicity and this must be very carefully handled. An individual should be designated to deal with press queries and present statements on behalf of the health authority.
6. Activities such as water play, sand play, use of playdough and cooking sessions should cease during the outbreak.
7. Consider the siblings of the affected children and advise other schools which they attend to ensure that they are aware of the possibility of secondary cases and to inform the CCDC of these. There is a strong possibility of a secondary wave of cases after a further two days, most commonly in siblings and close contacts of the first cases. The size of the wave will reflect the diligence of the control measures advised. A third or fourth wave, therefore, would be very concerning.
8. It is useful to seize this opportunity to emphasize the importance of infection control and conduct activities to enhance the hand washing practices of the children.
9. Anyone who handles food *must* be asymptomatic for 48 hours prior to returning to such duties.
10. Consider whether some of the children have behavioural problems which may lead them to smear faecal matter within the environment. This may create an increased problem with environmental contamination and cross infection. This soiling must be cleaned immediately with detergent and water. In the event of pupils with such behavioural problems having symptoms of diarrhoea and/or vomiting, they should be excluded from school until they have been symptom-free for 48 hours.

Case study three (School)

Mary is a five year old pupil at the local primary school. She did not attend school yesterday because she has had flu-like symptoms. She has returned to school today but is obviously unwell. Mary feels very sick, has a high temperature and appears apathetic and sleepy. Her mum is called and takes her to see her General Practitioner, who suspects bacterial meningitis and immediately admits her to the local hospital.

What action may be taken at this time?

Points to consider

- The GP suspects bacterial meningitis but it may be a viral type or something entirely different, e.g. appendicitis.

At this stage the CCDC may advise antibiotic therapy for close contacts within a period of seven days prior to Mary becoming ill.

- The risk of any member of the public becoming infected is 2 in 100 000 in any one year. The risk to close contacts is 2 in 100 (×1000). The risk to other contacts is 2 in every thousand, to ten thousand. Therefore, the side effects of sensitization and resistance problems is considered to outweigh the benefits of prescribing antibiotics.
- Meningococcal bacteria are found naturally at the back of the throat and nose of about 10 per cent of the general population.
- There are two common strains of meningococcal meningitis in the UK – B and C. (Other types are rare.) Group B is the most common form of bacterial meningitis in the United Kingdom and is responsible for two thirds of the cases reported.
- All cases of meningitis should be notified to the Consultant in Communicable Disease Control (CCDC). This is a legal responsibility of the doctor suspecting or diagnosing meningitis.
- The CCDC will determine who has been a close contact of Mary and arrange subsequent chemoprophylaxis for them.

- Close contacts include:
  - people living in the same household
  - those who have intimately kissed the infected person
  - people who have shared sleeping quarters
  - people who have given mouth-to-mouth resuscitation.
- Antibiotics may kill the bacteria at the back of the throat and reduce the risk of acquiring meningitis, but they cannot guarantee to prevent it.
- Some vaccines are available but
  - none are against type B, the most common
  - the vaccine against C type meningitis may be used for close contacts if Mary is found to have this strain.
- It is extremely important to ensure the staff at the school are given correct written and verbal information regarding meningitis.
- Contact numbers and information should also be made available to anxious parents and they should be advised to be vigilant.

Seven days later, Joshua and Rebecca, who both sit on the same table as Mary, do not attend school as they are unwell. The headmistress finds out later that day that Joshua has been admitted to hospital with suspected meningitis. She immediately informs the CCDC.

What action may be taken now?

Points to consider

- The CCDC's first task is to check Joshua's diagnosis. By this time a confirmed diagnosis should be available for Mary.
- The CCDC will probably convene an outbreak control group. This team will probably include:
  - Public Health
  - School staff
  - Infection Control Nurse
  - School Nurse
  - Microbiologist.

(continued)

Suggested action

1. Action that will be taken by the CCDC includes:
   — to seek advice from the Regional Epidemiologist and the Meningitis Reference Laboratory
   — to distribute information about meningococcal disease to all concerned
   — to make available chemoprophylaxis to all class contacts
   — to offer vaccination if cases are found to be Group C type meningococcal disease
   — to consider taking throat swabs.

2. Antibiotic treatment may be given by the GPs or, alternatively, the administration may be co-ordinated by the Public Health Department and given at the school. If this is the case, it is crucial to ensure the school is visited and the flow of work assessed prior to the actual administration of the medication. People involved in this process may include:
   — infection control nurses and doctors
   — school staff
   — parents
   — pupils
   — health care staff
   — school nurses
   — health visitors
   — practice nurses
   — community medical officers
   — pharmacists.

3. Other considerations include:
   — media coverage – a spokesperson is usually designated to discuss the situation with the Press. It is important to ensure the Press are kept fully informed whilst ensuring confidentiality of the infected individuals.
   — Control of crowds and Press. This emotive subject may invoke a huge public and media response.
   — A helpline may be useful.
   — Meetings held in the school for parents and staff.
   — Written and verbal information should be made available, including:
     a) protocols for staff
     b) consent forms
     c) information regarding the disease, antibiotics and vaccinations.
   — Records must be kept including:
     a) consent forms
     b) batch numbers of vaccines, etc.
     c) health history.

An unfortunate possibility is that a child may die. This happens once a year in an average district. Should this occur, there will be immense pressure from the public and media: for example, to close the school. From an infection control perspective, it is unnecessary to actually take any additional measures or precautions.

REFERENCES

Baker T P H 1987 Infection control for the day care facility. ASEPSIS – The Infection Control Forum 9(1): 7–11

Berg R 1988 Day care for children in the APIC curriculum for infection control practice. Kendall Hunt, Iowa, 1310–1324

Black R E, Dykes A C, Anderson K E et al 1981 Handwashing to prevent diarrhoea in day care centers. American Journal of Epidemiology 113: 445–451

Bonner A F, Dale R 1986 Giardia lamblia day care diarrhoea. American Journal of Nursing 86(7): 818–820

Chorba T L, Meriwether R A, Jenkins B R, Gunn R A, MacCormack J N 1987 Control of non-food-borne outbreak of salmonellosis: day care in isolation. American Journal of Public Health 77(9): 979–981

Department for Education and Employment 1998 Statistics of Education: Schools in England. Statistical Volume. DfEE, London

Department for Education and Employment 1999 Statistics of Education: Children's Day Care Facilities at 31 March 1998. DfEE, London

Department of Health 1990 The Children Act 1989 Consultation Paper No. 2. Policy and standard of day care educational services (Guidance). Department of Health, London

Department of Health 1999 Guidance on infection control in schools and nurseries (poster and leaflet). Department of Health, London

Early E, Battle K, Cantwell E, English J, Lavin J E, Larson E 1998 Effect of several interventions on the frequency of handwashing among elementary public school children. American Journal of Infection Control 263–269

Evans R 1992 Child's play. Nursing Times: Journal of Infection Control Nursing 88(Suppl.): 24

Gillis C L, Holaday B, Lewis C C, Pantell R H 1989 A Health Education Program for Day-care Centers. American Journal of Maternity and Child Nursing 14: 266–268

Health and Safety Executive 1995 SI 1995/3163 The Reporting of Injuries, Diseases and Dangerous Occurrences Regulations. HMSO, London

Health and Safety Executive 1999 Control of Substances Hazardous to Health Regulations. HSE Books, Sudbury

Holaday B, Pantell R H, Lewis C C, Gillis C L 1990 Patterns of faecal coliform contamination in day care centres. Public Health Nursing 7(4): 224–227

Jewkes R K, O'Connor B H 1990 Crisis in our schools: survey of sanitation facilities in schools in Bloomsbury Health District. British Medical Journal 301: 1085–1087

Kaltenthaler E C, Elsworth A M, Schweiger M S, Mara D D, Braunholt D A 1995 Faecal contamination on children's hands and environmental surfaces in primary schools in Leeds. Epidemiology and Infection 115: 527–534

Koopman J 1978 Diarrhoea and school toilet hygiene in Cali, Colombia. American Journal of Epidemiology 107: 412–420

Laborde D J, Weigle K A, Weber D J, Rotch D B 1993 Effect of faecal contamination on diarrhoeal illness rates in day care centers. American Journal of Epidemiology 138: 243–255

Landis S E, Earp J L, Sharp M 1988 Day-care center exclusion of sick children: comparison of opinions of day-care staff, working mothers and paediatricians. Paediatrics 81, 5: 662–667

Lopez J, DiLiberto J, McGuckin M 1988 Infection control in day care centers: present and future needs. American Journal of Infection Control 16: 26–29

Lopez J, DiLiberto J A L, Sharp M 1998 Infection control in day care centers: present and future needs. American Journal of Infection Control 16(1): 26–29

May H 1998 Now wash your hands … Nursing Times 94(4): 63–66

Osterholm M T 1987 Infection control for the day care facility. ASEPSIS – the Infection Control Forum 9(1): 2–5

Payne D 2000 Deadly risk from exotic pets. Nursing Times 96(24): 13

Russell B 1987 Infection control for the day care facility. ASEPSIS – The Infection Control Forum 9(1): 11–13

Suviste J 1996 The toy trap uncovered. Nursing Times 92(10): 56–59

Wilson J 2001 Infection Control in Clinical Practice, 2nd edn. Baillière Tindall, London

Wilson J, Breedon P 1990 Universal precautions. Nursing Times 86(37): 67–70

8

Residential and nursing homes

M. Whitlock
J. Lawrence

INTRODUCTION

Most of those living in care homes and nursing homes are elderly. Recent changes in healthcare provision mean that older people requiring care may receive it in a residential or nursing care home. The changes, which are taking place at the time of writing, are the re-shaping of services within communities in which Primary Care Trusts will have a leading role (DoH 2002). Currently the Health Authorities have the responsibility for nursing homes but in light of the changes, this may alter according to local needs and demographic factors.

The Office of Population, Censuses and Surveys (1991) estimates that the average lifespan is increasing by two years per decade. Older people have complex healthcare needs, often combining acute and chronic illnesses, compounded by problems of poverty and a lack of social support (DoH 2001a).

Advanced age means that residents are more vulnerable to infection as a result of multiple factors including a diminished immune response, co-existing chronic disease, malignancy and poor nutrition. In addition, sharing eating and living accommodation can increase the risk of cross infection occurring.

It is essential that infection control principles be applied in these settings in order to reduce the likelihood of cross infection. When appropriate infection control policies are adopted, the environment is safer for people to live and work in and in turn this can make it cost-effective (DoH 1996).

Care homes can be privately owned or managed by the local social service department. People living in a care home have their clinical nursing care provided by a district nurse. Nursing homes are usually privately owned by individuals or a company. There are a number of homes, privately owned, which have dual responsibility for both general care and nursing care.

Care homes providing nursing employ trained nursing staff to provide or supervise clinical nursing care. This ensures that those interventions are undertaken by staff with appropriate skill and expertise, thus helping to avoid the risk of complications such as infection. However, it is essential that *all* staff are adequately trained in the principles of infection control to ensure appropriate practice.

The vulnerability of the residents to infection arises through the ageing process and/or mental illness, which may result in an inability to maintain basic hygiene, thus increasing the risk. The clinical presentation of infection can be difficult, as residents may not always be able to express themselves or staff may incorrectly interpret symptoms. For example, chronic incontinence may mask symptoms of urinary tract infection (Nicolle et al 1996).

Responsibilities

Home owner

The owner of the care home is responsible for the health and safety of residents, staff and visitors under the current Health and Safety Act (1974). This includes maintaining a safe environment for residents, visitors and staff. In addition the Control of Substances Hazardous to Health (COSHH) regulations place a duty of care on employers to ensure risks are assessed with regard to micro-organisms and transmission of micro-organisms.

The person in charge of the care home is responsible for ensuring there is an effective infection control policy that is adhered to and understood by the staff and visitors (DoH 1996). They must also ensure that the home meets the requirements of the Registration Homes Act 1984.

Consultant in Communicable Disease Control (CCDC)

The CCDC is employed by the Health Authority with executive responsibility for the control of infectious disease in the community within a geographical area. The CCDC is usually also an officer of the local authority, which has statutory power for communicable disease control (Public Health Infectious Diseases Regulations 1988). An infection control service is not the responsibility of the CCDC, but ensuring that adequate measures are in place is, through the registration and inspection team within the Care Standards Agency.

Community Infection Control Nurses (CICN)

CICNs are appointed to provide infection control advice in community settings. They liaise closely with the CCDC, and are an expert source of practical infection control advice that should be used by managers and matrons of homes when writing and implementing infection control policy, auditing standards and training staff.

General Practitioner (GP)

People living in care homes access medical care from their GP, who is responsible for the diagnosis and prevention of infectious disease. The GP also has an ethical responsibility to consider the effect of the diagnosis on others. Liaison is essential between the GP and infection control teams when outbreaks are suspected within the home. Under the Control of Disease Act (1984), the GP is responsible for the formal notification to the CCDC of any resident suffering from a notifiable disease (see Chapter 3 on Public Health).

Environmental Health Officer (EHO)

EHOs are responsible for the inspection of food premises as well as the enforcement of the Food Safety Act 1990, and are employed by the local authority. They investigate complaints, advise on kitchen design, waste disposal and pest control, and collaborate with the CCDC investigating outbreaks of food- or water-borne disease.

Nursing and care homes are classed as food businesses, and the environmental health officer has the power to enter and inspect food premises at all reasonable hours under the Public Health (Control of Disease) Act 1984 (HMSO 1984).

Each local area will have their own arrangements for nursing and residential homes, which should contain a guide to include the following:

- food safety law
- food hygiene inspections
- hazard analysis

- critical points in purchasing, handling, storage, preparation, cooking, cooling and reheating
- design and structure of premises
- people and training, hygiene and illness
- general practices
- cleaning and disinfection
- pest control.

The Food Standards Agency has produced a booklet as a guide to food hazards for businesses (HMSO 2000). Figure 8.1 shows a sample local authority questionnaire to food business managers. If concerns arise following completion of this questionnaire, the nursing home manager should discuss them with the local environmental health department.

Staff

All staff should take reasonable steps to protect residents and themselves from infections acquired in residential and nursing homes (DoH 1996). This applies to day, night and agency staff.

A nominated senior nurse or another responsible individual can be nominated as an infection control liaison/link person. These nominated individuals can undertake training in order to be able to raise infection control awareness amongst staff and residents, identify problems and seek advice from the community infection control nurse or others.

ENVIRONMENT/FACILITIES

It is desirable that the residential or nursing home is non-clinical, thus ensuring that the environment is as near to a resident's expectation of a home from home that can be achieved safely. However, this needs to be balanced with the requirement to maintain an environment which is capable of being adequately cleaned and otherwise maintained in order to reduce the risk of cross infection.

Floors/surfaces

Non-carpeted areas must be covered with a surface that meets the needs of the residents and

---

How Does Your Food Business Measure Up?

Answer each question by ticking yes or no, then see the guide below to find out how well you are doing.

1. Have all the food safety hazards in your business been identified?	Yes/No
2. Are control measures in place for all the food safety hazards?	Yes/No
3. Are the floors, walls, ceilings and woodwork clean, in good condition and easy to keep clean?	Yes/No
4. Are the working surfaces clean, smooth, non-absorbent and without cracks or crevices?	Yes/No
5. Are there sufficient sinks and wash basins and can they be easily accessed by food handlers?	Yes/No
6. Is all raw food stored and handled in separate areas to other food?	Yes/No
7. As far as possible, is all perishable food kept either refrigerated or hot?	Yes/No
8. Are refrigerators and chillers checked regularly to ensure that they are operating below 5°C and are records of the checks kept?	Yes/No
9. Are the premises cleaned and disinfected (using approved materials) regularly, in accordance with a laid down plan?	Yes/No
10. Is food waste and other refuse stored hygienically and removed frequently and are all refuse containers kept clean?	Yes/No
11. Is there good lighting and ventilation in all parts of the premises?	Yes/No
12. Do all food handlers wear clean overclothing which is changed when necessary?	Yes/No
13. Do all food handlers always practice good personal hygiene and wash their hands frequently?	Yes/No
14. Have food handlers been given adequate training in food hygiene and are they properly supervised?	Yes/No

How many Yes answers did you score?

>10   You're doing all right, but don't be complacent – standards must not be allowed to fall.

8–10   You have a fair bit of work to do, but you have made a start.

≤7   You have big problems! Immediate action is necessary to get your business into shape.

Figure 8.1   A sample local authority questionnaire to food business managers. Reproduced by kind permission of Department of Housing and Environmental Health Services, Leeds City Council.

staff from an aesthetic as well as a health and safety perspective. The surface should be non-porous, and facilitate effective regular cleaning and disinfection. Non-carpeted areas should also be in place where there is a likelihood of spillage of blood/body substances, to facilitate effective cleaning. Non-carpeted rooms are desirable when the resident is suffering from diarrhoea and vomiting. Though a carpeted single room may be preferred, it is worthwhile ensuring that the carpets chosen facilitate regular steam cleaning and disinfection. They should have a waterproof backing, joints should be sealed, and pile fibres should preferably be water-repellent and non-absorbent (Ayliffe et al 2000).

Soft furnishings

Soft furnishing, for example chairs, should preferably be made of impervious or water-repellent surfaces to avoid harbourage of dust and dirt and to facilitate effective cleaning.

Wash hand basins

All residents' rooms and rooms where clinical care is carried out should be equipped with wash hand basins. The basin should be equipped with:

- mixer taps
- liquid soap in a dispenser
- disposable paper hand towels in a dispenser.

There should be a splashback at the wash hand basin to protect the surface, and a foot-operated waste bin. These facilities are regarded as clinical hand washing and should be separate from general facilities such as wash basins located in vanity units or in adjacent bath or shower rooms. Cleaning of the wash hand basins should take place at least once daily.

Bathrooms and showers

It is desirable that bath and shower rooms are located en-suite or adjacent to the residents' rooms.

Baths and showers must be cleaned after each use with a cream cleanser. (Daily routine cleaning with a detergent-based cleaner is usually all that is required.) A non-abrasive chlorine-releasing powder can be used for cleaning following use by a resident suffering from an infection or who has an antibiotic resistance problem (such as methicillin-resistant *Staphylococcus aureus*). The water supply must comply with relevant guidance and be properly maintained to ensure prevention of *Legionella pneumophila* which can affect the elderly vulnerable group (NHS Estates 1993).

Shower and bath equipment should be made of materials that meet the needs of the residents and have surfaces that facilitate effective cleaning.

Toilets

Toilets, toilet seats, fixtures and fittings must be cleaned daily and when visibly soiled. Toilet seats must be dried following cleaning. Colour-coded disposable cloths are recommended for cleaning. Toilet brushes should be rinsed well in the flushing water of the lavatory pan. Excess water should be shaken off and the brush stored dry (Ayliffe et al 2000).

A chlorine-releasing agent may be required for cleaning all surfaces if there is gross contamination or if a resident with a diagnosed gastrointestinal infection has used the toilet. If a resident has a diagnosed gastrointestinal infection, dedicating a toilet for their use alone or the use of their own commode is advisable. Pouring disinfectant into the toilet pan is unlikely to reduce infection risks (Ayliffe et al 2000).

Commodes

Commodes must be cleaned daily using a detergent-based cleaner. If visibly soiled the commode must be disinfected using a chlorine-releasing agent. It is desirable that commodes are allocated to individual residents. Where this is not possible, commodes must be cleaned in between each and every use. When cleaning takes place, staff should wear a disposable plastic apron and disposable gloves which must be discarded following use; then hands must be washed thoroughly.

Commode pans are either disposable or re-usable. The disposable type are disposed of after use via a macerator, and re-usable pans are processed using a washer disinfector specifically designed for the purpose. The washer disinfector rinse cycle must reach 80°C and hold at that temperature for one minute. This process is known as pasteurization and is used for equipment in a medium risk category (see Chapter 5), but cannot be used to sterilize (Wilson 2001).

After use of a commode, residents must be offered hand washing facilities and social cleaning of the external meatus should be undertaken when a urinary catheter is in situ.

Sluices

Sluices in residential and nursing care homes should be of sufficient size to allow for working space. Where the home is on more than one level, a sluice should be sited on each floor. This prevents body substances being transported over distances in commode pans and other containers, and prevents spillage. Sluices should be sited as close to the rooms as possible. Sufficient space should be available for the washer disinfector/macerator, shelving for equipment, waste bins and a wash hand basin. Flooring and surfaces should be easy to clean and impervious to blood and body substances.

Laundry rooms

The following points should be considered when setting up a laundry in the home:

- type of linen to be laundered
- amount of items to be laundered
- ventilation generally, and additionally for the tumble dryer
- shelving for individual containers for residents' clothing
- space for wash hand basin with liquid soap and disposable paper hand towels
- waste bins with foot pedals and lids
- adequate space and separate areas for soiled and foul linen
- first aid box
- area for ironing.

Basements are sometimes used as the laundry area, but care must be taken to ensure that adequate ventilation is available in the interests of health and safety for the laundry worker.

There must be clear separation of soiled and contaminated linen and clean, washed items. Soiled, infected or foul linen should be held in specific colour-coded containers which alert the laundry worker to the type of linen being dealt with (Table 8.1).

Sluicing of linen by hand must not take place, as it poses an infection risk to the operator. Any faeces should be removed from linen in the resident's room and disposed of into the clinical waste bag in accordance with the disposal of clinical waste.

Infected and foul linen is placed in a soluble membrane plastic bag at source, which is placed directly into an outer terylene bag. This prevents the laundry worker handling foul or infected linen as the soluble membrane bag is placed directly into the washing machine after removing from the outer bag.

The laundry worker must be provided with personal protective equipment (PPE) in the form of a disposable plastic apron and household gloves when handling soiled, infected or foul linen. PPE must be removed when the linen is in the wash and prior to its removal from the machine. For health and safety purposes and infection control, access to the laundry should be restricted to staff dealing with laundry only.

Before purchasing a washing machine, ensure that it is capable of washing at the recommended temperatures (NHS Executive 1995).

NOTIFIABLE DISEASE

Cases of infectious disease either known or suspected should be notified to the CCDC. Formal notification is undertaken by the general practitioner. This function is statutory under the Public Health (Infectious Diseases) Act 1988. Non-notifiable infections or infestations should also be reported to the CCDC or the community infection control nurse. Prompt notification of infection or infestation allows monitoring, investigation and control of spread. These infections include:

- suspected influenza
- post-operative wound infections
- conjunctivitis
- sore throats
- herpes simplex (e.g. cold sores)
- herpes zoster (shingles)
- chickenpox
- scabies
- lice/fleas
- rashes of unknown origin
- diarrhoea and/or vomiting (unknown cause/more than one resident)
- infections recorded by the GP but not understood by the home
- suspected food poisoning.

Investigation of food poisoning is carried out by the environmental health department in collaboration with the CCDC. The environmental health officer has statutory powers (HMSO 1984) to enforce co-operation from the home in complying with any recommendations made following such incidents. These incidents can also include

Table 8.1 Categories of linen (Source: NHS Executive 1995)

Category	Bag colour	Description	Recommended process
Used	White linen or clear plastic	Used soiled and foul linen	Washing at 65°C for 10 min or 71°C for 3 min
Infected	Water-soluble bag placed into red outer bag	Linen from clients with certain infections or as advised by the infection control nurse	Not sorted prior to washing as per used linen
Heat-labile	Orange stripe	Fabrics which can be damaged by thermal disinfection (e.g. wool)	Wash at 40°C and add hypochlorite to the penultimate rinse

investigation and follow-up of outbreaks with water-borne infections and viral diarrhoeal outbreaks.

OUTBREAK OF INFECTION

(Chapter 3, Public Health function, is directly relevant.)

An outbreak can be defined in the following way:

- Two or more individuals suffering with the same infection and linked in some way.
- More people than expected in the home suffering from the same infection or symptoms of infection.

Action required

Action by person in charge of the care home

- Record of all the people affected (staff and residents), including name, age, diagnosis, date and time of onset of symptoms.
- Type of specimens sent to the laboratory including the date collected and sent.
- Name of the general practitioner and date the resident was seen.
- All advice associated with the control of infection is documented.
- Staff and visitors are informed of the advice as given by the CCDC and infection control nurse.

Table 8.2   Management of infection

Infection	Inform/notify	Actions
Diarrhoea and/or vomiting, viral or bacterial. May be non-infectious in origin, but should be treated as infectious until proven otherwise	General Practitioner. CCDC when more than two people affected	Action for all cases. Standard infection control precautions. Undertake risk assessment taking into account residents' continence, personal hygiene, compliance and the susceptibility of others. Contact the ICN, CCDC, and GP for help and advice on any special precautions required. Keep a daily record of residents' symptoms, including onset date and specimen date. Retain any food samples for the EHO.
Respiratory infection, bacterial or viral	GP may request sputum specimen	Standard infection control precautions. Ensure residents are vaccinated against influenza and pneumococcal disease. Single room with door shut. Universal precautions.
Skin infection and infestations	Contact GP and CICN	Standard infection control precautions. Single room may be required. Universal precautions. Avoid skin to skin contact with any lesion.
Blood-borne infections	Contact GP and inform CCDC/CICN	Standard infection control precautions. Isolate residents with sudden onset of jaundice. Universal precautions. Rule out Hepatitis A. Chronic carriage of HCV, HBV or HIV does not usually require isolation.
MRSA (methicillin-resistant *Staphylococcus aureus*) Other drug-resistant organisms	Seek advice from CICN	Standard infection control precautions. Advice based on risk assessment. Cover all wounds. Isolation not usually necessary unless on the advice of the CICN.

Other actions

Following a report of illness to the environmental health department, the home may be advised to collate information pending investigation and results, should food poisoning be the suspected cause of the outbreak. The following are required to be retained for the environmental health officer:

- Food consumed where possible
- Menus of meals consumed by residents or others from three days prior to the first resident becoming ill
- Records of staff illness.

Environmental Health Officer actions

The EHO will interview residents about the food they have consumed and discuss with food handlers to check the level of knowledge, understanding, level of training and procedures for the safe handling of food and equipment. The EHO may also inspect the kitchen area and review the process for the safe handling and cooking of food.

Home staff

When staff are suffering from diarrhoea and vomiting they must not resume work till they are free of symptoms for at least 48 hours after the diarrhoea and vomiting has ceased. This exclusion time may vary in different regions, and it is always recommended to follow local practices and advice from the CCDC and infection control teams.

Staff employed within the affected home must not work in any other home during the outbreak. Advice should be obtained from the infection control team.

Specimens of faeces will be required from affected staff and they may be excluded until the result is known, and/or until asymptomatic. The person in charge of the home must ensure that staff are issued with specimen containers supplied through the infection control team or environmental health officer. Local arrangements should be checked in regard to collection of the specimens for delivery to the laboratory.

ISOLATION OF RESIDENTS

The decision to isolate residents to control infection in a residential or nursing home setting must not be taken lightly and should always be taken after assessing the risk to the individual, other residents and staff. When isolation precautions are required they should be tailored to meet the needs of each resident rather than the application of a ritual. When isolation nursing is being considered, contact should be made with the infection control nurse (Wilson 2001).

Key points for isolation

- Isolation in nursing and residential homes should be the exception rather than the rule.
- Viral illness is the most common infection that is likely to affect people living in residential or nursing homes.
- Vaccinating individuals can prevent viral illness such as influenza. Vaccines are modified annually to ensure that current strains are included.
- Viral diarrhoea caused by rotavirus or Norwalk virus are difficult to control without adequate isolation facilities.
- Single rooms with wash hand basins and en-suite facilities should ideally be available.
- Sluices equipped with a washer/disinfector or macerator will improve the health and safety of staff and assist in controlling the spread of infection.
- Two people who have the same infection can be cared for in one room, although single rooms may still be required.
- Residents nursed in isolation should not leave their room to use another toilet, unless dedicated for their use.
- In some care homes residents may be confused and wander; therefore it may be necessary to isolate the residents who are confused away from those who are not, to reduce the risk of cross infection.
- Verbal and written explanations should be given to the resident, relative and/or carer stating why the resident is being nursed in isolation.

- Visitors of residents suffering from infection should seek permission from the person in charge before visiting.
- Advice on the appropriateness of isolating residents should always be undertaken following advice from the infection control nurse and/or the CCDC. Isolation can cause anxiety, loneliness and fear of neglect (Ayliffe et al 2000).
- Cognizance must be given to the extra time required to care for residents who are nursed in isolation.

OCCUPATIONAL HEALTH

Each residential or nursing care home should have policies in place that ensure the health and safety of staff employed within the home. These policies should consist of current health and safety legislation, for example the Statutory Instrument SI (HMSO 1992) on Personal Protective Equipment (PPE), and Care of Substances Hazardous to Health (COSHH) Regulations (Health and Safety Commission 1998). All staff should be encouraged to read policies as part of induction/on-going training.

Pre-employment health questionnaires should be completed to allow information relating to previous illness and vaccination to be recorded.

A policy must be in place for inoculation incidents. This should include clear guidance on immediate actions, recording, reporting and referral. Guidance should give advice on post-exposure prophylaxis following incidents associated with residents who are known to be suffering from a blood-borne virus infection (DoH 2001b).

Vaccination against Hepatitis B should be given to all healthcare workers who have direct contact with blood or other potentially infectious body fluids or tissues (DoH 2001b).

Policies must be in place to protect the residents from staff who are suffering from a communicable disease. Staff should adhere to the following principles:

- Diarrhoea and/or vomiting require exclusion until fully recovered. Advice should be sought from the CICN regarding exclusion and for how long.

- Report any rashes/septic lesions to the home manager.
- Infective lesions must be covered and exclusion from certain duties may be required.
- Appropriate treatment must be sought from the GP of the staff member.
- Compliance with advice, e.g. providing samples for laboratory testing.
- Staff must not work in any other home during the exclusion period.
- Report illness to the home manager/matron as soon as possible (refer to Chapter 3, Public Health function, for list of notifiable diseases).
- Staff who are pregnant and have any concerns in regard to infection should discuss the issue with the infection control nurse and/or their general practitioner. Advice can then be given accordingly.

The requirement for exclusion from work should, when necessary, be confirmed by the CCDC. This allows for assessment of the susceptibility of the residents in the home to the illness.

Managers should note that exclusion from work without pay due to a communicable disease might discourage staff from reporting illness.

STANDARD INFECTION CONTROL PRECAUTIONS (SICP)

It must always be remembered that the blood or body fluids of any individual can be a source of infection. Following standard infection control precautions is a fundamental component of safe practice. SICPs are applied by the healthcare worker to all residents when in contact with blood and body fluids. Each individual member of staff is responsible for their own personal health and safety (Centers for Disease Control 1987).

The key principles are:

- The adoption of an effective hand washing technique between tasks and between resident contact. Alcohol hand rub for hand decontamination should be provided in areas which do not have ready access to a wash hand basin or where rapid decontamination of physically clean hands (i.e. unsoiled) is required.

- Staff who have moist lesions in their hands, e.g. eczema, should where appropriate, and following advice from the CICN/GP, avoid undertaking invasive procedures, handling clinical waste or performing an aseptic technique. The lesions must be covered with an impermeable dressing to ensure the health and safety of the affected staff member and residents. In addition, wearing appropriate disposable gloves can also reduce risk.
- Direct contact with blood and body fluids should be avoided by the use of personal protective equipment (PPE) in the form of disposable latex or vinyl gloves, disposable plastic apron and eye protection, which must be disposed of as clinical waste where the risk of splashing exists.
- The use of gloves is not an alternative to effective hand washing, which should be carried out following glove removal. Disposable gloves are single use items and must be discarded after each use or procedure (ICNA 2002b).
- The care home manager/matron must ensure that supplies of personal protective equipment are provided in sufficient quantities to meet the needs of the residents and staff.
- Spillage of blood or body fluids must be cleaned up as soon as possible, as they are a potential source of infection to others.
- Clinical waste, e.g. soiled dressings, must be incinerated in accordance with local policies.
- Sharps injuries must be avoided by ensuring that comprehensive policies are in place and adhered to (Royal College of Nursing 2001).
- Medical equipment must be appropriately decontaminated and re-processed (see Chapter 5).

Notes on spillages

The use of hypochlorite on urine spills may react with the urine causing a release of chlorine vapour (DoH 1990).

Hypochlorite solution is corrosive and must be handled with extreme care. Also refer to the COSHH regulations for handling.

Box 8.1 Spillage procedure (RCN 2000)

- Cover the spill with disposable paper towels to absorb excess liquid.
- Ventilate the area, e.g. open windows, doors.
- Put on disposable gloves and apron.
- Pour hypochlorite solution over the spill and leave for several minutes.
  Strength of hypochlorite should be 10 000 ppm for blood spills.
  Chlorine-releasing powders, granules or tablets can also be used, i.e. sodium dichloroisocyanurate (NaDCC), and all solutions must be discarded on completion of the task.

Powders and granules are less messy and will absorb spills, often without the need for paper towels.

- Clear away towels from the spillage and place in a yellow waste bag.
- Wash the area using detergent and water.
- Discard all used materials into a yellow waste bag.
- Wash hands thoroughly.

The use of hypochlorite solutions on carpeted areas should be avoided. Detergent and water can be used on carpets together with regular cleaning using a steam cleaner.

Specific advice on the use of appropriate disinfectants can be obtained from the local CICN.

Spills of other body fluids can be cleaned using detergent and water following soaking up the spill using paper towels (Box 8.1).

Disposal of sharps

Sharps injury

All incidents associated with sharps must be reported to the manager/matron and documented fully. If the injury involved a resident known to be a carrier of a blood-borne virus, the injured person should report to the local accident and emergency unit where an individual risk assessment will be undertaken. Additional vaccination may be required if the sharp injury involved exposure to Hepatitis B Virus. Although there is currently no prophylaxis for Hepatitis C Virus (HCV), local policy should outline immediate management including blood sampling.

If the sharps injury resulted in possible exposure to HIV, antiviral treatment may be offered, although this treatment is not without side-effects.

Box 8.2 Safe working practices

Prior to use ensure:

- Competence in the procedure
- Use of most appropriate device
- Sharps box is correctly assembled
- Sharps box complies with BS7320 and EN Standards
- Sharps boxes are available in correct size
- Sharps boxes are available at all locations required
- Sharps box is taken to point of use and placed on a level surface or wall mounted below shoulder height
- Box is out of reach of vulnerable people

During use:

- Use needleless safety devices where appropriate
- Wear appropriate protective equipment (e.g. powder-free gloves)
- Assemble device with care
- Do *not* disassemble device unless unavoidable
- If unavoidable, use device on sharps box or forceps to remove needle
- *Do not* re-sheathe needles
- Use vacuum blood collection devices where appropriate
- Use a container to carry sharp devices – do not carry by hand
- Keep sharps box closed between use
- Use handle to carry box

After use:

- Safe disposal is the responsibility of the user
- Dispose of sharps directly into sharps box
- Fill sharps box to 'fill line' only and lock
- Label sharps box with source
- Dispose of sharps box securely as clinical waste
- Do not put box in clinical waste bag
- Waste storage areas must be lockable, pest-proof and easy to clean.

Healthcare workers are advised to become familiar with their local arrangements for obtaining post-exposure prophylaxis (PEP). This allows staff to make an informed decision as to whether they may wish to receive PEP in the case of a high-risk incident occurring.

The manager of the healthcare worker should ensure that mechanisms are in place allowing the healthcare worker to obtain PEP within two hours of receiving the injury, whether day or night. Attempts must also be made to explore the circumstances surrounding the injury, such as how, why and when. This assists in risk identification, allowing prevention strategies to be put in place, thus reducing risks of subsequent injuries.

Where staff have no access to occupational health support, blood testing should be undertaken by the general practitioner of the healthcare worker.

Managers/matrons should be aware that under RIDDOR (Reporting of Injuries, Diseases and Dangerous Occurrences Regulations 1995) employers may be required to report significant exposure to blood-borne viruses.

Waste management

Each residential and nursing care home must have a waste management policy that demonstrates to all staff employed within the residential or nursing home how waste is handled and controlled. The waste management policy should be written in conjunction with the infection control policy.

Key points

- Waste containers should have foot-operated lids.
- Waste awaiting collection must be held in locked containers when unattended.
- Waste must be collected by a licensed contractor.
- Clinical waste should be managed in accordance with current guidance – Environmental Protection Act 1991 (HMSO 1991).
- Safe management is the responsibility of the care home owner/manager.
- Safe disposal of waste is the responsibility of the user.
- Obtain advice when required from the CICN.

For categories of waste in accordance with HSAC guidance, please refer to Chapters 6 and 10.

CLINICAL PROCEDURES
Asepsis

The principles of asepsis must be observed when undertaking any clinical procedure (Box 8.3). The term aseptic technique is a collective term for the methods used to prevent microbial contamination of living tissue/fluid or sterile articles. The technique prevents contamination of susceptible sites.

Urinary catheter care

Urinary tract infection (UTI) is a major problem in nursing homes and rehabilitation centres where the elderly, debilitated and others catheterized for prolonged periods are at greater risk of acquiring recurrent UTIs and of developing the long-term

complications associated with the infection (Warren et al 1982, reprinted in Wilson 2001).

Bacteria can enter the bladder during insertion. (See also Chapter 6, Home nursing, section on urinary catheter care.)

Key principles for a urinary drainage system

- Assess each resident for the appropriateness of the drainage system.
- The catheter size should be the smallest that will facilitate free drainage.
- The balloon size should be the smallest to facilitate retention of the catheter.
- Material should be appropriate for the anticipated length of the urinary drainage (see Table 8.3).
- All components of the system must be sterile.
- Use a sampling port for obtaining specimens of urine.
- Maintaining a sterile, continuously closed urinary drainage system is central to the prevention of catheter-associated infection (DoH 2001b).
- Avoid disconnecting/introducing system parts, in order to reduce the risk of micro-organisms entering the closed system.
- Adopt an aseptic technique at weekly bag changes.
- Avoid drained urine or air bubbles re-entering the bladder by keeping the drainage bag lower

---

Box 8.3 Key principles of asepsis

- Keep the exposure of the susceptible site to a minimum (e.g. keep wounds covered)
- Ensure an appropriate hand decontamination technique prior to the procedure
- Consider the availability and use of alcohol hand rub during the procedure (Ayliffe et al 2000)
- Use sterile or non-sterile gloves depending on the nature of the susceptible site and the procedure being undertaken (ICNA 2002b)
- Protect uniform or clothing with a disposable plastic apron (RCN 2000)
- All fluids and materials must be sterile
- Sterile packs should be checked for evidence of damage or moisture penetration and that the item is sterile
- Contaminated/non-sterile items must not be placed in the sterile field
- All disposable items should be disposed of in accordance with the waste management policy
- Single use items must not be reused (Medical Devices Agency 2000)
- Reduce activity in the immediate vicinity of the area in which the procedure is to be performed

---

Table 8.3 Selection of urinary catheters (reproduced with permission from Wilson 2001)

Catheter material*	Indication	Comments
Plastic	Very short term use only; avoid if possible	Rigid material, irritates mucosa and causes trauma
Latex (thin silicone coat)	Short-term use; up to 14 days	Prone to encrustation, associated with trauma and strictures
Latex coated with Teflon	Short-term use; up to 28 days	Minimal mucosal irritation, resistant to encrustation
Latex with bonded silicone coating	Long-term use; up to 12 weeks	Minimal mucosal irritation, resistant to encrustation
Latex with hydrogel coating	Long-term use; up to 12 weeks	Minimal mucosal irritation, resistant to encrustation
All silicone	Long-term use; up to 12 weeks	Minimal mucosal irritation, but D-shaped lumen prone to encrustation

Note: examine the packaging carefully for a description of the catheter material.

than the bladder but not on the floor (Ayliffe et al 2000).

- Empty the drainage bag when full or if the resident becomes uncomfortable.
- Container for emptying should be for individual use only and decontaminated in a washer disinfector after use or washed in hot water and detergent, rinsed and dried.
- Use a plastic disposable apron and disposable gloves when emptying the drainage bag as there is an anticipated risk of contact with a body substance and possible risk of splashing (McDougall 1999).

Catheterization technique

Catheterization should only take place when alternative methods of management have been considered (DoH 2001b). Reasons for carrying out catheterization include the following:

- chronic or acute retention
- incontinence in those who are debilitated
- post-surgery
- measuring accurate output
- administration of drugs, for example cytotoxic
- irrigation of the bladder.

The type of catheter used will depend on how long urinary drainage by this route is required. Within the residential and nursing homes it is likely that long-term use will be the most common (see Table 8.3).

Insertion of a catheter

- Ensure that the resident is prepared and comfortable.
- Observe the principles of asepsis: effective hand decontamination and use of sterile gloves.
- All equipment must be sterile.
- Use soap and water or saline to clean the external meatus and perineal area.
- Use an appropriate lubricant from a sterile single-use container to minimize urethral trauma (DoH 2001b).

- Insert the catheter that has been selected.
- Use sterile water to inflate the balloon.

The catheter can be secured to the thigh, making it comfortable when in position. There is no scientific evidence to support this practice but it can prevent a telescoping effect in the urethra which may encourage migration of micro-organisms into the urethra.

When the catheterization is complete, ensure that a record is made in the care plan of the following:

- type of catheter
- size of catheter
- balloon size and amount of water in the balloon
- date and time inserted
- signature of person carrying out the procedure.

Meatal cleansing

Daily bathing/showering is sufficient as part of cleaning the meatus (Wilson 2001). Always ensure that cleaning takes place after any bowel movement/faecal incontinence to prevent contamination. Hands must be decontaminated before and after the procedure. Report and record any skin reactions or discharge around the urethral meatus.

Bladder installations

There is no evidence to suggest that this procedure contributes to the prevention of urinary tract infection. It may however be carried out in specific circumstances, such as during urological surgery and associated interventions.

Urinary sample collection

The integrity of the closed drainage system must be maintained and the principles of asepsis adhered to. The following key points should be observed:

- Indiscriminate sampling should be avoided and only carried out to meet the needs of the resident.
- Sampling must take place using the sampling port.

- A sterile syringe and small bore needle should be used. (Some systems employ the use of a needle-free sampling port, which avoids the risk of an inoculation injury.)
- Transfer the urine sample to a sterile specimen container, avoiding environmental contamination.
- Label the specimen, complete the request form and place in the dedicated plastic specimen bag for transport to the laboratory.

Catheter removal

The following key points should be observed:

- Remove the catheter as soon as the resident's condition allows.
- Use disposable non-sterile procedure gloves for the procedure.
- Deflate the catheter balloon in accordance with the manufacturer's instructions.
- Hand decontamination must be carried out after glove removal and disposal of waste.
- Monitor urinary output and document same. Normal urination should occur within six hours.

Use and care of intravenous devices

Intravenous (IV) therapy is used to administer intravenous solutions, blood products and total parenteral nutrition (TPN). The use of IV catheters is associated with complications which are both non-infectious and infectious (ICNA 2001).

It is advised that the home has policy/guidelines for the insertion of catheters and care of residents receiving IV therapy. The community infection control nurse can assist in developing procedures. Principles of asepsis must be applied for insertion of the IV catheter. All details regarding the catheter type, solutions used and date and time of insertion must be recorded in the resident's care plan.

Managing the IV site (ICNA 2001)

Daily inspection of the site is essential to ensure that the device has not become dislodged and to observe for any signs of infection (Box 8.4).

Table 8.4 Infectious and non-infectious complications

Non-infectious	Infectious
Trauma	Entry site infection
Haematoma	Tunnel infection
Thrombosis	Blood stream infection related to the catheter
Air embolism	Endocarditis

Box 8.4 Signs of infection

- Erythema
- Tracking (redness along the line of the vein)
- Oedema/swelling
- Heat
- Pain/tenderness
- Purulent drainage

If any of the above are noted, the line requires to be removed.

Other key points for IV management

- Keep number of manipulations of the system to a minimum.
- Always decontaminate hands before and after handling.
- Use of gloves dependent on local policy.
- Accurate documentation on equipment, date of insertion, site, daily observations and care carried out.

IV site dressings

The use of a dressing for the site is to prevent contamination, trauma to the site and to keep the catheter secure. The type of dressings recommended (Table 8.5 and ICNA 2001) include:

- Transparent to allow continuous visual inspection of the catheter and site.
- Self-adhesive to ensure greater stability, reduce risk of trauma, mechanical phlebitis and external contamination.
- Semi-permeable to protect from bacteria and liquid while allowing the site to 'breathe'.
- Sterile to prevent external contamination of the catheter site.

The dressing should be changed when it becomes soiled, loosened, damp or if the site is not visible.

Table 8.5 IV dressing types

Dressing	Suggested use	Comments
Sterile gauze	Short-term use (less than 24 hours)	Poor visibility of exit site and no protection from moisture Limited security
Transparent film dressing	Cannula in place for more than 24 hours	Can be expensive Semi-permeable Good security Early inspection recommended Recommended dressing type
Material adhesive dressing (sterile)	Cannula in place for more than 24 hours	Cheap Poor visibility at exit site and little protection from moisture

Table 8.6 IV administration and change times (from Wilson 2001)

Type of infusion	Change times
Clear fluids	72 hours
Total parenteral nutrition	24 hours
Lipids/blood	After each infusion
Line accessed frequently (filter recommended)	24–48 hours

Administration sets

There are different types of administration sets that may be used. This will depend on the type of fluid being administered. Table 8.6 suggests types and change times.

Parenteral nutrition

This type of feeding is employed when residents are unable to have a sufficient intake of nutrients by any other method. A central venous catheter is used for this type of administration, usually via the subclavian, femoral or jugular veins.

The central venous catheter will normally be inserted within the hospital setting in an operating theatre or similar environment. Tunnelled central venous catheters are mainly used for those requiring long-term chemotherapy or total parenteral nutrition. It is advised to record the temperature and pulse 4-hourly to detect any signs and symptoms of sepsis during administration of total parental nutrition (Wilson 2001). See Chapter 6,

and Figure 6.9, for extrinsic and intrinsic sources of infection, routes of access of contamination and related factors.

Enteral feeding

Enteral tube feeding is an increasingly common method of nutritional support. However, feeds contain nutrients which can make them a source for the growth of micro-organisms, and thus it is essential to take the necessary steps to reduce risks of contamination. Bacteria, including salmonella, Klebsiella, enterobacter, *E. coli* and *S. aureus* have been found in high concentrations in enteral feeds. These may cause gastro-enteritis and, through colonization of the gut, may result in septicaemia and pneumonia (Thurn et al 1990, Wilson 2001).

Research has clearly shown that 'poor handling' is the main cause of bacterial contamination of sterile enteral feeds (Anderton 2000).

Enteral feeding equipment

When selecting equipment the aim is to use a system with a hazard-reducing design, for example with no parts easily touched during assembly that come into contact with the feed. A delivery system that requires a minimal number of connections is recommended (Box 8.5) (Anderton 1994).

Pre-packaged, sterile, ready-to-use feeds should be used in preference to feeds requiring

---

Box 8.5 Equipment for enteral feeding

- Feed (bag, cartoon or can)
- Feeding pump
- Syringe
- Bolus giving set
- Giving set
- Bag sets for decanted feeds
- Extension tubes and sets
- Dedicated containers and utensils
- Connectors

NB: Choose a system with a minimum number of connections to reduce handling.

Box 8.6 Enteral feeding: documentation

- Type of feed
- System and device used
- Date and time commenced
- Duration of feed
- Fluids used to flush the tube and amount
- Time of feed completion
- Any adverse affects
- Time feed stored in refrigerator (if appropriate)

---

reconstitution, dilution or additions (Aidoo and Anderton 1990).

Equipment labelled with the symbol for single use (Fig. 6.11) indicates that the device is intended to be used once, then discarded (MDA 2000).

Some syringes currently used for bolus feeding are designed for reuse, but it is important to check that they are specifically recommended for the purpose for which they are used.

Always follow the manufacturer's instructions for decontamination and ensure also that a policy is in place locally for all staff.

Preparation – key points

- Store the feed as per the manufacturer's instructions.
- Always check the expiry dates of the feeds.
- Use pre-filled containers to reduce handling.
- Do not decant feeds unless no other system is suitable or available.
- Powdered modular feeds must be mixed using utensils which have been disinfected in a dish-washer. Alternatively they may be thoroughly washed and dried, using paper towels, and designated for this use only.
- Sterile water is the preferred option for mixing feeds and is *essential* for immunocompromized patients (ICNA 2002a). Alternatively, cool boiled water may be used and can be stored, covered, in the refrigerator to be used within 24 hours.
- Before opening, the outside surface of bottles, cans or cartons should be thoroughly disinfected using 70% isopropyl alcohol (Anderton 1995).

- Use full-strength formulas which avoid adding water, medication or other substances directly into the feed container.

Administration – key points

- All persons dealing with enteral feeds should be suitably trained/educated in all aspects of enteral feeding and the systems in use. Records should be kept of training.
- Hands must be thoroughly washed and dried prior to preparing and administering feeds.
- Avoid touching any inner surfaces of the equipment.
- Adopt a 'non touch' technique when preparing a feed, priming and connecting the administration set to the feeding tube.
- Protective clothing such as plastic aprons and disposable gloves are not required unless splashing of blood/body fluids is anticipated.
- When setting up feeds always ensure that the feed is labelled with the resident's name, date and time of the feed.
- Document information in the resident's care plan (Box 8.6).
- Discard single-use equipment after use.

Drug administration via the enteral route

The tube must be flushed with water before and after administration of medicines:

- Thoroughly decontaminate hands before and after handling.
- Use sterile or cool boiled water.
- Use a separate syringe to flush the system.

Aqueous solutions are preferable to elixirs and crushed tablets as they may adhere to the wall of the tube and result in blockage that will encourage bacterial growth. When elixirs are required to be used, dilute with the same volume of cool boiled or sterile water. If more than one drug is being administered, flush with 5–10 ml of water between each drug bolus.

Hanging times of feeds

Once a feed is opened but not connected to a sterile giving set it should be treated as a non-sterile feed and the hangtime limited to 4 hours. Where possible, use feeds which are ready to hang, thus avoiding decanting. If decanting is necessary it must be undertaken in a clean environment using an aseptic technique, and hangtime limited to 12 hours (Payne-James 1991). A recent publication states a hangtime of 24 hours (ICNA 2002a), but local risk assessment may reduce this time.

Modified or mixed feeds have a maximum hangtime of 4 hours (ICNA 2002a).

Gastrostomy site care

The site should be kept clean and dry. Any discharge from the site can be removed using sterile normal saline and an aseptic technique. A loose key-hole absorbent dressing can be applied if required.

Signs of infection around the site must be reported and documented. A swab for culture should be taken and sent for testing, and the result will indicate if antibiotic treatment is required.

Wound management

The care and management of wounds is fully discussed in Chapter 14.

Within the nursing and residential home setting it is essential that guidelines be in place for managing wounds. Many residential and nursing homes will have access to the services of a tissue viability nurse specialist in the community. This nurse can be contacted to provide advice on all aspects of wound care.

The types of wounds being managed in the care home setting include:

- venous and arterial ulcers
- pressure-related wounds
- traumatic wounds (e.g. following a fall)
- post-operation following discharge from hospital.

Following audit conducted in nursing homes during 1996 to 1998, 72 standards were devised, one of which stated 'there is evidence that staff are aware of the infection risks associated with the management of wounds' (PHLS 2000).

Staff should also be suitably trained/educated to enable effective wound management to take place.

REFERENCES

Aidoo K E, Anderton A 1990 Decanting – a source of contamination of enteral feeds? Clinical Nutrition 9: 157–162

Anderton A 1994 What is the HACCP (hazard analysis critical control point) approach and how can it be applied to enteral tube feeding? Journal of Human Nutritional Diet 7: 53–60

Anderton A 1995 Reducing bacterial contamination in enteral tube feeds. British Journal of Nursing 4: 368–377

Anderton A 2000 Microbial contamination of enteral tube feeds: How can we reduce the risk? Nutricia Clinical Care, Trowbridge

Ayliffe G A J, Fraise A P, Geddes A M, Mitchell K 2000 Control of Hospital Infection: A Practical Handbook, 4th edn. Arnold, London

Centers for Disease Control 1987 Recommendations for the prevention of HIV transmission in healthcare settings. Morbidity and Mortality Weekly Report 36: 2S

Department of Health 1988 Public Health Infectious Diseases Regulations 1988. HMSO, London

Department of Health 1990 Spills of Urine: Potential Misuse of Chlorine-releasing Disinfecting Agents. SAB59 (90) 41. Medical Devices Agency. DoH, London

Department of Health 1996 Guidelines on the Control of Infection in Residential and Nursing Homes. Public Health Medicine Environmental Group (PHMEG), London

Department of Health 1997 Guidance on Post-exposure Prophylaxis for Health care Workers Occupationally Exposed to HIV. PL/CO(97)1. DoH, London

Department of Health 2001a Caring for Older People: a Nursing Priority. Integrating knowledge, practice and values. Standing Nursing Midwifery Advisory Committee (SNMAC). DoH, London

Department of Health 2001b The *epic* Project: Developing National Evidence-based Guidelines for Preventing Healthcare Associated Infections. Journal of Hospital Infection 47(Suppl.)

Department of Health 2002 Shifting the Balance of Power: the Next Steps. DoH, London

Health and Safety Commission 1998 Control of Substances Hazardous to Health Regulations. HSE Books, Sudbury

Health and Safety Commission Health Services Advisory Committee 1999 Safe Disposal of Clinical Waste. HSE Books, Sudbury

Health and Safety Executive 1998 The Reporting of Injuries, Diseases and Dangerous Occurrences Regulations 1995: Guidance for employers in the healthcare sector. HSF Information Sheet No. 1 4/98. HSE Books, Sudbury

HMSO 1974 The Health and Safety Act (1974). HMSO, London

HMSO 1984 The Public Health (Control of Diseases) Act (1984). HMSO, London

HMSO 1988 The Public Health (Infectious Diseases) Regulations (1988). HMSO, London

HMSO 1990 The Food Safety Act (1990). HMSO, London

HMSO 1991 The Environmental Protection Act (1991). HMSO, London

HMSO 1992 Statutory Instrument on Personal Protective Equipment. HMSO, London

HMSO 1998 The Food Standards Agency. A Force for Change. HMSO, London

HMSO 2000 The Food Standards Agency. A Guide to Food Hazards and Your Business. HMSO, London

Infection Control Nurses' Association 2001 Guidelines for Preventing Intravascular Catheter-related Infection. ISBN 09-515-62053. ICNA, Bathgate

Infection Control Nurses Association 2002a Enteral Feeding Guidelines (in press). ICNA, Bathgate

Infection Control Nurses Association 2002b Glove Usage Guidelines. ICNA, Bathgate

McDougall C 1999 A clean sheet. Nursing Times 95(Suppl.): 28

Medical Devices Agency 2000 Single-use Medical Devices: Implications and Consequences of Reuse. MDA DB2000(04). Department of Health, London

NHS Estates 1993 The Control of Legionella in Healthcare Premises – A Code of Practice. Health Technical Memorandum 240. HMSO, London

NHS Executive 1995 Hospital Laundry Arrangements for Used and Infected Linen. HSG(95)18. HMSO, London

Nicolle L E, Strausaugh L J, Garibaldi R A 1996 Clinical microbiology reviews 9(1): 1–17. American Society for Microbiology, Washington DC

Office of Population, Censuses and Surveys 1991 Census. HMSO, London

Payne-James J J 1991 Enteral nutrition and the critically ill: infection risk minimization. British Journal of Intensive Care Sept/Oct, 135–141

Public Health Laboratory Service (PHLS) 2000 Audit of Infection Control Practice in Nursing Homes 1996–1998. PHLS, London

Royal College of Nursing 2000 Universal Precautions (poster). RCN, London

Royal College of Nursing 2001 Be sharp – be safe! Avoiding the risk. RCN, London

Thurn J, Crossley K, Gerdts A 1990 Enteral hyperalimentation as a source of nosocomial infection. Journal of Hospital Infection 15: 203–218

Warren J W, Tenney J H, Hoopes J M, Muncie H L 1982 A prospective microbiological study of bacteriuria in patients with chronic indwelling urethral catheters. Journal of Infection and Disinfection 146: 719–723

Wilson J 2001 Infection Control in Clinical Practice, 2nd edn. Baillière Tindall, London

FURTHER READING

Department of Health 2000 Care Standards Act 2000. HMSO, London

Department of Health 2002 Care Homes for Older People. National Minimum Standards. HMSO, London

9

General practice

D. Khan

INTRODUCTION

General practice is often the first contact the public has with the health service, with over 750 000 consultations with healthcare staff occurring every day (Morgan et al 1990). The risk of infection being transmitted within the general practice environment is related to the large numbers of people using the facilities, sharing equipment and their contact with each other and staff. More recently the increase in investigations and invasive procedures, including minor surgery, has added to the risk.

A number of people attending the surgery will be at particular risk of acquiring infection. These include patients who are immunocompromised by way of disease or drug therapy, the very old and the very young and those with chronic debilitating conditions such as diabetes. Staff are also at risk, including those non-immune to childhood infectious diseases or Hepatitis B virus.

Some patients may be a risk to others if they are incubating or showing signs and symptoms of infection. These patients may well not be aware that they have obvious signs of infection when they attend surgery. Finally, patients may be asymptomatic. These patients, for example those with blood-borne viruses, may pose a particular risk if routine infection control procedures are not in place.

Infection may be spread directly from person to person, mainly from the hands of staff. Infection may also be spread indirectly through contact with contaminated equipment, or less commonly by a contaminated environment. Invasive procedures such as minor surgery breach the body's defence systems exposing the patient to a risk of infection as well as the operator to potential contamination with blood and body fluids. Airborne transmission of viruses via coughs and sneezes is an important route of spread of viral infections, especially in crowded surgeries.

INCIDENCE OF INFECTION WITHIN GENERAL PRACTICE

Incidence and prevalence rates of infections acquired whilst in hospital are well documented (Emmerson et al 1996). At present there is limited data available on incidents of infection within the general practice setting particularly related to wound infections from minor surgery. This is thought to be attributed to infections mainly going unnoticed and not being reported (BMA 1989). However, outbreaks of infection have occurred in settings with similarities to general practice, highlighting the potential risk. An outbreak of Hepatitis B virus occurred in a dermatology clinic where fifty patients developed the infection (Hlady et al 1993). Investigations showed areas where inadequate infection control practices and procedures were followed. These included the use of a contaminated electrocautery tip and repeated use of a cotton bud for application of liquid nitrogen, repeated use of vials of local anaesthetic and failure to wear gloves or wash hands during procedures. All of these were thought to have contributed to the outbreak.

Similarly, four patients were thought to have been infected with the Human Immunodeficiency Virus (HIV) following operations from a single minor surgical operation list in Australia (Chant et al 1993). All the patients had minor operations performed after the suspected index case. Attributing factors were believed to have been inadequate decontamination of instruments and lack of nursing support for the doctor performing the surgery.

Theoretical risks of infection have also been highlighted in relation to patient examinations. These include risks from vaginal specula where human papillomavirus (HPV), the cause of cervical dysplasia, could be transmitted if not decontaminated adequately after use (BMA General Medical Services Committee 1994). One study of auriscopes found over a third were contaminated with bacteria (Overend et al 1992).

PRACTICE SETTINGS AND STAFF

Practice design

The design of any healthcare setting is crucial in preventing the potential for cross infection (Ayliffe et al 2000). General practice often has the advantages of premises being purpose built, but also the disadvantage of some practices being housed in older buildings not designed for that purpose.

It is important to consult the Infection Control team at an early stage, whenever refitting, refurbishment or major capital bids are planned (NHS Estates 2001a).

All the rooms should be well ventilated and well lit. The size of the doctors' room, nurses' room and other clinical rooms should all be large enough to allow staff and patients to move freely without bumping into couches, trolleys and equipment. The walls and ceiling should all be painted with a product that can be easily washed and disinfected if contaminated. Flooring should have a washable covering such as non-slip sheet vinyl, coved to the edges. Carpet should be avoided as it is not easily cleaned and should not be used in clinical areas. Work surface should be seamless and washable, and should allow enough space for separate areas of clerical and clinical work such as preparation of equipment. Storage of equipment should be in washable cupboards to avoid contamination by dust and splashing.

Hand wash sinks should be available in all rooms. These should be separate from sinks for cleaning instruments and should be large enough to physically wash hands with elbow-operated taps.

A 'dirty' room should be available for cleaning and decontaminating equipment and for disposal and storage of general equipment, clinical waste and used linen. This should have a large deep sink suitable for washing equipment, a separate hand wash sink, and washable storage space. No clean or sterile equipment should be stored here.

Segregation of patients waiting to see the doctor should be possible for those with known or suspected infections such as chickenpox. Preferably a designated room not occupied during surgery time should be used. Within the waiting room a procedure should be in place to deal with body fluid spillage such as vomit. Staff responsible for dealing with the incident should be aware of the correct procedure.

Multi-use rooms

As space is limited within the practice environment, maximum use of rooms usually occurs. For example, a room may be used for minor surgery, chiropody and ulcer and other wound dressings. Multi-use of rooms leads to many problems. Cleaning of the rooms between each use is generally not feasible and could lead to heavily contaminated rooms, creating infection risks especially if minor surgery is to follow. Cleaning of contaminated equipment might not be possible due to lack of facilities. Storage space needs to be found for specialized equipment for occasional clinics, and may lead to inadequate decontamination of equipment if additional supplies are not available. Clinics may alternatively be held in rooms where inadequate facilities exist, such as no hand wash sink or where cleaning facilities are positioned well away from the room.

When planning specialized clinics in general rooms, adequate provision for cleaning the rooms after use, storage of specialized equipment and additional facilities need to be taken into account. Careful planning and management of room usage is also needed to ensure that the patient is not put at additional risk of infection by having dirty procedures followed by clean or surgical procedures – for example, removing sutures from a clean surgical wound following the dressing of a leg ulcer wound known to be colonized with bacteria.

Other premises

The use of general practice sites other than the main surgery, such as branch surgeries and out-of-hours co-operatives and primary care centres, is also required to follow local infection control policies and procedures.

BASIC PRINCIPLES IN INFECTION CONTROL

General infection control principles have changed very little over the years, even with changes in disease patterns and new infections emerging. Principles are based on the use of practices and procedures that prevent or reduce the likelihood of infection being transmitted from a source, such as a person, contaminated body fluid or equipment (UK Departments of Health 1998).

Since it is impossible to identify most infected patients – especially those with HIV or Hepatitis B – a system of standard (universal) infection control precautions has been adopted in healthcare world-wide, and these apply equally in general practice. These principles are designed to protect healthcare staff from infection, for instance as a result of a needlestick injury, and also to protect the patient from potential cross infection.

The following summarizes the principles forming the basis of standard (universal) infection control precautions:

- Apply appropriate basic hand hygiene practices with regular hand decontamination.
- Avoid contamination of self and clothing by appropriate use of protective clothing.
- Protect open wounds and skin lesions with waterproof coverings.
- Dispose of clinical waste and sharps safely.
- Prevent inoculation injury to yourself and others.
- Use approved procedures for cleaning, disinfection and sterilization of equipment.
- Apply effective basic environmental cleaning procedures.
- Clean up blood and body fluid spillage promptly.
- Ensure all staff are aware of, understand, and adhere to infection control policies and procedures.

Hand decontamination

As other chapters have pointed out, hand washing is the single most important means of preventing the spread of infection (Reybrouck 1986). Hands become contaminated with a wide variety of organisms, which are acquired by everyday activities including handling and touching people, contact with secretions and excretions, contaminated equipment and the environment. Effective hand decontamination removes these transient organisms, thus preventing their transmission to others. Hands can be decontaminated using warm water and a liquid soap solution. Alternatively, visibly clean hands can be decontaminated using an alcohol-based solution.

Within the practice environment **each clinical area should have**:

- an accessible sink separate from sinks used for cleaning equipment
- elbow-operated taps
- liquid soap in a dispenser
- disposable paper towels in a dispenser
- a poster demonstrating the correct procedure

- antimicrobial soap for invasive procedures/minor surgery
- alcohol hand rub/gel/wipes.

The sink should be designated for hand washing only, and should not be used for cleaning equipment, disposing of specimens or for making tea and coffee.

Nails should be kept short and clean, and no jewellery should be worn other than a wedding ring. Nailbrushes should not be used, as these become contaminated (Ayliffe et al 2000). If it is necessary to use a nailbrush, particularly before clinical procedures, then these should be sterile single use only and disposed of after application. Comprehensive guidance on hand decontamination is available (ICNA 2002a).

Drying of hands

The drying of hands is also an essential part of hand washing (Gould 1994). Washing hands effectively will remove large numbers of transient organisms but drying them thoroughly afterwards will continue to remove more. The best way to dry hands is by the use of disposable paper towels or hand dryers. However, in the clinical setting hand dryers are not recommended (Ansari et al 1991). The use of cotton hand towels is also not recommended as these become heavily contaminated during use and remain moist. Even if a good standard of hand washing is achieved, the use of a cotton towel will only replace organisms on the hand from the towel, not reduce them. Audits into infection control standards within general practice have shown that effective hand washing and drying is often not achieved. This is mainly due to a lack of facilities and the use of cotton hand towels (Dawson et al 1995, Finn and McCulloch 1996).

Protective clothing

All members of staff should wear appropriate protective clothing at work and there should be plenty of readily accessible supplies (Health and Safety Executive 1992).

Employers have a duty to provide:

- Non-sterile, powder-free, disposable gloves, e.g. latex or vinyl

- Sterile, powder-free, latex surgeons' gloves (variety of sizes)
- Low allergenic and latex-free gloves (e.g. nitrile) for those with correctly diagnosed latex allergy
- General household gloves for cleaning of equipment
- Single use, disposable plastic aprons
- Plastic protective goggles, spectacles or face visors.

Gloves

In general there are three distinct reasons for wearing gloves (ICNA 2002b):

- To protect the hands from becoming contaminated with organic matter and micro-organisms

- To protect the hands from certain chemicals that will adversely affect the skin condition of the user
- To minimize cross infection by preventing the transfer of micro-organisms from staff to patients and vice versa.

Glove choices (ICNA Guidelines 2002b)

Figures 9.1 and 9.2 illustrate reasons for the choice from a variety of alternatives. Gloves should always be changed between patients, and hands washed even though gloves have been worn. Gloves are an addition to, not a substitute for, hand washing. Gloves should not be washed or disinfected for reuse. Examination (procedure

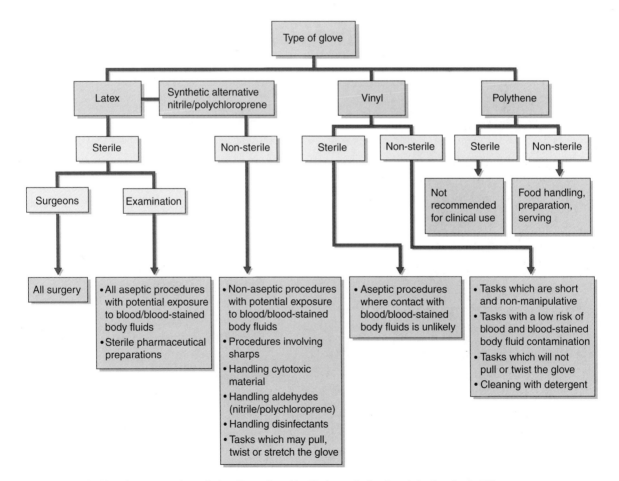

Figure 9.1 Making the correct glove choice. Reproduced by kind permission from Infection Control Nurses Association 2002b.

TASK EXAMPLES	TYPE OF GLOVE								
	Sterile				Non-sterile				
	1	2	3	4	5	6	7	8	9
All surgical procedures	◯	⊘							
Sterile pharmaceutical preparations Aseptic invasive procedures with potential exposure to blood/blood-stained body fluids			◯	⊘					
Personal protection from potential exposure to blood/blood-stained body fluids					◯	⊘			
Administration of cytotoxic drugs/chemicals					◯	⊘			
Aseptic procedures with low risk of contamination							⊘		
Low risk of contamination Non-invasive clinical care Environmental cleaning								⊘	
Food handling/preparation/serving									⊘

1. Surgeons' gloves sterile latex or combination latex/hydrogel

2. Surgeons' gloves sterile synthetic

3. Examination gloves sterile latex

4. Examination gloves sterile synthetic

5. Examination gloves non-sterile latex

6. Examination gloves non-sterile synthetic

7. Procedure gloves sterile vinyl (PVC)

8. Procedure gloves non-sterile vinyl (PVC)

9. Polythene glove (non-sterile plastic)

◯ Latex

⊘ Synthetic

All gloves should be powder-free and have the lowest levels possible of extractable proteins and chemical accelerators

Figure 9.2 Making the correct glove choice for a particular task. Reproduced by kind permission from Infection Control Nurses Association 2002b.

gloves) and surgeons' gloves are manufactured as single use items and must not be reused (MDA 2000).

After direct contact with a patient's secretions or excretions, if treatment of the client has not been completed, gloves should still be changed. Care should be taken not to contaminate articles such as notes, surfaces and telephones if the gloves have become soiled.

General purpose gloves, such as household rubber gloves, should be used for cleaning used instruments after use and prior to sterilization or when coming into contact with contaminated surfaces or items. These gloves may be reused but should be washed whilst on the hands with detergent and warm water and hung to dry. These gloves should be discarded if punctured or torn, or if there is evidence of deterioration.

Protective aprons

Plastic aprons are indicated for use when treating patients if clothes are likely to be contaminated with secretions or excretions, or when performing minor surgery, to protect the patient from potential cross infection. Aprons should be single use and disposed of when treatment has been completed.

Face protection

Masks are generally ineffective against airborne infection, but they may offer protection against potential dust and splashing of the mouth and face during certain procedures such as minor surgery and nail drilling. Face visors, goggles or spectacles are recommended when there is a risk of splashing body fluids onto the face, for example when cleaning instruments. These can be washed with general-purpose detergent, rinsed and dried after each use unless they are designated for single use only.

Clinical waste

Waste categories

Disposal of waste is governed by the Environmental Protection Act (duty of care) Regulations (1991). Within healthcare settings the Health and Safety Commission (1999) give guidance on waste management. Waste is divided into categories as set out in Box 9.1.

Other items of waste which are generated include:

- **General waste**: This includes waste from offices (inclusive of hearing-aid and other batteries), kitchens, residential accommodation, paper and small amounts of waste food. Dispose of in black plastic bags.
- **Aerosols, glassware and cans**: These items should be placed in a rigid container such as a specific cardboard container. Aerosols must not be placed in clinical waste sacks for incineration, as they may cause explosion.
- **Cytotoxic waste**: This includes any residue in sharps, swabs, syringes, gloves, containers, infusion sets, tubing, filters, disposable sheets, drapes and any item that comes in contact with the administration process. The waste must be disposed of in a specifically designated container for cytotoxic waste. Collection is required as soon as possible and a consignment note must accompany the waste when being collected by the disposal agent.
- **Pharmaceutical waste**: This includes waste products such as out-of-date medicines and is classified as Special Waste (HSC 1999). It also includes anaesthetic gases, anaesthetic cartridges not fully discharged, aerosol containers not fully discharged, vaccines out of date, and not fully discharged vaccines. They are disposed of by placing in a sharps container labelled 'Special Waste' and arrangements must be in place with the disposal agent in conjunction with the community pharmacy.

Box 9.1 Clinical waste: categories (HSC 1999)

- **Group A** includes identifiable human tissue, blood, animal carcasses and tissue from veterinary clinics, hospitals or laboratories; soiled surgical dressings, swabs and other similar soiled waste; other waste materials, for example from infectious disease cases, excluding any in category B or E.
- **Group B** includes discarded syringe needles, cartridges, broken glass and any other contaminated disposable sharp instrument or item.
- **Group C** includes microbiological cultures and potentially infected waste from pathology departments and other clinical or research laboratories.
- **Group D** includes drugs or other pharmaceutical products.
- **Group E** includes items used to dispose of urine, faeces and other bodily secretions or excretions which do not fall within group A. This includes used disposable bed pans or bed pan liners, incontinence pads, stoma bags and urine containers.

Clinical waste bags

All clinical waste should be placed in yellow clinical waste bags. Each bag should be no more than two thirds full, securely fastened with tape or grips and labelled to identify source. The bag should be clearly labelled with the surgery name and if the surgery is part of a clinic or houses more than one surgery in a building then the particular surgery name should be used. This will enable any problems identified with waste to be traced back to the actual generator of the waste.

Clinical waste bins

Clinical waste bins should be easily accessible in dirty areas, clinical rooms and treatment rooms where clinical waste is generated. The clinical waste bags should be placed in sack holders or bins suitable for the size of the bag, the bin should be clearly identified to indicate its contents, be fitted with a close-fitting lid and be foot-operational. This will allow the safe disposal of waste without contamination of the individual's hands and the bin lid. During certain clinics, additional waste bins may be needed and placed closer to the patient having treatment.

Clinical waste storage

Storage of waste can lead to particular problems in general practice. There is often limited storage space and waste has been left in alleyways or at the back of the premises (Dawson et al 1995). The clinical waste storage area should be a designated area that is separate from domestic refuse to avoid any mix-up of waste leading to incorrect disposal. It should be locked and inaccessible to animals, vermin and unauthorized persons and free from infestations.

Clinical waste disposal

Disposal of waste should take place at least weekly and the practice should ensure that the waste is transferred to an authorized person, that a description of the waste is produced, and that the carriers of the waste hold the appropriate registration and licence to dispose of the waste. Clinical waste produced at the surgery should be disposed of by incineration only (HSAC 1999).

Sharps management

A 'sharp' is defined as any object which can pierce or puncture the skin and which is potentially contaminated with blood or body fluids. Sharps injuries pose a real risk to health, particularly from blood-borne virus transmission such as Hepatitis B and C viruses, HIV, etc.

Sharps injuries are most likely to occur during and after use, or during and after disposal. Examples of these include the following:

- During use, injuries occur whilst detaching needle from syringe; during cannulation;

emergency care such as resuscitation, and lack of concentration. In addition a restless, frightened patient may be the cause of the injury.
- After sharps use injury can occur when re-sheathing the needle, transporting the sharp to a container, leaving sharps on a surface or to be disposed of by someone else, especially untrained staff such as reception staff. Injury can also occur from overfilled sharps containers and any devices that require disassembling prior to disposal.
- Injury can occur as a result of careless disposal, e.g. overfilling of the sharps container. Easily accessible and 'attractive' sharps containers have caused injury to children. Careful positioning of the sharps container is required, and storage on narrow windowsills can lead to containers being knocked off.

To avoid sharps injury the following practices should be observed:

- Never re-sheathe a needle manually. Where re-sheathing is unavoidable a re-sheathing device or single handed method should be used (UK Departments of Health 1998).
- Dispose of needle and syringe as one unit into a specific sharps container. If needles require separation from a syringe, e.g. when using non-disposable syringes for local anaesthesia, then use the needle-removing device on the sharps container.
- Sharps, needles and syringes must be placed into the sharps container by the person who used them.
- Blades should not be fixed to the handle until or unless they are to be used as part of the treatment.
- **Never leave sharps to be disposed of by someone else**.
- Sharps containers should be disposed of when no more than three-quarters full.
- ALL sharps must be disposed of by incineration.
- Sharps containers should comply with the British Standard BS3720 (1990) and European standard EN 3291 (1998).
- Sharps boxes must be securely assembled prior to use according to the manufacturer's instructions.

- Sharps boxes must not be placed into yellow bags prior to disposal.
- Sharps boxes must be labelled with their source prior to disposal.
- Sharps boxes in use should be positioned out of reach of patients, especially children, but close at hand when procedures are being performed.
- Portable sharps boxes designed for community use are readily available and should be used by all staff who generate sharps outside of the practice building.
- Ideally, sharps boxes in use (and where accessible by children) should be closed between use to deter/discourage inappropriate handling.

Inoculation injuries

Each practice should have a written policy on the prevention and management of inoculation injuries including exposure to blood and body fluids. Staff should follow the above practices at all times to minimize the risk of injury.

In the event of an injury occurring:

- Dispose of the sharp as indicated above.
- Encourage the wound to bleed but **do not suck it**.
- Wash the affected areas with running water and soap and cover with a waterproof occlusive dressing (do not use an alcohol swab).
- If splashes of the mouth or eye occur, irrigate with copious amounts of clean or sterile water or saline.
- Note the name, address and contact details (e.g. telephone number) and diagnosis of the source patient, if known.
- Report the incident to the designated person or GP in the practice without delay, in order that a risk assessment of the source patient can be undertaken. Further guidance may be required from the local A&E department or microbiologist.
- Ensure completion of an accident/incident form.
- Report to Occupational Health in accordance with local policy.

All staff members should know their Hepatitis B immune status, so that in the event of an inoculation incident they will be able to give this information to the person treating them in occupational health, A&E staff, etc. Staff should have access to occupational health facilities.

All high-risk blood/body fluid contamination incidents will require immediate attention as treatment, if necessary, may need to be instigated within a very short period of time. This includes incidents where the source patient is known to be, or suspected of being, infected with a blood-borne virus. Post-exposure prophylaxis (PEP) for management of sharps injuries contaminated with HIV may be required within 2 hours of injury to ensure maximum benefit (UK Departments of Health 2000). Further action should follow locally defined policy and be in line with national recommendations and guidance (UK Departments of Health 1998). All staff must be familiar with local policy and where to seek advice, particularly out of normal working hours.

Staff protection

The Health and Safety at Work Act (1974) governs general practice premises. The main aim of this act is to ensure that the employer and employee do all that is possible to ensure a safe working environment and that this safety is extended to anyone who enters the practice. The main infection risks for staff come from the potential contact with blood and body fluids and especially from contaminated sharps injury. Consequently general practitioners should ensure that all staff members who are at risk are immunized against Hepatitis B with the necessary follow-up to ensure seroconversion. However, in infections such as HIV and Hepatitis C there is no vaccine available to protect staff. It is essential therefore, that staff be provided with training and education to avoid the risk of potential cross infection such as handling specimens, venepuncture and sharps disposal.

Cleaning of body fluid spillage

All blood and body fluids spillage should be considered potentially infectious, and spillages should be cleaned up immediately. There is potential for a body fluid spillage such as vomit to occur any-where within the surgery. All members of staff should be instructed on what action to take, and the appropriate equipment should be readily available.

National guidelines issued by the HSE Advis-ory Committee on Dangerous Pathogens (1995) recommend the use of a high-concentration chlorine-releasing agent (such as sodium dichloro-isocyanurate (NaDCC) to disinfect blood and body spills prior to cleaning. However, the use of chlorine-releasing agents is not recommended for use on carpeted areas as the surface will be damaged.

Guidelines for recommended practice

Please refer to Chapter 10, Health centres, for a full description of methods.

Decontamination of equipment

Decontamination is a term used to cover methods of cleaning, disinfection and sterilization for the removal of microbial contamination from medical equipment and the environment. Within general practice decontamination is a process which ensures reusable medical items are rendered safe to reuse, and certain processes need to be in place to ensure this. All medical items must be adequately decontaminated between **each** patient use. The following section describes the decontam-ination process. Further information and advice on decontamination of individual items is avail-able in Chapter 5.

Definitions of cleaning, disinfection, sterilization

Cleaning The removal of accumulated deposits by washing with a cleaning solution fol-lowed by adequate drying. This will give a pre-liminary reduction in numbers of organisms and remove dirt, grease and organic matter which might protect organisms from heat or chemical disinfection.

Disinfection The removal of some types of pathogenic organism but not spores, which will give a partial reduction in the total number of organisms present. This will reduce the number of organisms to below that required to cause infection.

Sterilization The **complete** removal of all organ-isms including spores. This concept is absolute, that is, an item is either sterile or not sterile.

Categorization of equipment by risk assessment

(See also Chapter 5 on Cleaning, Disinfection and Sterilization.)

Medical devices should be categorized accord-ing to the risk they pose to patients. The proced-ure rather than the instrument governs the risk. Certain medical devices have specific require-ments on the method of decontamination, for example vaginal speculae (NHS General Medical Services Safety Information 1994).

Table 9.1 summarizes the classification of infec-tion risk associated with decontamination of medical devices.

Table 9.1 Classification of infection risk associated with decontamination of medical devices (Based on the risk assessment from Medical Devices Agency/Microbiology Advisory Committee 1996)

Risk	Application	Recommendation
High	Items in close contact with a break in the skin or mucous membrane or introduced into a sterile body area	Sterilization
Intermediate	Items in contact with intact skin, mucous membranes or body fluids, particularly after use on infected patients or prior to use on immunocompromized patients	Sterilization or disinfection Cleaning may be acceptable in some agreed situations
Low	Items in contact with healthy skin or mucous membranes or not in contact with the patient	Cleaning

Cleaning

Cleaning is a process that physically removes contamination but does not necessarily destroy micro-organisms. Cleaning is a pre-requisite of equipment decontamination to ensure effective disinfection or sterilization.

Instruments should be cleaned in a deep sink, designated for that purpose, in a solution of warm water and general-purpose detergent. If a brush is required to loosen debris it should be used whilst the instrument is below the surface of the water to avoid splashing. Brushes used in the process should be autoclavable, and autoclaved at the end a session. After washing, items should be rinsed well in clean water and dried on disposable paper towel.

Cleaning and decontamination of instruments should take place as soon as possible after use. Gloves, plastic apron and (when splashing is a risk) face and eye protection should be worn.

The use of an ultrasonic cleaner is preferred to manual cleaning as handling is reduced, cleaning is more efficient and thermal disinfection can be achieved (Miller and Palenik 1998). Current bench-top models are fully portable and do not require any fixed services. They incorporate automatic timers, have thermostatically-controlled heating and are extremely effective at removing surface soil. **N.B.** following removal from the cleaner, instruments must be rinsed well and dried before being processed through the sterilizer.

Disinfection

Disinfection with chemicals or heat has limited value within general practice.

Chemical disinfection is an unreliable process depending on the user's knowledge of concentration and immersion times. Items of equipment awaiting decontamination should not be stored in disinfectant but cleaned as soon after use as possible. Most reusable equipment used in general practice can be autoclaved. This method should always be used in preference to disinfection. Disinfectants should not be used as routine cleaning agents.

The use of water boilers is no longer recommended for disinfection in general practice (DoH HTM 2010 1994).

Sterilization

Sterile instruments such as those required for minor surgery can be obtained by using a hospital CSSD, purchase of single-use sterile equipment, or use of a steam sterilizer.

Hospital Central Sterile Service Departments (CSSDs) offer consistent quality and economies of scale. Availability of this facility, however, will depend on hospital CSSDs meeting the European standard EN46002 (1997). Strategies are currently being devised in regions for decontamination facilities to comply with current guidance (DoH 2000).

A suitable means of storage, collection and transport of both contaminated and sterile items would need to be developed if using this system.

Purchase of single-use sterile items may be the most cost-effective method if relatively small numbers of procedures are being undertaken. This may also be the best option for use at branch surgeries or similar where reprocessing facilities like deep sinks and autoclaves are not readily available.

Single-use sterile items must not be reprocessed unless the reprocessor can ensure the integrity and safety of the item (MDA 2000). Attempting to reuse without this guarantee will transfer legal liability for the item's safe performance from the manufacturer to the reprocessor.

Benchtop steam sterilizers are designed to sterilize unwrapped solid instruments for immediate use. They are unsuitable for bagged or wrapped instruments, or those with narrow lumens or cavities.

Benchtop vacuum steam sterilizers are now available, which are capable of sterilizing bagged and wrapped instruments (for storage and future use) and items with narrow lumens and cavities.

The users of the autoclave have a duty to ensure they are instructed on the correct use of the machine. This includes purchasing the machine most suited to their needs, loading the machine correctly, and ensuring it is maintained as recommended by the manufacturer. Routine monitoring and periodic testing of sterilizers is fully described in Chapter 5.

The use of hot air ovens is no longer recommended for sterilization in general practice (DoH HTM 2010 1994). Additionally, sterilizers that do not conform to the following MDA guidelines should not be used: (MDA DB(96)05 1996; MDA DB(98)04 1998).

Decontamination of healthcare equipment prior to inspection, service and repair

All medical equipment that has been contaminated with blood, body fluids or known infections must be decontaminated before being dispatched for inspection, service or repair (NHS Management Executive 1993). A certificate will need to be completed detailing the method of decontamination prior to work being carried out on the item, and further advice may be needed from the local engineers or the manufacturer prior to despatch.

Environmental cleaning

A clean environment is necessary to provide the required background to good standards of hygiene and asepsis and to maintain the confidence of patients and the morale of staff.

The practice environment should be kept clean, dry and well ventilated. Cleaning should be carried out in a planned manner and a cleaning schedule should be drawn up to include all equipment, fixtures and fittings. Careful planning is required when moving to new premises or when changes are made, ensuring new items/areas are added to the schedule.

The cleaning schedule should specify the method, frequency, timing where relevant, the equipment to be used and how it is to be cleaned. The responsibility for each task should also be indicated (NHS Estates 2001a).

General-purpose detergent and warm water and drying are all that is required for environmental cleaning. Chemical disinfectants have limited value and should only be used for blood or body fluid contamination. Ceramic or cream cleaner may be used for sinks and toilets. Mops and buckets should be stored clean, dry and inverted. Mop heads should be launderable or

disposable, and cleaning cloths should be disposable after use.

Linen

Where possible the use of linen should be avoided. Couches should be covered with paper rolls specifically designed for that use and changed after each patient use. Blankets should be avoided where possible, with paper covers being used to maintain patient dignity. If linen is to be used then an appropriate laundry facility should be found. Linen should not be carried home and laundered in a member of staff's domestic washing machine.

CLINICAL PRACTICE
Specimen handling

A specimen is defined as any bodily substance taken from a person for the purpose of analysis, such as blood or urine. Specimens can therefore pose a risk to all staff handling them, from reception staff to laboratory staff. To reduce this risk, persons who handle specimens should be kept to a minimum, should be trained to handle specimens and should be covered by the appropriate immunization.

Patient information

Within the practice environment patients also need to be advised on appropriate specimen collection and should always be given the appropriate container. Ideally a designated specimen return area should be available, such as a plastic box that can be easily cleaned in case of spillage or contamination. The patient should be encouraged to place the specimen in the container, thus reducing potential staff contact. Leaking and broken specimens should be placed into the clinical waste system and any spillage cleaned up promptly. Specimens should not be stored near food or drink.

Collection and storage

For accurate results to be obtained, specimens should be received by the laboratory within

Table 9.2 Collection and storage of microbiological specimens for general practice

Specimen	Refrigerate	Container	To lab within
Wound swab	NO – store at room temperature	Blue top swab containing transport medium DO NOT USE GREEN TOP FOR VIRAL SWABS	ASAP or within 24 hours
Viral swab	YES	Viral transport medium	ASAP or within 24 hours
Chlamydia swab	YES – overnight only May be frozen for five days	Chlamydia kit	ASAP Test within 7 days
Tissue/pus	NO – send directly to lab	Plain universal container	Immediately
Urine	YES – overnight only	Universal container with boric acid	ASAP or within 24 hours
Sputum	NO – store at room temperature	Plain universal container	ASAP or within 24 hours
Faecal	Can be stored at room temperature or refrigerated	Stool specimen container	ASAP or within 24 hours
Blood cultures	NO – send directly to lab for incubation	Specific bottles as supplied by the manufacturer	Immediately
Bloods for virology	YES – overnight only	Clotted specimen tube	Within 24 hours
CSF	NO – send directly to lab	Plain universal container	Immediately

24 hours maximum. After this time the dominant or more virulent organisms, such as staphylococci, will flourish, and the weaker organisms, for instance anaerobes, will die off and a false result may be obtained. The laboratory will generally discard specimens over 48 hours old. For the correct collection and storage of specimens see Table 9.2.

Transfer to the laboratory

Specimens sent to the laboratory often cause concern for laboratory staff by either being sent in the incorrect packaging or by not including the correct patient information. The patient's details must be placed on both the specimen container and the specimen request form. The specimen must be placed in a plastic bag with the request form in the separate pouch which is attached. Specimens known or suspected to contain high-risk pathogens, such as blood-borne viruses, tuberculosis, *Salmonella typhi*, should be marked 'risk of infection' using a biohazard sticker. The diagnosis need not be specified, but adequate patient details should be provided by the general practitioner, by telephone if necessary.

Transportation of specimens is usually by a courier service to the local hospital laboratory. Specimens may be sent by the postal system provided they comply with the Prohibited and Restricted Goods packaging requirements issued by the Royal Mail (Public Health Laboratory Service 1993, Health Service Advisory Committee 1991). Only first class post or Datapost may be used. The definition of infectious substances includes:

- infectious substances
- genetically modified micro-organisms and organisms
- biological products
- diagnostic specimens
- wastes.

The following is an extract from the 602 packaging specification:

Infectious substances may only be transported in packaging which meets the U.N. Class 6.2

specifications and the 602 packaging requirements. This ensures that strict performance tests which include a nine-metre drop test and a puncture test have been met. The outer shipping package must bear the U.N. packaging specification. (PHLS 1993, HSAC 1991)

Packaging system

- The primary receptacle must be a watertight, leakproof receptacle containing the sample and wrapped in enough absorbent material (e.g. wadding or cotton wool) to absorb all fluid in case of breakage.
- The secondary receptacle must be durable, watertight and leakproof to enclose and protect the primary receptacle. Several primary containers may be wrapped in one secondary receptacle. Enough absorbent material must be used to cushion multiple primary receptacles.
- The secondary package is then placed in an outer package which protects it and the contents from outside influences such as physical damage and water whilst in transit (e.g. a padded bag is recommended by the Royal Mail).
- Information concerning the enclosed sample/s and the identity of the sender and receiver should be attached to the outside of the secondary receptacle. The package must be labelled 'PATHOLOGICAL SPECIMEN – FRAGILE WITH CARE'.

Personnel who are permitted to send specimens or who ask members of the public to do so include:

- recognized laboratory or institution
- qualified medical practitioner
- registered dental practitioner
- registered nurse
- registered osteopath
- veterinary surgeon.

It should be noted that under no circumstances may members of the public post any pathological specimen except at the specific request of the above personnel (Royal Mail 1994).

Should staff have any concerns regarding the correct methods for local systems it is recommended that the local pathology laboratory be contacted for up-to-date advice.

Onsite testing of specimens

For specimens tested onsite, such as urine, the operator should wear disposable gloves and apron and wash hands thoroughly after handling specimens. Samples tested onsite should be disposed of in an appropriate sluice facility, not down a hand wash sink in clinical rooms.

Use of analytical equipment

Use of analytical equipment, for example blood glucose and cholesterol monitoring, are widely undertaken procedures within general practice. Failure to follow correct and safe practices during their use can put staff at risk of infection and can result in incorrect diagnosis for patients (HSE 1991).

Managers responsible for the day-to-day care of analytical equipment should ensure it is in good working order to ensure safe working practice. If any equipment is not performing correctly it should be withdrawn immediately. Maintenance and decontamination of the equipment must be carried out according to manufacturer's instructions and to comply with guidance on the decontamination of equipment prior to inspection, service and repair (NHS Management Executive 1993).

Recommended safe practice (HSE 1991) for analytical equipment

- To prevent any unnecessary spread of infection any patients known to be carrying, or strongly suspected of carrying, a blood-borne virus should not have blood monitoring carried out this way.
- Only those trained to do so should operate the analyser.
- As with any clinical procedure, hands should be decontaminated before and after completion of the task.

- The operator should wear gloves to prevent any skin contamination.
- The patient's skin should be clean and dry.
- Surfaces should be protected with a paper towel.
- All blood spillage should be cleaned up immediately following the body fluid spillage procedure.
- The patient's finger should be wiped with clean gauze or cotton wool after blood letting and the gauze disposed of as clinical waste.
- Any lancet, reagent strip, used needles or syringes should be disposed of into a sharps box immediately after use.
- If mechanical devices are used they should be cleaned following manufacturer's instructions after becoming contaminated.

MINOR SURGERY IN GENERAL PRACTICE

Introduction

Minor surgery is now performed in the majority of general practices. Procedures undertaken include injections, aspirations, incisions, excisions, curette, cautery and cryocautery. Other procedures such as vasectomy and endoscopy are also being performed (BMA General Medical Services Committee 1994).

Patients undergoing invasive procedures such as minor surgery will have an increased risk of infection. It is essential, therefore, that appropriate infection control procedures are in place to ensure protection of both patients and staff.

Preventing infection such as post-operative wound infection is dependent on provision of an appropriately-designed environment and procedure room, adequate supplies of sterile equipment and access to reprocessing facilities and a good knowledge of infection control procedures. In addition, a good operative technique is essential in reducing risks, including post-operative infection.

Types of procedures

Some procedures that are classed as minor surgery such as injections, cautery and cryocautery do not usually require additional standards of provision. Other procedures such as endoscopy require additional input from an infection control team before they can be instigated. For all other invasive procedures, the following provisions should be noted. Further information on infection control issues within healthcare environments is detailed in 'Infection Control in the Built Environment' (NHS Estates 2001b).

Environment for minor surgery

The following provision needs to be made:

- a designated procedure (minor surgery) room
- patient preparation and recovery area
- equipment/instrument decontamination and reprocessing facilities
- written infection control procedures.

Procedure room

Room size

The room should be large enough to allow access for the operator and assistant(s) to move freely around the patient, instrument trolley and other fixed or mobile equipment. Equipment and furniture should be kept to a minimum to reduce the risk of dust accumulation and allow for easy cleaning. A typical minimum room size would be $4\,m \times 5.5\,m$.

Walls and ceilings

Walls and ceiling should be intact and painted with a product (such as oil-based 'eggshell finish' paint to a British Standard) able to withstand regular cleaning with detergent and hot water and the occasional chemical disinfection with a chlorine-releasing agent (for blood or body fluid splashes). Walls should be washed when visibly soiled, otherwise at least once a year. Tiling is an alternative, but tiles must be replaced if they become cracked or damaged and grouting should be in good condition with no obvious soiling or mould growth. Areas behind basins, sinks or work surfaces may be protected with tiling or plastic or stainless steel splash-backs.

Flooring

Flooring should be intact, impervious, washable and visibly clean. Non-slip sheet vinyl with welded seams is recommended. Ideally the vinyl should be coved at the edges to provide a continuous surface with the walls. Floors should be cleaned after each session, or daily, using detergent and warm water.

Work surfaces

Work surfaces should be intact, seamless and easily washable. They should be kept clear of unnecessary items. Extraneous items such as paper work, books and pot plants *should not* be housed in the procedure room. Surfaces should be free of open fissures, open joints and crevices that will retain or permit the passage of dirt particles, and all joints must be sealed (NHS Estates 2001b). Separate designated work surfaces should be available for the preparation of equipment or sterile supplies, specimen receipt, instrument processing and clerical work. A stainless steel, free-standing dressing trolley designated for use in minor surgical procedures should be available. The trolley top should be routinely cleaned with detergent and hot water and dried. If it becomes contaminated with body fluids, clean in the normal manner then disinfect with an alcohol wipe.

The patient couch

The patient couch covering must be intact and of a material impervious to body fluids. During procedures the couch should be covered with disposable paper towelling which is changed between patients. Linen couch covers are not recommended.

Storage of equipment

Storage of equipment, instruments and consumable supplies should preferably be within washable cupboards. Open shelving may be suitable for wrapped or covered items, providing that shelves are regularly cleaned with a damp cloth and detergent solution and that items are not at significant risk of contamination by splashing with blood or body fluids.

Refrigerator

A separate refrigerator may be required for chemical reagents or drugs. The refrigerator must be defrosted regularly and the seals and internal surfaces kept clean using hot water and detergent. A separate refrigerator thermometer should be used to ensure a satisfactory temperature of 0–5°C. No food, beverages or specimens should be kept in this refrigerator.

Lighting

Lighting in the room should allow good visibility for the procedure. Natural lighting from windows is preferred. To ensure privacy for patient and operator, obscure glass should be used in clinical and changing areas. Blinds should be used in preference to curtains and should be of the vertical-vane type which can be adjusted to maintain privacy, allow a good supply of natural light, and can be easily cleaned with detergent and water when visibly soiled.

Artificial lighting, whether fixed or mobile, should be of suitable construction that allows easy cleaning and does not allow a build-up of dust or insects. It should be cleaned using a cloth moistened in detergent solution. Light diffusers from strip lamps should be dismantled for cleaning when visibly soiled.

Ventilation

Ventilation in the procedure room should aim to ensure the comfort of both patients and staff. Mechanical ventilation may be required and can be provided in the form of an electric inlet or extractor fan. Air movement induced by any form of mechanical ventilation must flow from 'clean' to 'dirty' areas. The vanes and surfaces of the fan must be regularly cleaned. When using free-standing fans, ensure they are clean and dust-free before use and that they are sited in such a way as to prevent airborne contamination of the operation site or sterile operation field.

Heating

Heating should be provided to ensure the comfort of both patients and staff. This will usually be in the form of radiators. Radiators quickly accumulate dust and must be cleaned regularly with a damp cloth, detergent and warm water or by vacuum cleaning. Positioning of radiators should allow for adequate space below them to ensure access for satisfactory cleaning of the floor surface.

Hand wash facilities

A designated wash hand basin with running hot and cold water, preferably with a mixing faucet, should be sited in the procedure room. Elbow taps should control the water. An adjacent wall-mounted cartridge-type soap dispenser for general hand hygiene and an antiseptic/detergent or an alcohol hand rub for preparation for an aseptic procedure should be available. A disposable paper towel dispenser should also be provided. Nail brushes, when used for preparation for an aseptic procedure, should be sterile and single-use.

Patient preparation and recovery area

An area or room providing privacy should be available near to the procedure room for patient changing, preferably with ready access to toilet and hand wash facilities. The recovery area should be supervised, and depending on the procedure may need to accommodate a couch or trolley. Equipment for the management of body fluid spillage should be made available in these areas.

Equipment decontamination and reprocessing facilities

Facilities for instrument processing, the collection and disposal of used single-use equipment, clinical waste, sharps and contaminated linen should be provided in a separate, well-ventilated room adjacent to the procedure room.

Separation of 'clean' and 'dirty' tasks

If instrument decontamination and reprocessing is undertaken in the procedure room, designated space is required to undertake this safely. Separation of 'clean' tasks (such as preparation of sterile items) and 'dirty' tasks (for example instrument cleaning) is essential to prevent cross contamination.

A deep sink with draining facilities and hot and cold running water is required for instrument cleaning and decontamination (wash hand basins **must not** be used for this purpose).

Staff changing facilities

A room for staff to change into suitable clothing should be sited near to the procedure room. Hand washing and toilet facilities should be readily accessible from the staff changing area.

Infection control procedures

Staff preparation

All staff involved in minor surgical procedures should have been vaccinated against Hepatitis B and have documented proof of immunity.

Hand decontamination

Hands should be decontaminated between each patient activity with warm running water and liquid soap and dried thoroughly on paper towels. Alternatively, an alcohol hand rub may be used on visibly clean hands. Prior to minor surgical procedures a more thorough hand wash with an antiseptic detergent preparation is required. As stated above, nail brushes, if used, should be sterile and single-use.

Wrist jewellery and stoned rings should not be worn, and fingernails should be short with only clear varnish being used. Further guidance on hand decontamination prior to surgical procedures is available (ICNA 2002a).

Surgical hand wash

Surgical hand washing prior to minor surgery or invasive procedures will remove the transient organisms and reduce levels of resident flora from hands. This can be achieved using aqueous antiseptic – detergent such as chlorhexidine 4%

or povidone-iodine 7.5%. This requires a thorough two-minute application and should then be rinsed and dried using sterile towels. Alternatively, an alcoholic solution with or without antiseptic can be used, such as chlorhexidine in 70% alcohol. This will provide a more rapid effect and can be used between cases on visibly clean hands. Two 5 ml applications are required, which should be rubbed around the hands and wrists following the standard method until the hands are dry (ICNA 2002a).

Protective clothing

All personnel should wear disposable plastic aprons when anticipating contact with blood and body fluids. Single-use, sterile, non-powdered latex surgeon's gloves should be worn by the person/s performing minor surgical procedures. Latex-free alternative products must be available for those staff with a confirmed latex allergy. In addition single-use, non-sterile, non-powdered procedure/examination latex gloves should be worn for all anticipated contact with blood and body fluids (ICNA 2002b). Plastic goggles and masks or full-face visors should be available for use if splashing of body fluids is likely.

Surgical instruments

Instruments used for minor surgical procedures **must be sterile at the point of use**. Options available for the supply of sterile equipment are discussed in the section on decontamination, pp. 156–158, and in Chapter 5.

The workload should be managed to ensure adequate time for infection control procedures to be effectively carried out between patients. This may require varying intervals of time between cases to allow for decontamination and re-sterilization of equipment.

Patient preparation

Preoperative information

Advice and a risk assessment should be sought on patients who are at a higher risk of infection. These include those who have heart valve disease or who have had valve replacement, patients who have had splenectomy, those patients receiving steroid treatment, and diabetics. These patients may require prophylactic antibiotic cover or similar. Advice should also be sought on those patients known to be suffering from, or suspected to be at risk from, Creutzfeldt–Jakob disease (CJD).

Skin preparation

The agents recommended for disinfection of the operation site are:

- 0.5% chlorhexidine
- 1% iodine in 70% alcohol
- alcoholic povidone-iodine 4%.

All are applied with friction for two minutes and allowed to air dry. Alcoholic solutions are more effective and rapidly acting than aqueous solutions (Ayliffe et al 2000).

Shaving the operation site should be avoided where possible (Cruse and Foord 1980, Simmons 1998). If it is necessary it should be done as close to the operation as possible. Clipping of the site is preferable to shaving.

Postoperative information

Patients should be supplied with both verbal and written instructions on the management of wounds following minor surgery. This should include:

- bathing instructions
- care of the wound and dressing
- when and how to contact the surgery if a problem occurs.

An operation register must be maintained and should include the date, patient details, the surgical intervention and the names of those undertaking and assisting in the procedure. Mechanisms must be in place for the reporting, recording and follow-up (including microbiological examination as necessary) of infections resulting from minor surgery.

CONCLUSION

Within the practice environment, infection control is everybody's business and is both an individual and collective responsibility. Policies and procedures for infection control and a good basic level of education and knowledge are essential to ensure protection for patients and all staff. Additionally, emerging diseases, antimicrobial resistance (DoH 1999) and the development of new technologies make an effective and manageable infection control programme within general practice essential.

REFERENCES

Ansari S A, Springthorpe U S et al 1991 Comparison of cloth, paper and warm air drying in eliminating viruses and bacteria from washed hands. American Journal of Infection Control 9: 243–249

Ayliffe G A J, Fraise A P, Geddes A M, Mitchell K 2000 Control of Hospital Infection: A Practical Handbook, 4th edn. Chapman and Hall Medical, London

British Medical Association 1989 A Code of Practice for Sterilisation of Instruments and Control of Cross Infection. BMA, London

British Medical Association General Medical Services Committee 1994 Minor Surgery in General Practice: A Review. BMA, London

British Standards Institution (1990) Specification for Sharps Containers. BS7320. BSI, London

Chant K, Lowe D, Rubin G et al 1993 Patient to patient transmission of HIV in private surgical consulting rooms (letter). The Lancet 342: 1548–1549

Cruse P J E, Foord T 1980 The Epidemiology of Wound Infection: A Ten Year prospective study of 62,939 wounds. Surgical Clinics of North America 60, 27

Dawson J, Khan D A, Dawson K, Hemmings C 1995 Auditing infection control. Practice Nursing 6(3): 13–17

Department of the Environment 1991 Environmental Protection Act – Duty of Care (1991). A Code of Practice. HMSO, London

Department of Health 1994 Health Technical Memorandum HTM 2010. Steam Sterilisers, Parts 1–4. HMSO, London

Department of Health 1999 Health Service Circular (HSC) 1999/049 Resistance to Antibiotics and other Antimicrobial Agents. DoH, London

Department of Health 2000 HSC 2000/032 Decontamination of Medical Devices. NHSE

Emmerson A M, Enstone J E, Griffin M, Kelsey M C, Smyth E T M 1996 The second national prevalence survey of infection in hospitals – overview of results. Journal of Hospital Infection 32: 175–190

European Union 1997 European Standards for Sterile Supply Departments. EN 46002 (1997). EU, Luxembourg

European Union 1998 European Standards for Sharps Containers EN 3291 (1998). EU, Luxembourg

Finn L, McCulloch J 1996 Infection control in GP surgeries: safe practices. British Journal of Nursing 5(6): 341–348

Gould D 1994 The significance of hand drying in the prevention of infection. Nursing Times 90(47): 33–35

Health and Safety Commission Health Services Advisory Committee 1999 Safe Disposal of Clinical Waste. HSE Books, London

Health and Safety Executive Health Service Advisory Committee 1991 Safe working practices and the prevention of infection in clinical laboratories. HMSO, London

Health and Safety Executive 1992 Personal Protective Equipment at Work Regulations. HMSO, London

Health and Safety Executive Advisory Committee on Dangerous Pathogens 1995 Protection against blood borne infections in the workplace: HIV and Hepatitis. HMSO, London

HMSO 1974 Health and Safety at Work Act (1974). HMSO, London

Hlady W H, Hopkins R S, Ogilby T E, Allen S T 1993 Patient to patient transmission of Hepatitis B in dermatology practice. American Journal of Public Health 83(12): 1689–1693

HMSO 1990 Recommendations of the Expert Advisory Group on AIDS and the Advisory Group on Hepatitis. HMSO, London

Infection Control Nurses Association 2002a Hand Hygiene Guidelines. ICNA, Bathgate

Infection Control Nurses Association 2002b Glove Usage Guidelines. ICNA, Bathgate

Medical Devices Agency 1996 Sterilization, Disinfection and Cleaning of Medical Equipment. Guidance on decontamination from the Microbiology Advisory Committee to the Department of Health. ISBN 1 85839 518 6. DoH, London

Medical Devices Agency 1996 The Purchase, Operation and Maintenance of Benchtop Steam Sterilizers. Device Bulletin (DB) (96) 05. DoH, London

Medical Devices Agency 1998 The Validation and Periodic Testing of Vacuum Steam Sterilizers. Device Bulletin (DB) (98) 04. DoH, London

Medical Devices Agency 2000 Single-use Medical Devices: Implications and consequences of re-use. Device Bulletin (DB) 2000 (04). DoH, London

Miller C H, Palenik C J 1998 Infection Control and Management of Hazardous Materials for the Dental Team, 2nd edn. Mosby, St. Louis

Morgan D R, Lamont T J, Dawson D J, Booth C 1990 Decontamination of instruments and control of cross infection in general practice. British Medical Journal 300: 1379–1380

National Audit Office 2000 The Management and Control of Hospital Acquired Infection in Acute NHS Trusts in England. HMSO, London

National Health Service 1994 NHS FPN 654 General Medical Services Safety Information. Instruments and Appliances used in the Vagina and Cervix: Recommended Methods for Decontamination. HMSO, London.

NHS Estates 2001a Standards for Environmental Cleanliness in Healthcare. HMSO, London

NHS Estates 2001b Infection Control in the Built Environment. HMSO, London

NHS Management Executive 1993 Decontamination of Equipment Prior to Inspection, Service and Repair HSG (93) 26. HMSO, London

Overend A, Hall W W, Goodwin P G 1992 Does your earwax lose its pathogens on your auriscope overnight? British Medical Journal 305: 1571–1573

Public Health Laboratory Service 1993 Safety Precautions; Notes for Guidance, 4th edn. PHLS, London

Reybrouck G 1986 Handwashing and hand disinfection. Journal of Hospital Infection (1): 5–23

Royal College of Nursing 2000 Good Practice in Infection Control: Guidance for Nurses Working in General Practice. RCN Publication Code 000 866. RCN, London

Royal Mail 1994 Prohibited and Restricted Goods (Leaflet). Royal Mail, London

Simmons M 1998 Pre-operative skin preparation. Professional Nurse 13, 7

UK Departments of Health 1998 Guidance for Clinical Health Care Workers: Protection Against Infection with Blood-borne Viruses. DoH, London

UK Departments of Health 2000 HIV Post Exposure Prophylaxis: Guidance from the UK Chief Medical Officers' Expert Advisory Group on AIDS. DoH, London

Health centres

D. Khan

INTRODUCTION

Until recently infection control issues have focused on hospitals and hospital-acquired infection. Guidelines, research-based practices and education have been well developed for the hospital setting. In the past these guidelines have been extended to the community but the uniqueness of the services provided, the many disciplines involved and the variety of settings in which treatment is provided has meant these guidelines are not always suitable. The development of designated community infection control nurses has led to a more individual, tailored approach to specifically meet the community healthcare infection control needs (Community Infection Control Nurses Network 1999).

Although community infection control guidelines differ from those in hospitals, the basic risk of infection remains the same. Healthcare undertaken in the community, particularly in health centres, involves many invasive procedures such as dental surgery, nail surgery, insertion of intrauterine devices and minor surgery. As Chapter 9 illustrated, these invasive procedures breach the body's defence systems, exposing the patient to a risk of infection as well as the operator to potential contamination with blood and body fluids.

Decontamination and supplies of sterile equipment are not as readily available in the community, and there is often limited access to a sterile supplies department. Consequently sterilization of equipment is undertaken as an additional task of the healthcare worker, involving purchase, testing and maintenance of equipment as well as training and education of the operator.

In the community, patient treatment often takes place out of the healthcare setting and in outreach clinics, residential homes and the patient's home. This requires additional guidelines and policies to deal with practices in these settings such as hand washing, sharps disposal, and return to base of used instruments for decontamination.

Staff treating patients following discharge from hospital encounter additional problems relating to infection control. Patients recovering from severe illness are often left debilitated and prone to infection. A number of patients may have acquired or been colonized with multi-resistant organisms such as methicillin-resistant *Staphylococcus aureus* (MRSA), requiring specific instructions on care. Many patients are discharged with wounds requiring further care, and earlier discharge into the community means subsequent wound infections may not develop until the patient is home (Mishriki et al 1990).

Minor surgery, including injections, incisions, excisions, aspirations, curette, cautery and cryocautery are now performed in health centres. Procedures such as vasectomy and endoscopy are also being performed. Those patients undergoing invasive procedures such as minor surgery will have an increased risk of infection. It is essential therefore that comprehensive infection control procedures are in place for protection of patients and to ensure staff involved are protected from occupational risk.

In summary, community settings have their own specific requirements for infection control and these are best met by specific research-based guidelines. See Chapter 9, General practice, in particular the section Basic principles in infection control, for details.

BASIC PRINCIPLES IN INFECTION CONTROL

Hand decontamination

Hand decontamination (Box 10.1) is dealt with in several chapters of this book: see Chapter 9 for full details.

Chapter 9 lists the essential equipment required for hand decontamination in every clinical area, and its designation for hand washing only and no other purpose. Requirements for drying of hands in the clinical setting are also given in Chapter 9.

Protective clothing

All members of staff should wear appropriate protective clothing at work and there should be plenty of readily accessible supplies (Health and Safety Executive 1992). Staff should have an adequate number of supplies to last when working outside of the health centre building.

Box 10.1 Hand decontamination

All staff should decontaminate hands:

- at the beginning and the end of all clinical duties
- when hands are visibly soiled
- after wearing gloves
- before aseptic procedures
- before serving food
- after going to the toilet
- after every physical contact with patients, even if hands remain visibly clean. This has implications for all health centre sites where clinical work is undertaken, as not all centres currently provide adequate facilities
- by keeping nails short and clean. No stoned rings, wrist watches or jewellery should be worn other than a wedding ring
- using a nailbrush only if necessary before clinical procedures and only if sterile, single use only and disposed of after use.

Please see the Protective clothing section of Chapter 9 for a list of items which employers have a duty to provide.

Glove choices (ICNA Guidelines 2002)

Chapter 9 illustrates (Figs 9.1 and 9.2) the many alternatives available and reasons for the choice. As Chapter 9 emphasizes, gloves should **always be changed between patients**, and hands washed even though gloves have been worn. Gloves are an addition to hand washing, not a substitute. Gloves should not be washed or disinfected for reuse. In addition, examination (procedure gloves) and surgeon's gloves are manufactured as single use items and must not be reused (MDA 2000).

After direct contact with body fluids, if treatment of the client has not been completed, gloves should still be changed or removed. Care should be taken not to contaminate articles such as notes, surfaces and telephones if the gloves have become soiled.

Instructions for the use of general purpose gloves are given in Chapter 9.

Protective aprons

Plastic aprons are indicated for use when treating patients if clothes are likely to be contaminated with secretions or excretions, or when performing invasive procedures such as nail surgery, to protect the patient from potential cross infection. Aprons should be single use and disposed of when treatment has been completed.

Face protection

Details are given in Chapter 9.

Clinical waste

Disposal of waste is governed by the Environmental Protection Act (Duty of Care) Regulations (Department of the Environment 1991). All clinical waste generated within the health centre and outside should be dealt with in line with the relevant guidelines (Health and Safety Commission 1999). Box 9.1 (p. 153) gives details, and is supported by information on other varieties of waste for disposal and methods of dealing with it (pp. 153–155).

Sharps management

Please refer to page 154 for comprehensive guidelines on avoidance of sharps injury.

Sharps safety offsite

Portable sharps boxes designed for community use are readily available and should be used by all staff who generate sharps outside of the practice building. These should all be fitted with a sealable safety lid to prevent spillage during transit.

The healthcare worker should only leave sharps boxes in patients' homes following individual assessment. Care should be taken if there are children in the home, as the sharps box may attract attention.

Inoculation injuries

Each health centre should have a written policy on the prevention and management of inoculation procedures including exposure to blood and body fluids. Staff should follow the practices outlined in Chapter 9 at all times to minimize the risk of injury. Procedure in the event of an injury occurring is repeated here:

- Dispose of the sharp safely into container.
- Encourage the wound to bleed but **DO NOT SUCK IT**.
- Wash the affected areas with running water and soap and cover with a waterproof occlusive dressing. Do not use an alcohol swab.
- If splashes of the mouth or eye occur, irrigate with copious amounts of clean or sterile water or saline.
- Note the name, address and contact details (e.g. telephone number) and diagnosis of the source patient, if known.
- Report the incident to the designated person, e.g. line manager, without delay in order that a risk assessment of the source patient can be undertaken. Further guidance may be required from the local A&E department or microbiologist.
- Ensure completion of an accident/incident form.
- Report to Occupational Health in accordance with local policy.

All staff members should know their Hepatitis B immune status, so that in the event of an inoculation incident they will be able to give this information.

All high-risk blood/body fluid contamination incidents require immediate attention, as treatment, if necessary, may need to be instigated within a very short period of time. This includes incidents where the source patient is known to be or suspected of being infected with a blood-borne virus. Post-exposure prophylaxis (PEP) for management of sharps injuries contaminated with Human Immunodeficiency Virus (HIV) may be required within two hours of the injury to ensure maximum benefit. Any further action should follow the locally-defined policy and be in line with national recommendations (DoH 2000a). All staff must be familiar with the local policy and where to seek advice, especially out of hours.

Cleaning of body fluid spillage

All blood and body fluid spillage should be considered potentially infectious and spillages should be cleaned up immediately. All members of staff should be instructed on what action is required, and appropriate equipment should be readily available.

Recommended practice for cleaning of blood or body fluid spills (RCN 2000)

For spillage of high-risk body fluids such as blood, follow Methods 1 or 2. For spillage of low-risk body fluids such as excreta, vomit, etc., use Method 3.

Method 1 (hypochlorite method)

- Wear protective clothing and soak up excess fluid using disposable paper towels.
- Cover the area with paper towels soaked in 10 000 parts per million of available chlorine (liquid or tablet form) and leave for two minutes.
- Remove organic matter using the towels and discard as clinical waste.
- Clean area with detergent and hot water and dry thoroughly.
- Clean the bucket/bowl in fresh soapy water and dry.
- Discard the protective clothing as clinical waste.
- Wash hands thoroughly.

Method 2 (sodium dichloroisocyanurate (NaDCC) method)

- Wear protective clothing and cover the spillage with NaDCC granules.
- Leave for at least two minutes.
- Scoop up the debris with paper towels and/or cardboard.
- Wash the area with detergent and hot water, and dry thoroughly.
- Dispose of all materials as clinical waste.
- Clean the bucket/bowl with fresh soapy water and dry.
- Discard protective clothing as clinical waste.
- Wash hands thoroughly.

Method 3 (detergent and water)

- Wear protective clothing and mop up organic matter with paper towels or disposable cloths.
- Clean the surface using a solution of detergent and hot water and paper towels or disposable cloths.
- Rinse the surface and dry thoroughly.
- Dispose of materials as clinical waste.
- Clean the bucket/bowl in fresh soapy water and dry.
- Discard protective clothing as clinical waste.

Staff protection

The main infection risks for staff come from the potential contact with contaminated blood and body fluids, especially from sharps injury, as Chapter 9 outlines. Consequently all staff members who are at risk should be immunized against Hepatitis B with the necessary follow-up to ensure immunity has been achieved. However, in infections such as HIV and Hepatitis C there is no immunization to protect staff. It is essential therefore that staff be provided with training and education to avoid the risk of potential infection such as in handling specimens.

All staff should have access to appropriate occupational health services.

Decontamination of equipment

The decontamination and re-processing of medical devices is explained in Chapter 5. Specialist equipment is dealt with separately under individual sections.

HEALTH CENTRE ENVIRONMENT, EQUIPMENT AND FACILITIES

The design of any healthcare setting is crucial in preventing the potential for cross infection (Ayliffe et al 2000). Within health centres, clinics such as those for dentistry and podiatry require specialist design and equipment, and further advice should be sought.

General clinical rooms are used for numerous purposes, such as ulcer clinics, family planning and physiotherapy. Careful planning and management of room usage is needed to ensure that the patient is not put at additional risks of infection by having dirty procedures followed by clean or surgical procedures. A risk assessment should be undertaken to enable the planning of clinics to be appropriate pertaining to facilities and nature of the clinic.

Within the health centre there also needs to be a differentiation between office space and clinical space. Office work taking place in designated clinical rooms can lead to a build-up of dust and extraneous items such as paper, books and journals and equipment such as photocopiers, making adequate cleaning difficult.

Clinical rooms

As suggested in Chapter 9 in relation to general practice, all the rooms should be well ventilated and well lit. The size of clinical rooms should be large enough to allow staff and patients to move freely without bumping into couches, trolleys and equipment.

The walls and ceiling should be painted with a product that can be easily washed and disinfected if contaminated. Flooring should have a washable covering such as non-slip sheet vinyl, and carpet should be avoided as it is not easily cleaned. Work surfaces should be seamless and washable.

Chapter 9 also makes the following points about the essential components of the general practice hand wash sink, which apply equally to the health centre setting:

- an accessible hand wash sink separate from the sink used for cleaning equipment
- elbow-operated taps
- liquid soap
- disposable paper towels
- a poster demonstrating the correct hand washing procedure
- antimicrobial soap for invasive procedures/ minor surgery.

The sink should be designated for hand washing only and should not be used for cleaning equipment, disposing of specimens or for making tea and coffee. The drying of hands is also an essential part of hand washing (Gould 1994). The best way to dry hands is by the use of disposable paper towels. In the clinical setting, hand dryers are not recommended (Ansari et al 1991).

Storage of equipment

Storage of equipment, instruments and consumable supplies should preferably be within washable cupboards. Open shelving may be suitable for wrapped or covered items, providing shelves are regularly cleaned with a damp cloth and detergent solution and that items are not at significant risk of contamination by splashing with blood or body fluids.

Due to the wide variety of services and equipment that is used within the health centre, adequate facilities must be provided to store all equipment safely. Specialist clinics such as ulcer clinics may require numerous large items of equipment (for example, buckets which require storage inverted and in pyramids), and additional space and shelving will be required.

The patient couch and chairs

The patient couch or chair covering must be intact and of a material impervious to body fluids. During procedures the couch should be covered with disposable paper towelling which is changed between patients. Linen couch covers and pillowcases are not recommended.

Linen

Where possible the use of linen should be avoided. Couches should be covered with paper rolls specifically designed for that use and changed after each patient. Blankets should be avoided where possible, with paper covers being used to maintain patient dignity. If linen is to be used then an appropriate laundry facility should be used. Linen should not be carried home by members of staff and laundered in their domestic washing machine.

Refrigerator

A refrigerator may be required for chemical reagents or drugs. The refrigerator must be defrosted regularly and the seals and internal surfaces kept clean using hot water and detergent. A separate refrigerator thermometer should be used to ensure a satisfactory temperature of 0–5°C. No food, beverages or specimens should be kept in this refrigerator.

Heating

Heating should be provided to ensure the comfort of both patients and staff. This will usually be in the form of radiators. Radiators quickly accumulate dust and must be cleaned regularly with a damp cloth, detergent and warm water or by vacuum cleaning. Positioning of radiators should allow for adequate space below them to ensure access for satisfactory cleaning of the floor surface.

Patient waiting area

The patient waiting areas should allow segregation of patients who may be infected.

An area or room providing resting facilities should be available near to procedure rooms for patients who have had treatment such as dental or minor operations. This area should provide changing facilities with access to toilet and hand wash facilities. The area should be supervised, and depending on the procedures undertaken may need to accommodate a couch or trolley as well as chairs. Equipment for the management of body fluid spillage should be made available in these areas.

Toys for children's play, if required, should be washable to allow easy cleaning. It is useful to clarify who is responsible for cleaning toys and frequency of cleaning. Soft fabric toys should be avoided.

Baby changing facilities should be provided. This should include a changing mat with an intact waterproof covering. Cleaning equipment to allow the mat to be cleaned should be provided, along with hand wash facilities and clinical waste bins for disposal of nappies.

Equipment and supplies

Supplies of medical equipment will be required and dependent on the use will need to be sterile and/or reusable. The professional using the equipment is responsible for ensuring that it is sterile at time of use if required and that reusable equipment has been decontaminated appropriately.

Hospital Central Sterile Service Departments (CSSDs)

Hospital Central Sterile Service Departments (CSSDs) offer consistent quality and economy of scale, and facilities must meet recently-introduced standards for service provision (EN 46002 1998). Regional strategies are currently being devised in England and Wales for decontamination facilities (DoH 2000b).

Obtaining supplies from hospital CSSDs may be the best option for occasional use equipment and items required to be sterile at the time of use, such as for nail surgery and intrauterine device insertion. A suitable means of storage, collection and transport of both contaminated and sterile items would need to be developed with this system.

Single use sterile items may be the most cost-effective method if relatively small numbers of procedures are being undertaken. Purchase of such items may be the best option where reprocessing facilities such as deep sinks and autoclaves are not available and for items used in a patient's home.

Single use sterile items must not be re-processed (MDA 2000). Product Liability will be assumed by an individual reprocessing equipment (under The Product and Consumer Protection Act 1987) for any failure of process or harm resulting from such reprocessing.

Benchtop steam sterilizers are designed to sterilize unwrapped solid instruments for immediate use. They are unsuitable for bagged or wrapped instruments, or those with narrow lumens or cavities. Benchtop vacuum steam sterilizers are now available, however, which are capable of sterilizing bagged and wrapped instruments (for storage and future use) and items with narrow lumens and cavities.

Routine monitoring and periodic testing of the sterilizer's performance is required to give assurance that sterilizing conditions are being consistently met. Guidance on this can be found in two Medical Devices Agency documents (MDA DB 9605 1996, MDA DB 9804 1998a).

Benchtop steam sterilizers or benchtop vacuum steam sterilizers are the best option when reprocessing on site is required due to a rapid turnover of equipment. This occurs in specialisms such as dentistry and podiatry.

Chapter 5 of this book, on Cleaning, disinfection and sterilization, offers more detail.

Environmental cleaning

All information under this heading relating to general practice (Chapter 9, p. 158) is relevant in health centres.

PODIATRY

During the course of a day the podiatrist will see many patients and during busy clinics can move from patient to patient every twenty minutes. During their treatment, wounds are exposed and patients are handled, therefore providing opportunities for infections to be spread. Infection from patients with wounds, skin lesions or fungal infections may be transferred via couches, chairs and equipment, and from the hands of staff. Contamination with body fluids will put staff at risk of infection as well as other patients if good infection control procedures are not in place.

Certain people who attend for podiatry will be at risk of infection. These include the elderly, diabetics, those with existing ulcers or wounds and any patient who is immunocompromised.

Patients presenting with foot problems will also be at increased risk. They may have reduced sweating ability, making the feet dry and likely to crack; they may have pressure points likely to cause pressure wounds and consequently poorly fitting shoes, adding to the risk of open lesions and thus potential infection. These characteristics make it essential that good infection control procedure, staff education and awareness exist within all podiatry departments.

Environment and facilities

Procedure room

See Chapter 9, section on Procedure room, for the requirements for a clean working environment in clinics.

Privacy curtains

Curtains used for patient privacy should be hung so as not to come in contact with the operator's workstation or the patient. Curtains should be washed every six months or if visibly stained.

Podiatry chair

The patient couch covering must be intact and of a material impervious to body fluids. The foot extension or stool should be protected with a paper cover, changed between each patient. After each patient the stool should be cleaned paying particular attention to joints and hinges.

Workstation

The workstation should be arranged so as to allow the operator adequate space to move around the patient and equipment trolley or surfaces. Clinical waste and sharps disposal bins should be close by. The operator's work unit or trolley should be made of a suitable surface such as laminate that can be decontaminated between use. Unprotected wood surfaces should not be used. Only the equipment used for one patient at a time should be laid onto the work unit, as excess equipment could become contaminated.

Hand wash facilities

A designated wash hand basin with elbow taps, running hot and cold water, preferably with a mixing faucet, should be sited in the podiatry room. An adjacent wall-mounted cartridge-type soap dispenser for general hand hygiene and an antiseptic/detergent or an alcohol hand rub for preparation for an aseptic procedure should be available. A disposable paper towel dispenser should also be provided.

Equipment decontamination and reprocessing facilities

Facilities for instrument processing, the collection and disposal of used single use equipment, clinical waste, sharps and contaminated linen should be provided separate from the working field. Separation of 'clean' tasks (such as preparation of sterile items) and 'dirty' tasks (for instance instrument cleaning) is essential to prevent cross contamination.

A deep sink with draining facilities and hot and cold running water is required for instrument cleaning and decontamination. As stated elsewhere, wash hand basins **must not** be used for this purpose.

Surgical instruments

All reusable instruments such as nippers, burrs or files need decontamination between use. This is best achieved by sterilization via an autoclave (Society of Chiropodists and Podiatrists 1998). Cleaning and drying is required prior to sterilization.

The use of an **ultrasonic cleaner** is recommended by the Society of Chiropodists and Podiatrists (1998). As stated in Chapter 9 for general practice, this is preferred to manual cleaning as handling is reduced, cleaning is more efficient and thermal disinfection can be achieved (Miller and Palenik 1998). Current benchtop models are fully portable and do not require any fixed services. They incorporate automatic timers, have thermostatically-controlled heating and are extremely effective at removing surface soil.

N.B. following removal from the cleaner, instruments must be rinsed well and dried before being processed through the sterilizer.

If an ultrasonic cleaner is not available, items should be cleaned using warm water, general-purpose detergent and a brush. The items should be cleaned under the surface of the solution to prevent splashing, then dried thoroughly using disposable paper towelling prior to sterilization.

Instruments used for all nail surgery **must be sterile at point of use**. The instruments should either be prepacked or used immediately from the autoclave.

The workload should be managed to ensure adequate time for infection control procedures to be effectively carried out between patients. This may require varying intervals of time between cases to allow for decontamination and re-sterilization of equipment. For correct use of sterilizers, see Chapter 5.

Hand decontamination

Hands should be washed well between each patient activity with warm running water and liquid soap, and dried thoroughly on paper towels. Alternatively, an alcohol hand rub can be used on visibly clean hands. Prior to nail surgery a more thorough hand wash with an antiseptic is required.

Protective clothing

Gloves should be worn to reduce the risk of staff infecting patients, particularly during nail surgery, and to reduce the risk of staff becoming infected or colonized whilst treating patients. For non-surgical work, if there is no contact with blood or body fluids gloves need not be worn.

Gloves should always be changed between patients, and hands washed even though gloves have been worn. Gloves should also be changed if they become punctured or torn during a procedure.

General purpose gloves such as household rubber gloves should be used for cleaning instruments after use and prior to sterilization, or when coming into contact with contaminated surfaces or items. These gloves may be reused but should be washed whilst on the hands with detergent and warm water and hung to dry. These gloves should be discarded if punctured or torn or if there is evidence of deterioration.

Face protection

Podiatrist and close support staff must protect their eyes and respiratory tract against foreign bodies, splatter and aerosols during procedures. Research has shown that nail work such as clipping and drilling can cause ocular infections, and in the case of dust can be inhaled (Millar et al 1996, Burrows et al 1996). When nail drills are used, dust control facilities should be available. Dust extraction systems should have regular maintenance and suitable filters should be fitted. Dust bags should be emptied on a regular basis or when full.

Eye protection should be worn for nail clipping and drilling. Eye spectacles should conform to BS2092 (1992a) and EN 166 (1996).

Disposable dust masks should also be used for all nail drilling, conforming to standard EN 149 (1996). These should be single use and disposed of after each session.

Protective aprons

This topic is covered earlier in this chapter under Basic principles in infection control.

Sharps management

All blades must be sterile at the point of use and are **single use only**. The bullet list under Sharps Management earlier in this chapter is a useful guide.

Skin preparation and treatment

If feet are visibly dirty they should be washed prior to treatment. Before starting treatment, feet should be wiped with an alcoholic antiseptic. The solution should be allowed to dry prior to treatment starting.

Care of wounds

For care of wounds, see also Chapter 14.

When dressing or assessing wounds it is imperative that a good aseptic technique is adopted to reduce the risk of infection and transfer of infection to staff or other patients (Thomlinson 1987).

Guidelines for best practice

- Open wounds should not come into contact with any item which is not sterile.
- Scissors for wound dressings should be sterile.

- Any item in contact with the wound should be discarded or appropriately decontaminated after use.
- The procedure should be performed using gloved hands and sterile gauze.
- Any medication or solution applied to the wound must be from a single-use sachet. Multi-use tubes and pots should not be used.
- At the follow-up appointment there should be an assessment for any signs of infection.
- If there are any signs of infection, i.e. redness, heat, swelling or discharge of pus, then a swab should be sent.

Patient information

Patients should be supplied with both verbal and written instructions on the management of wounds following nail surgery. This should include bathing instructions, care of the wound and dressing, and when and how to contact the podiatrist if a problem occurs.

Equipment decontamination guidelines for podiatry staff

The list (Table 10.1 at the end of this chapter) is not exhaustive and should be used in conjunction with manufacturers' recommendations, locally defined policies and additional information provided within this chapter and Chapter 5.

ULCER CLINICS

See also Chapter 14 (Wound care). The effectiveness of ulcer clinics within community settings has been well documented. Ulcer clinics which are predominately nurse-led have proved to be a cost-effective service, improving healing and being of great benefit to the patient (Moffatt et al 1992, Simon et al 1996).

During the course of the clinic there are opportunities for transmission of infection to occur. Bacteria present in the wounds are likely to contaminate used dressings, buckets and staff hands. Several patients having wound dressings taken down and exposed at the same time can lead to cross contamination, and the fast turnover of patients can put pressure on staff to perform infection control procedures inadequately.

Guidelines for good practice

The environment

- Ulcer clinics should only take place in clinical rooms that are a suitable size, where there is an easily cleanable floor (no carpets) and, if applicable, with access to sluicing facilities to empty water used for soaking legs.
- The environment should be arranged in order to allow staff to move around the patient without bumping into equipment.
- Adequate distance between each patient treatment section should be ensured to prevent cross contamination.
- The environment should be protected from potential contamination with water.
- Supplies of equipment should be available in each section to avoid the use of one central trolley where potential contamination can occur.

Clinical practice

- Hands should be decontaminated prior to treatment and between patients.
- Gloves and aprons must be worn for dressing changes and always changed between patients.
- Wounds should be exposed for only the minimum amount of time to promote healing and prevent cross contamination.
- Use single-use medication and dressings per patient.
- Dispose of waste via clinical waste system.
- Dispose of used water in a sluicing facility only; hand wash sinks must not be used.
- Wound swabs (when required) should be taken with swabs containing transport medium, stored at room temperature and sent to the laboratory as soon as possible.

Equipment decontamination guidelines for ulcer clinics

Table 10.2 at the end of this chapter is not exhaustive and should be used in conjunction with manufacturers' recommendations, locally defined policies and additional information provided within this chapter and Chapter 5.

FAMILY PLANNING AND WELL WOMAN CLINICS

The main risks of infection within the family planning clinic relate to staff exposure to body fluids and the risks from invasive procedures and the reuse of medical equipment for patients.

Theoretical risks of infection have been highlighted from the reuse of vaginal specula where viruses causing cervical cancer could be spread if adequate decontamination is not undertaken. Consequently this risk, together with the risk from blood-borne viruses, has led to specific guidelines being issued for any item entering the vagina (National Health Service 1994).

Decontamination guidelines for equipment and the environment

The list (Table 10.3 at the end of this chapter) is not exhaustive and should be used in conjunction with manufacturers' recommendations, locally defined policies and additional information provided within this chapter and Chapter 5. Items may alternatively be sent to local sterile supplies departments for decontamination.

PHYSIOTHERAPY

Physiotherapists are involved in hands-on patient care, have potential contact with wounds and open lesions, and use a variety of equipment during treatments. Additionally, treatment is likely to occur following recent inpatient care in hospital, such as following hip replacement or a stroke, where colonization or infection with multi-resistant organisms may have occurred.

The risk that infection could be transferred between staff, patients and equipment during physiotherapy is considered high (Ayliffe et al 2000). The risks are related to contamination of hands and equipment following contact with body fluids, including lesions and wounds.

Other risks include reuse of equipment between patients, such as flotron pressure cuffs and interferential.

Hand decontamination

As with all healthcare professionals hand washing is essential in reducing the risk of cross infection (Reybrouck 1986). Hands should be decontaminated after all patient contacts, after gloves have been used, before and after contact with wounds, and after dealing with contaminated equipment. In the patient's home, hand wash facilities may not be of a suitable standard. All physiotherapists should carry an alcoholic hand rub, gel or wipes.

Protective clothing

Gloves should be worn to protect the physiotherapists if contact with body fluids is likely, for example when collecting a sputum sample or using an internal interferential. Gloves should be worn when handling wound dressings or if undertaking any invasive procedure.

When wearing gloves for procedures involving use of equipment such as an internal interferential, care must be taken not to touch or handle equipment with contaminated gloves in order to reduce the likelihood of contamination.

Carrying and transporting equipment

Facilities should be available to allow easy transportation of used equipment from the health centre to other outreach clinics and the patient's home when using a person's own car. The use of a washable plastic container is recommended.

Decontamination of equipment

Table 10.4 (placed at the end of the chapter) is not exhaustive and should be used in conjunction with manufacturer's recommendations, locally defined policies and additional information provided within this chapter and Chapter 5.

MEDICAL LOANS

Basic principles

Basic principles of infection control are based on the use of practices and procedures that prevent or reduce the likelihood of infection being transmitted from contaminated body fluid or equipment (UK Health Departments 1998). They should be followed by all staff involved in healthcare, and apply equally to persons working with home loan equipment.

Protective clothing

Personal protective clothing should be supplied for all those involved in handling and decontaminating medical loaned equipment.

General purpose gloves such as household rubber gloves should be used for cleaning returned equipment or when coming into contact with contaminated surfaces or items. These gloves may be reused and should be washed whilst on the hands with detergent and warm water and hung to dry. They should be discarded if punctured or torn, or if there is evidence of deterioration. Single use disposable plastic aprons should be worn to protect clothing when there is a risk of clothes becoming wet. Face visors, goggles or spectacles are recommended when there is a risk of splashing body fluids onto the face, for example when cleaning instruments. These can be washed with general-purpose detergent, rinsed and dried after each use unless they are designated for single use only.

Environment

One of the major problems encountered by the medical loans service is having the facilities and a large enough environment to adequately decontaminate returned medical equipment for reuse such as wheelchairs and beds.

The medical loans system should be arranged in order for dirty and clean equipment to be kept separate and for cleaned stored equipment to be kept away from the decontamination area.

The medical loans environment should have designated areas and facilities for returned equipment, decontamination and drying of equipment, maintenance, and storage.

Returned equipment

The return area should be large enough to receive equipment and should be easily cleanable. Hand wash facilities and supplies of protective clothing should be readily available for staff.

Decontamination and drying of equipment

The decontamination area should be of a suitable size to house decontamination equipment. A deep sink separate from the hand wash sink should be provided for washing smaller items that cannot go through a heat washer. This should have an adjacent draining area to allow items to dry.

For larger items such as mattresses an easily cleanable rest surface should be provided. This should be cleaned and dried between each use. Some areas now have automated systems in use for larger items like bed frames, chairs and commodes.

Maintenance

A clean area should be set aside for inspection, repair and maintenance of equipment. All equipment should be adequately decontaminated prior to maintenance, and certificates demonstrating the method of decontamination should accompany the item (MDA 1995). This includes equipment that is returned to the manufacturer.

Storage

A damp-free storage area is required with shelving large enough to allow inverted storage of equipment. All items should be stored above floor level and the area kept free from pests and vermin.

Decontamination processes

See also Chapter 5.

Categorizing of equipment by risk

Medical loans should be categorized according to the risk they pose for patients. The usage rather than the item governs the risk. **Minimal or low-risk items** include those which are in contact with healthy skin or not in contact with patient (such as stair rails, bathroom equipment and wheelchairs). These require cleaning and drying. **Medium-risk** items are those which are in contact with mucous membranes (such as commodes, bedpans and respiratory equipment). Medium risk equipment should be either disposable or able to withstand heat or chemical disinfection. **High-risk** items are those in contact with a sterile part of the body. (High-risk items are not generally dealt with through the loan store.) These should be disposable, or if decontamination is required further advice should be sought from the infection control team.

Cleaning and disinfection

Cleaning

Instruments should be cleaned in a deep sink, designated for that purpose, in a solution of warm water and general-purpose detergent. If a brush is required to loosen debris it should be used whilst the instrument is below the surface of the water to avoid splashing. After washing, items should be rinsed well in clean water and dried with a disposable paper towel.

Disinfection

Disinfection with chemicals has limited value. Chemical disinfection is an unreliable process depending on the user's knowledge of concentrations and immersion times. Chemical disinfection should only be used if a heat treatment cannot be used. The disinfectants used should be those of proven value only (see Chapter 5). Disinfectants should not be used as routine cleaning agents.

Heat is the best method for decontamination of equipment and is most efficient in the presence of water as this will conduct the heat evenly over an item (Ayliffe et al 2000). For fabric items this is best achieved with a washing machine. A temperature of 65°C for ten minutes is required to achieve disinfection (DHSS 1987). A dryer should be available to dry equipment. For non-fabric smaller items, an automated washer should be used. The temperature required to disinfect is 90°C held for at least one minute (Ayliffe et al 2000). A steam cleaner should be used for decontaminating intricate areas of equipment.

Any item that is marked for single use only must not be re-processed unless the reprocessor can ensure the integrity and safety of the item (MDA 2000). Attempting to reuse without this guarantee will transfer legal liability for the item's safe performance from the manufacturer to the reprocessor.

Mattresses need to be checked on return prior to re-issuing for signs of leakage into the mattress material. All mattresses should be totally enclosed within a launderable cover that prevents leakage into the mattress.

Transportation

Systems need to be in place during transportation of the loaned equipment to ensure clean and dirty equipment do not come into contact with each other. Protective plastic bags or wrapping should be used for items leaving a patient's home. The transport vehicle design should be such that it allows easy cleaning and should be cleaned on a daily basis or after each return delivery.

The Medical Devices Agency (1998b) recommends a delivery programme whereby the vehicle is used for delivery only one day (or morning), and then for return of equipment the next day (or afternoon), followed by cleaning after each round. Facilities for hand washing and dealing with body fluid spillage should be available to the drivers.

VACCINATION CLINICS

Immunization of children and occasionally adults is carried out within the health centre. Additionally, Heaf testing, BCG and childhood immunizations are carried out in schools and influenza and pneumococcal immunization in residential homes.

For all procedures regarding vaccinations, please follow instructions given in the current Department of Health publication 'Immunization against Infectious Disease' (1996).

Prior to immunization taking place, the following procedures need to be established to ensure a successful immunization programme:

- Consent must be obtained and suitability for immunization established.
- Doctors and nurses providing immunization should have received training and be proficient in the appropriate techniques.
- Preparations must be made for the management of anaphylaxis and other immediate reactions.
- Vaccines should be stored in conditions that maximize their potency and assist vaccine efficacy rates (the cold chain).

The cold chain

The cold chain is a system designed to ensure that each vial of vaccine is maintained under appropriate conditions until its use. The effect of adverse temperatures on vaccines is cumulative, and failure to maintain the temperature anywhere along the chain from delivery to storage will decrease the vaccine potency.

Transport

Vaccines are transported from regional depots to health centres or general practice via this cold chain system. During transport refrigerated vans should be used. Vaccines may be sent through the postal system but should not be accepted by the health centre if more than 48 hours have elapsed since the time of posting, which should be clearly labelled. On arrival at the clinic or surgery the vaccines should be checked to ensure the cold chain has been maintained and that no damage has occurred to the vaccines. Within each area there needs to be a designated person who receives the vaccines and takes responsibility for their storage and handling. This person should have specific training for this, and in their absence there needs to be a nominated deputy.

Specific care should be taken not to over-stock on vaccines and to ensure a stock rotation to avoid wastage and reduced effectiveness from expired vaccines.

Storage

When vaccines are received, they should be immediately placed in the refrigerator that is specifically designed to store vaccines. Domestic fridges are not suitable for vaccine storage, and food, milk or specimens should not be placed in the vaccine fridge. Manufacturer's instructions should be observed at all times on storage requirements. Vaccines must not be stored below 0°C, as freezing can damage them. Storage in the refrigerator should allow air to circulate between packages, and vaccines should not be stored on shelves or in storage compartments on the fridge door. Defrosting of the fridge should take place regularly, while the vaccines are stored in an alternative fridge or insulating cool boxes.

Storage temperature

Accidental or unannounced disconnection of the electrical supply to the fridge can cause a break in the cold chain. Measures need to be in place to prevent this, such as switchless sockets and notices on switches not to switch them off. To keep an accurate measure of the temperature of the fridge, particularly overnight and over the weekends, a maximum and minimum thermometer should be used. This applies irrespective of what type of built-in mechanism is present within the fridge. The maximum and minimum temperature should be recorded daily, or if the fridge is used infrequently, at the start of any immunization session.

Vaccine usage

Reconstituted vaccines should be used according to manufacturers' instructions and used within the recommended period. Only the vaccine required for a session or part of a session should be taken out of the fridge. Single dose containers are preferred, but once opened, multi-dose vials should be disposed of at the end of the session. The skin does not need to be cleaned with alcohol or antiseptic before administration of the vaccine, but if it is to be used then the skin should be allowed to dry first.

Unused or partly used vials should be disposed of in the sharps containers and sent for incineration (HSC 1999). Outdated vaccines can be returned to the pharmacy.

Any vaccine spillage should be cleaned up immediately. The spillage should be treated as body fluid spillage and cleaned up using a hypochlorite solution (see body fluid spillages) and cleaned with general-purpose detergent. Any waste should be disposed of into the clinical waste system.

Vaccination offsite

When it is necessary to take vaccines to another venue such as a residential home or school, then a cool box or insulated container with frozen ice packs may be used. The vaccines must not be allowed to come into contact with the ice packs as this can cause the vaccine to freeze. During this session it is advised to work out of the cool box in order to keep the vaccine cool.

BCG clinics at schools

Heaf gun

- Use disposable plastic plates.
- The disposable plastic plates **must** be changed between each patient use.

- If the six needles are protruding from the head prior to use, the head must not be used and disposed of immediately in the sharps box.
- The Heaf gun handle should be cleaned at the end of each session with an alcohol wipe or if the handle becomes contaminated.

CONCLUSION

Within health centres infection control is everybody's business and is both an individual and collective responsibility. Policies and procedures for infection control and a good basic level of education and knowledge are essential to ensure protection for patients and all staff. Additionally, a shift towards a primary care-led service, emerging diseases, antimicrobial resistance (Health Service Circular 1999) and the development of new technologies all make an effective and manageable community infection control programme within community settings essential.

Table 10.1   Podiatry clinics: equipment decontamination guidelines

Item	Method of decontamination
Blacks file	Clean with general purpose detergent and warm water. Remove debris with a brush, then autoclave between each use. Store dry.
Blades	Single use only. Change between each patient use. Remove blades using suitable blade remover only. Dispose of in sharps box only.
Blade handles	After each use, clean with brush, warm water and general purpose detergent. Autoclave and store dry.
Cartridges (local anaesthetic)	Single use only. Change between each patient use. Store dry. Dispose of in sharps box only.
Cleaning brushes	After use on instruments, the brush should be rinsed under running water and autoclaved along with the instruments.
Debris tray	After each use, wipe with general purpose detergent and warm water. If visibly contaminated wipe with alcohol wipe.
Foot rests	These should be cleaned at the start and after each session or when visibly contaminated, using water and general purpose detergent.
Nail instruments: burrs, nippers, files	Clean with general-purpose detergent and warm water. Use scrubbing brush to remove debris, rinse and autoclave. Store dry. Ultrasonic cleaner can be used, if available, prior to autoclaving.
Nail surgery	Sterile packs must be used.
Needles	Single use. Do not resheath unless needle guards are used. Dispose of in sharps containers.

(continued)

Table 10.1   (*continued*)

Item	Method of decontamination
Scissors for wound dressings	Use sterile only. After use wash in warm water and general purpose detergent, rinse, dry and autoclave.
Surfaces/instrument trays	These should be cleaned at the end of each session and prior to nail surgery. They should be wiped with alcohol wipes.
Skin preparation (patient's skin)	Use alcohol with chlorhexidine, allow to dry. For nail surgery/skin surgery, an iodine solution may also be used.
On domiciliary visits	
Hand hygiene	Use alcoholic hand rub, wipe or gel on physically clean hands and between tasks. A soap and water wash followed by drying is required to remove dirt, soil and alcohol solution build-up.
Instruments	Instruments should be placed in an instrument tray with lid. On return to clinic, wash instruments tray and lid using running water and general purpose detergent; dry, rinse and autoclave. Store dry. Ultrasonic cleaner may be used.
Nail surgery	Use sterile packs only.
Operator's bag	Should be kept clean, tidy and free from debris. Wipe with warm water and detergent after each session. Whilst working keep bag closed to prevent contamination.
Sharps disposal	All sharps must be disposed of safely in an approved sharps container. A transportable, securely sealed box must be used.

Table 10.2   Ulcer clinics: equipment decontamination guidelines

Item	Method
Blood pressure cuffs	Where possible protect the leg with a plastic sheet. Use only washable, detachable sleeves. If visibly contaminated, and after each session, send to laundry for cleaning.
Buckets	Use only with liners. After each session rinse with warm water and general purpose detergent, dry thoroughly using disposable paper towels, and store dry, inverted and in pyramids.
Bucket liners	Single use only. Change between each patient use – dispose of in a clinical waste bag.
Doppler machines	After each use wipe with large alcohol wipe.
Scissors (nursing, bandage, cutting)	Clean after each use with alcohol wipe and allow to air dry.
Swabs (from ulcers)	Swabs can be taken when the wound dressing is removed. Wounds do not need to be cleaned prior to swabbing.
Environment	
Floor protection	Prior to commencement of each clinic the floor should be protected with plastic sheets. If excessive splashing, the sheet must be changed between patient use.
Footstools	Between each use, these should be cleaned with general purpose detergent and hot water and dried.
Water (disposal)	Water used for soaking bandages prior to removal must be disposed of in a designated sluice area in a separate sink, other than that designated for handwashing.

Table 10.3 Family planning/well woman clinics: decontamination guidelines

Equipment	Method
IUD insertion	Sterile gloves must be worn. Use only packs that are sterile prior to use. Prepacked sterile packs are recommended. Do not autoclave on site.
Instruments	If single use, discard into clinical waste system. If re-usable, wash in warm water and general purpose detergent, rinse and dry. Autoclave and store dry.
Vaginal diaphragms (caps)	Wash in warm water and general purpose detergent, rinse and dry. Autoclave and store dry.
Vaginal specula	Use disposable where possible. If re-usable, immediately wash in warm water and general purpose detergent after use, rinse and dry. Autoclave and store dry.

Table 10.4 Physiotherapy clinics: decontamination guidelines

Item	Method
Flotron pressure machine cuffs	Send for laundering after each use.
Interferential: internal application	A disposable sleeve must be used to protect the internal applicator. After use it should be disposed of as clinical waste. The holder of the internal applicator should be wiped with a large alcohol wipe after each use.
Interferential: external application	Sponges used should be single patient use only. The electrodes should be wiped with a large alcohol wipe after each use.
Perinometers	Where manufacturers recommend the probe is for reuse, a condom should be used and removed after use. The probe should then be cleaned with an alcohol wipe after use.
Suction machines:	
Catheter	Disposable, single use.
Tubing	Single patient use only. Replace regularly.
Machine	After patient use return machine for decontamination via medical loans.
Splints	Wash with warm water and detergent, rinse and dry.
Vaginal cones	Single patient use is preferred. Any reusable item placed in the vagina is subject to specific decontamination guidelines and must be sterilized in between use (General Medical Safety Information 1994). The cones must be sterilized after use on individual patients. During use for an individual, the cones can be washed in detergent and water.
Vaginal cone shells	Single patient use only. Dispose of after use.
Vaginal cone weights	If reusable, wash in warm water and detergent, rinse and dry. Then sterilize. *Patient information*: Patient should be advised to wash the cone after each use with warm water and detergent and dry using disposable tissue/paper towel.
Ultrasounds	Wipe head with alcohol wipe between use.
Wax therapy	Patient's hands must be washed prior to insertion in the wax. Remove jewellery such as rings. Patients with open lesions must not use the wax. Any wax that is removed should be heated prior to return to the bath.

REFERENCES

Ansari S A, Springthorpe U S, Sattar S A et al 1991 Comparison of cloth, paper and warm air drying in eliminating viruses and bacteria from washed hands. American Journal of Infection Control 9: 243–249

Ayliffe G A J, Fraise A P, Geddes A M, Mitchell K 2000 Control of Hospital Infection. A Practical Handbook, 4th edn. Chapman & Hall Medical, London
British Standards Institution 1992 British Standard BS 2092 Specification for eye protectors

for industrial and non-industrial uses. BSI, London

Burrows J G, Millar N A, Hay J, Stevenson R 1996 Health and Safety issues in the use of podiatry nail drills. Journal of British Podiatric Medicine 51(11): 161–164

Community Infection Control Nurses Network 1999 Survey of Community Infection Control Nurses in the United Kingdom 1998. CICNA, Bathgate

Department of Health 1987 Product and Consumer Protection Act. DoH, London

Department of the Environment 1991 Waste Management – duty of care. A code of practice. HMSO, London

Department of Health 1996 Immunisation against infectious disease. HMSO, London

Department of Health 1999 Health Service Circular HSC 1999/049. Resistance to Antibiotics and other Antimicrobial Agents. HMSO, London

Department of Health and Social Security 1987 Hospital laundry arrangements for used and infected linen. HSC (37) 30. HMSO, London

Department of Health 2000a Guidelines on post exposure for health care workers occupationally exposed to HIV. HMSO, London

Department of Health 2000b HSC 2000/032 Decontamination of Medical Devices. DoH, London

European Commission 1996a European Standards Specification for Personal Eye Protectors. Industrial and non industrial. EN 166. EC, Brussels

European Commission 1996b European Standards. Specification for Personal Facemask Protectors. Industrial and non industrial. EN 149. EC, Brussels

European Commission 1997 European Standards for Sterile Supply Departments EN 46002. EC, Brussels

European Commission 1998 European Standards for Sharps Containers EN 3291. EC, Brussels

Gould D 1994 The significance of hand drying in the prevention of infection. Nursing Times 90(47): 33–35

Health and Safety Commission, Health Services Advisory Committee 1999 Safe Disposal of Clinical Waste. HSE Books, Sudbury

Health and Safety Executive, Health Service Advisory Committee 1991 Safe working and the prevention of infection in clinical laboratories. HMSO, London

Health and Safety Executive 1992 Personal Protective Equipment at Work Regulations. (EEC Directive): HMSO, London

Health and Safety Executive, Advisory Committee on Dangerous Pathogens 1995 Protection against blood borne infections in the workplace: HIV and Hepatitis. HMSO, London

HMSO 1974 Health and Safety at Work Act (1974). HMSO, London

Infection Control Nurses Association 2002 Glove Usage Guidelines. ICNA, Bathgate

Medical Devices Agency 1995 Decontamination of medical devices and equipment prior to inspection service or repair. MDA SN 9516. DoH, London

Medical Devices Agency 1996 The purchase, operation and maintenance of benchtop steam sterilizers (MDA DB 9605). Medical Devices Agency, London

Medical Devices Agency 1998a The validation and periodic testing of benchtop vacuum steam sterilizers (MDA DB 9804). Medical Devices Agency, London

Medical Devices Agency 1998b Medical device and equipment management for hospital and community organisations (MDA DB 9801). Medical Devices Agency, London

Medical Devices Agency 2000 Single use medical devices: implication and consequences of re-use (MDA DB 2000(04)). Medical Devices Agency, London

Millar N A, Burrows J G, Hay J, Stevenson R 1996 Putative risks of ocular infection for chiropodists and podiatrists. Journal of British Podiatric Medicine 51(11): 158–160

Miller C H, Palenik C J 1998 Infection Control and Management of Hazardous Materials for the Dental Team, 2nd edn. Mosby, St. Louis

Mishriki S F, Law D J W, Jeffery P J 1990 Factors affecting the incidence of post operative wound infection. Journal of Hospital Infection 11: 253–262

Moffatt C J, Franks P J, Oldroyd M et al 1992 Community clinics for leg ulcers and their impact on healing. British Medical Journal 305(5): 1389–1392

National Health Service 1994 FPN 654 General Medical Services Safety Information. Instruments and appliances used in the vagina and cervix: Recommended methods for decontamination. DoH, London

NHS Estates 2001 Standards for environmental cleanliness in healthcare. HMSO, London

NHS Management Executive 1993 Decontamination of equipment prior to inspection, service or repair. HSG (93) 26. HMSO, London

Parker L J 1999 A practical guide to glove usage. British Journal of Nursing 8(7): 420–424

Reybrouck G 1986 Handwashing and hand disinfection. Journal of Hospital Infection 8(1): 5–23

Royal College of Nursing 2000 Good practice in infection control: guidance for nurses working in general practice. Publication code 000 866 RCN. RCN, London

Simon D, Frsak L, Kinsella A et al 1996 Community Leg Ulcer Clinics: a comparitive study in two health authorities. British Medical Journal 312: 1648

Society of Chiropodists and Podiatrists 1998 Statement on Instrument Sterilization. Society of Chiropodists and Podiatrists, London

Thomlinson D 1987 To clean or not to clean? Nursing Times 83(9): 71–75

UK Health Departments 1998 Guidance for Clinical Health Care Workers: Protection Against Infection with Blood-borne Viruses. Recommendations of the Expert Advisory Group on AIDS and the Advisory Group on Hepatitis. DoH, London

11

Dental practices

A. Fuller

INTRODUCTION

In recent years, there has been increasing concern in dentistry with regard to how infection control and universal precautions are integrated into clinical practice.

Implementing safe and realistic infection control procedures requires the full compliance of the whole dental team. It is the responsibility of the individual dentist to ensure that all members of the dental team understand and implement infection control strategies (Coates and Gaffney 1996).

Infections such as Hepatitis B and C, together with the public concern over Human Immunodeficiency Virus, have been highlighted through incidents of cross infection between dental personnel. These transmissions have led to the close examination of how infection control principles are employed within dentistry.

In an attempt to standardize the dental profession's approach to infection control, the USA Centers for Disease Control first published 'Recommended Infection Control Practices for Dentistry' in 1986 (CDC 1986). In response the British Dental Association (BDA) addressed the issue within the UK and adopted the use of Universal Precautions. These precautions apply to blood and other body fluids containing visible blood. Therefore, blood and certain body fluids of all patients are considered potentially infectious from blood-borne pathogens. Universal precautions are intended to prevent parenteral, mucous membrane and non-intact skin exposures of healthcare workers to blood-borne pathogens.

However, the impetus to actually acknowledge these recommendations came following the famous Acer–Bergalis case in which transmission of human immuodeficiency virus occurred in dental practice (Ciesielski et al 1992). The reporting of this case in the media caused generalized patient fear and paranoia. Handpieces and their lack of sterilization were implicated in this case as the first possible transmission of HIV to a patient from a healthcare worker.

Since this, a number of publications have been made available to increase the knowledge and compliance in the control of infection within dental practice. To support the adoption of universal precautions and infection control protocol, legislation such as the Control of Substances Hazardous to Health (COSHH) (1999), and directives from the Department of Health and governing dental bodies have been developed.

PROTECTIVE CLOTHING

Glove use

Risks have become apparent with the recognition that certain dental procedures are potential sources of transmission of blood-borne viruses. Therefore, increased awareness of the need to wear gloves as part of universal precautions has become part of normal clinical practice.

Gloves protect not only team members from direct contact with micro-organisms in the patient's mouth, but also from contaminated surfaces, and offer protection to patients from micro-organisms found on the hands of the dental team. Instituting the general use of gloves also demonstrates to the patient that the dental team is taking infection control precautions.

Intact skin is an excellent barrier. However, a study conducted by Allen and Organ (1982) discovered that 40% of dentists had micro-lesions on their hands and that patient's blood could be retained under the fingernails of a dental team member for several days.

The selection and use of gloves is an issue which requires thorough assessment, not only by the dentist and dental personnel, but also the patients exposed to the latex. The major risks relate to sensitization from the proteins, accelerators and cornstarch used to assist in the donning and removal of gloves. It is therefore essential that purchasers are aware of the risks, subsequent management and alternatives if significant risks of litigation are to be avoided (ICNA 2002).

Gloves used for patient care are not to be reused on a subsequent patient. Gloves are a single use item only (MDA 1995). Surgical or examination gloves should not be washed before use; nor should they be washed or disinfected for reuse. Washing of gloves causes the penetration of liquids through undetected holes in the gloves and a deterioration of the glove material by disinfecting agents (CDC 1993, Miller and Palenik 1994).

As a general rule, **sterile gloves** are to protect the patient whereas the use of **non-sterile latex gloves** protects dental personnel. These are suitable for the following procedures (CDC, 1993):

- examinations
- routine restorative procedures
- prophylaxis
- prosthetic and endontic treatments
- radiography
- laboratory work – handling impressions, etc.

On leaving the chair-side during patient care, gloves should be removed and a fresh pair donned. This prevents contamination of any surfaces and possible contamination to the patient's mouth.

Torn or punctured gloves must be removed as soon as possible, hands washed, and the gloves replaced by a new pair.

Heavy-duty gloves should be worn for the handling and processing of instruments following use. These are reusable and stored dry.

Gloves should be worn when there is a potential to be in contact with items contaminated with pathogenic micro-organisms such as when handling contaminated waste, tissue, or teeth and containers of blood, saliva and other infectious material, or there is a risk of spillage or splash.

Gloves should not be seen as a substitute for basic infection control measures. Appropriate hand washing and handcare are particularly important in order to reduce risk and maintain skin integrity.

Face protection

Visors, face shields, masks and protective eye-wear are essential protective agents. Occasions when they are required appear in Box 11.1. They provide protection to the operator's face from micro-organisms that may be present in sprays, splashes and aerosol particles of body fluids or other potentially infectious materials and cause injury (Garrett et al 1993, Miller and Palenik 1994). Procedures which generate particles via the turbine handpiece, ultrasonic scaler and air/water syringe may damage the eyes of the operator during dental procedures (Wood 1992). Although dentists may wear their own glasses, these do not offer the same protection as safety glasses or visors.

For patients who are known to be pulmonary tuberculosis positive, the use of a particulate filter respiratory mask, which offers optimum protection, should be considered.

Aprons/gowns

As described in BDA Guidelines 1996, 'a wide variety of clothing is worn in many practices and usually represents the corporate image'. Short-sleeved gowns or tunics allow the forearms to be washed as part of the hand washing routine. Surgery clothing is required to be removed on leaving the clinical area or surgery premises. Surgery clothing should not be worn in eating areas. Use of disposable plastic aprons is advisable for the cleaning of instruments, or if there is a risk of

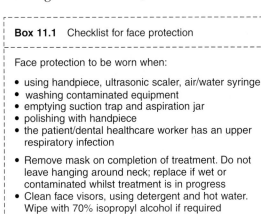

Box 11.1 Checklist for face protection

Face protection to be worn when:

• using handpiece, ultrasonic scaler, air/water syringe
• washing contaminated equipment
• emptying suction trap and aspiration jar
• polishing with handpiece
• the patient/dental healthcare worker has an upper respiratory infection

• Remove mask on completion of treatment. Do not leave hanging around neck; replace if wet or contaminated whilst treatment is in progress
• Clean face visors, using detergent and hot water. Wipe with 70% isopropyl alcohol if required

spillages or blood splashes contaminating clothing. Uniforms and gowns should be changed at least daily and when they become visibly contaminated with blood. Clothing should be made from a material which can withstand washing with detergent using the hot wash cycle of a domestic washing machine at 65° and above.

Hand washing

For many routine dental procedures such as examinations, and for non-surgical procedures, hand washing with plain soap and water is adequate. The use of liquid soap dispensers is preferred. Soap and water with thorough drying will remove transient micro-organisms acquired directly or indirectly from patient contact (Horton 1995). For surgical procedures an antimicrobial surgical handscrub is recommended, such as chlorhexidine 4%. Hand washing facilities should be designed or identified solely for this use to avoid cross contamination.

SURGERY DESIGN

A number of considerations are required for the layout of the dental surgery. Zoning (Fig. 11.1) is a recognized method of function, and one which influences the design of the surgery and working arrangements. Zoning uses a model identifying three areas of the dentist's working space. The primary source of contamination being the oral cavity, items entering this area are by definition critical or semi-critical, whilst the third area of the zone is the outer area and is defined as a lower priority and therefore facilitates the use of low-level disinfection. Using this identified method of working allows for a one-way flow of contaminated instruments and other items.

Structural considerations consist of:

• Appropriate work surfaces which are seamless, with covered ends which prevent the accumulation of contaminated material and facilitate cleaning.
• Two wash basins identified – one for hand washing and the second for dirty procedures. Elbow- or foot-operated taps are necessary.

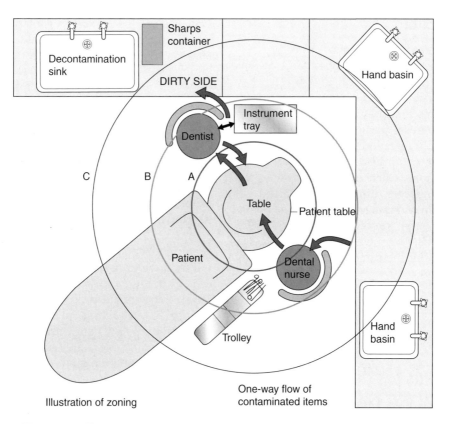

Figure 11.1 The dental surgery: zoning to ensure one-way flow of contaminated items.

- Access for the operator to essential equipment, e.g. bracket table, suction lines, and three-in-one syringe.
- A recognized separate area for the decontaminating and sterilizing of equipment. This should be away from the surgery and must include a sink ultrasonic washer autoclave and work on the principle of 'dirty to clean' (Wood 1992).
- Floor coverings that are impervious, seamless and easy to clean. Carpeting should be avoided.

Reducing environmental contamination

During dental procedures aerosol and environmental contamination can be limited by ensuring that the surgery is well ventilated, preferably by a mechanical means. When selecting suction and aspiration equipment it is best practice to purchase apparatus which will discharge directly into a waste outlet in order to reduce the potential for accidental spillage. High-speed aspirators should be exhausted externally so as to avoid the spread of potentially infectious material into the surgery (UK Health Departments 1998). External discharge vents need to be sited in such a way as not to compromise the general public. These must be maintained as directed by the manufacturer's guidance. Using this system during use of rotary equipment and air/water reduces the escape of salivary aerosols and splatter from the patient's mouth as well as reducing contamination to the dental team and nearby surfaces.

Use of the rubber dam has been recognized as reducing the number of micro-organisms escaping a patient's mouth via aerosol or splatter. Simultaneous use of the high-speed aspirator and rubber dam provides the best approach to minimizing dental aerosol (Marshall 1998).

In association with the above evidence it is suggested that antimicrobial mouth rinse such as chlorhexidine gluconate be used (Molinari and Molinari 1992), which can reduce the number of micro-organisms on the surface of mucous membranes prior to surgery or injection, therefore reducing the incidence of septicaemia or local infection.

DENTAL EQUIPMENT AND INSTRUMENTS

The dental unit and other items of equipment may become contaminated with blood and saliva during their use. When purchasing the equipment it is important that:

- it is easy to clean and maintain
- dental chairs have seamless surfaces
- controls are membrane-covered
- non-retraction valves are in place
- easy-clean filters are in place.

Instruments and other items that normally penetrate soft tissue or bone, for example scalers and surgical burrs, are generally reusage and must be sterilized after each use, or be discarded if single use. Instruments and equipment that come into contact with intact skin, which may be exposed to contamination either by hands or body fluids, should be disinfected as directed by the manufacturer's instructions. It is therefore essential that all equipment be processed as directed by the manufacturer and according to risk assessment. Inappropriate use of disinfectants and antiseptics must be discouraged. (Refer also to Chapter 5.)

Where disposables are possible, these include:

- burrs
- scalpels
- matrix bands
- aspirator tips
- saliva ejectors
- three-in-one tips
- bibs
- impression trays
- beakers.

These items **must not** be reprocessed but disposed of as single use.

The dental unit water supply

Water lines and airlines should be fitted with anti-retraction valves, which help prevent contamination. When water is allowed to stand within the line, some bacteria may attach to and accumulate on the inside of the lines forming a biofilm; therefore as water is released through the handpiece, ultrasonic scaler and air/water syringe bacteria are subsequently released into the patient's mouth. Good practice directs the dental team to discharge all water lines for at least two minutes prior to their use at the start of the day. This will remove any stagnant water left overnight; there should be a thirty-second discharge following the treatment of each individual patient (Samaranayake 1993).

Lewis and Boe (1992) advocate three minutes running time to decontaminate the water lines between individual patient treatments. The latter recommendation is somewhat impractical and time-consuming should there be a busy clinical session, but is a consideration when the clinic has ceased, for example at lunch.

The presence of micro-organisms within the dental water supply has been implicated as a potential for cross infection in the immunocompromised patient. Jensen et al (1997) investigated the presence of *Pseudomonas aeruginosa* in dental water supplies and the possible association of positive sputum to the organism of patients with cystic fibrosis. A reservoir for sterile water can be inserted into the existing water line at the base of the high-speed handpiece and air/water syringe. Using this system bypasses the unit water and provides sterile water through the handpiece and syringe (Fayle and Pollard 1996, Williams et al 1996). The Centers for Disease Control (CDC) recommended this method be adopted as common practice within the USA, and it has been adopted by the American Dental Association (ADA) since 1995 (Waggoner 1996).

Installation of this system also allows for the disinfection of the system and reduction of biofilms within the tubing of the unit. Disinfection should be carried out as per local policy, although a hypochloride solution is generally recommended.

Suction systems

It has been postulated that evacuation or suction systems in dentistry have been implicated as a source of cross infection between patients via the back flow of bacteria dislodged in the salivary ejector tubing. A study conducted by Barbeau et al (1998) examined the effect of back pressures upon the evacuation system tubing. Pathogens such as staphylococci and *Pseudomonas aeruginosa* were isolated from the biofilm. They concluded that despite evidence to support cross contamination, there was a potential for pathogens to shed from tubing biofilms following back flow. The management and subsequent care of these systems by regular disinfection was deemed essential.

Decontamination of the aspiration equipment should be conducted at the end of the day, using a non-corrosive, non-foaming disinfectant as recommended by the manufacturer and aspirated via the tubing. Certain dental units have detachable aspirator tubing, which can be removed and cleaned within the sluice or designated dirty area. This involves washing, rinsing and ensuring the equipment is in working order.

Most aspirator systems are plumbed into the main sewer system. However, mobile aspirator and older equipment systems require their contents to be emptied manually using a controlled method to avoid unnecessary aerosol contamination. Appropriate protective clothing must be used and the contents emptied into an allocated sluice sink or directly down the toilet. The surgery sink **must not** be used for this procedure. Suction bottles are kept clean and dry prior to and during use. No disinfectant should be added. Where possible, disposable suction liners should be used and disposed of as clinical waste.

Air/water syringe

The air/water syringe is one of the most used instruments within the dental unit. It is necessary for irrigating, removing debris, and drying cavities and teeth. This instrument becomes contaminated after use, particularly within the lumen of the syringe tip. Syringes are available with detachable and autoclavable tips. However, their fine lumen makes this equipment difficult to reprocess in a benchtop autoclave. The cleaning process for syringe tips prior to sterilization is complicated by their fine internal lumen (Martin 1998, Merchant and Molinari 1991). Disposable three-in-one tips are available and should be considered.

Dental handpieces

During use they are in contact with blood and saliva which collects on the external handpiece casing and may enter the handpiece chamber via the bur mounting causing internal contamination (Kellet and Holbrook 1980). The Lewis and Boe (1992) study investigated the behaviour of a dye solution, simulating patient material, when either injected into high-speed dental handpieces or waterlines or externally applied to the equipment. They identified that dye remained within the turbine chamber and was expelled during subsequent uses. Consequently **sterilization is essential** for reprocessing. However, Anderson et al (1999) evaluate the use of benchtop autoclaves for the reprocessing of hollow instruments such as high-speed turbines. Once cleaned and when lubrication had taken place prior to autoclaving, a level of reduction was observed.

Handpieces should be flushed with clean water, cleaned, dried, lubricated and autoclaved after each use according to manufacturer's instructions.

Light curing unit

Light curing units include a fibre-optic tip and have the potential to become contaminated during use. For those unable to be processed via the autoclave, the tip must be cleaned using a damp cloth containing detergent prior to disinfection. This should include both the handle and the light-curing tip.

Barriers may be applied to the equipment. Chong et al (1998) examined five methods of barrier. Cellophane wrap and plastic gloves were recommended since these barriers allowed the highest light intensity output. Once the barrier has been used it must be removed and disposed of as clinical waste.

Endontic and rotary instruments

Thorough cleaning and storage of all equipment is essential. All equipment must be cleaned using detergent and water prior to sterilization. All reusable burrs should be cleaned via an ultra-sonic bath. Quality control checks should be made to observe for damage and rusting.

Radiology

Following use of the X-ray machine all surfaces must be disinfected, and equipment used to develop radiographs cleaned as appropriate. Care should be taken when taking radiographs – gloves should be worn.

Cleaning of surfaces and equipment

During patient care, surfaces and equipment have the potential to become contaminated either as a result of direct contact or by aerosol parti-cles. Effective cleaning and disinfection are aided by zoning (Fig. 11.1). Therefore, cleaning of areas most likely to be contaminated is carried out following individual patient treatment. It must be stressed that the use of disinfectants and anti-septics must be controlled for cleaning purposes. A solution of detergent and water is adequate in most instances and may be followed by an alcohol (such as 70% Isopropanol) wipe. Blood spillage requires the use of 1% hypochlorite granules or solution (10 000 ppm available chlorine) applied directly to the area followed by detergent and water.

Impervious disposable coverings may be used on equipment which is difficult to clean such as air/water syringe tubing, non-flush chair controls. These must be changed between seeing patients and the underlying surface cleaned. However, their use can be costly and is not always necessary.

Spittoon and waste filters are decontaminated using a 1:10 000 hypochlorite solution at least daily or following heavy blood contamination. The bowl should be mechanically rinsed after each patient use.

Suction traps are cleaned as required and at least daily; adherence to body substance isolation precautions is essential.

Sharps

Used needles and other sharp instruments should not be sheared, bent or broken or re-sheathed by hand. Unique to dentistry is the reusable syringe; these are required to deliver local anaesthetic, and rely on re-sheathing the needle to remove the needle and cartridge safely. All dental personnel should be immunized for Hepatitis B and made aware of Hepatitis C should a needlestick or sharps injury occur. A local sharps policy must be made available incorporating information to access medical intervention. For the potential of occupa-tional exposure to HIV, ensure there is a mecha-nism in which to access post-exposure prophylaxis for the potential acquisition of HIV. Always ensure incidents are documented.

See Box 11.2 for a comprehensive list regard-ing sharps safety.

Decontamination of impressions

Any piece of equipment used within the oral cav-ity, orally soiled prosthetic devices or impressions are a potential source of cross infection. Conse-quently, impressions, prosthetic and orthodontic appliances must be carefully cleaned and disin-fected (Box 11.3) before they are sent to the labora-tory (BDA 1996). Most prostheses and appliances cannot withstand standard heat sterilization procedures, due to potential altering of the

---

Box 11.2 Prevention of inoculation injuries

- Avoid hand contact with rotating instruments
- A disarmed or a one-handed technique must be used to re-sheathe syringes
- Take care when passing syringes with needle
- Take care handling extracted teeth. Dispose of into designated sharps box
- Ensure burrs are firmly attached to handpiece
- Between use ensure local anaesthetic is rendered safe and cannot become contaminated. Dispose of immediately into a designated sharps box
- Take care when handling orthodontic bands and matrix
- Ultrasonic scalers, handpieces are positioned inwards on the bracket table whilst not in use
- Do not bend needles
- Place endontic files directly into designated receiver
- Ensure sharps box is not overfilled, is correctly closed and labelled with place of origin

---

Box 11.3 Disinfection of impressions and prostheses

- Rinse under running water (not in a hand wash basin) to remove debris, saliva and blood
- Repeat the process if necessary
- Immerse into solution used, e.g. Hypochlorite or commercially prepared as per manufacturer's directions
- Rinse and handle as normal
- Ensure a statement of decontamination accompanies the article prior to sending to the laboratory
- Solutions are freshly made daily and changed throughout the day when used excessively
- Containers are rinsed and stored dry when not in use

---

impression. As an alternative, articles are immersed into a suitable disinfecting solution as directed by the manufacturer. These are now generally commercially-prepared solutions. Disinfectants should not be sprayed onto the surface of the impression as contact is not guaranteed and spraying also creates an inhalation risk.

This procedure is not universally acknowledged throughout dental practice. Blair and Wassell (1996) conclude that there is no universally recognized impression disinfection protocol and this is reflected in the diverse decontamination procedures currently carried out.

CONCLUSION

The application of infection control to dentistry is one which is paramount and which requires the compliance of all the dental team in implementing safe and realistic practices. This ensures that issues of infection control are addressed and every effort is made to achieve a safe environment for both the patient and the individual operator.

REFERENCES

Allen A L, Organ R J 1982 Occult blood accumulation under fingernails: a mechanism for the spread of blood borne infections. Journal of American Dental Association 105: 455–459

Anderson H K, Fiehn N E, Larsen T 1999 Effect of steam sterilization inside the turbine chambers of dental turbines. Oral Surgery, Oral Medicine, Oral Pathology, Oral Radiology and Endontics 87(92): 184–188

Barbeau J, Ten Bokum L, Gauthier C, Prévost A P 1998 Cross contamination potential of saliva ejectors used in dentistry. Journal of Hospital Infection 40(4): 303–311.

Blair F M, Wassell R W 1996 A survey of the methods of disinfection of dental impressions used in the UK. British Dental Journal 108: 369–375

British Dental Association 1996 Infection Control in Dentistry Advice Sheet A12. BDA, London.

CDC 1986 Recommended infection control practices for dentistry. Morbidity and Mortality Weekly Report 35(15): 237–242

CDC 1993 Recommended infection control practices for dentistry (update). Morbidity and Mortality Weekly Report 42(RR-8): 1–12

Chong S L, Lam Y K, Lee F K et al 1998 Effect of various infection control methods for light cure units on the cure of composite resins. Operative Dentistry 23(3): 150–154

Ciesielski C, Marianos D, Chin-Yih O U et al 1992 Transmission of Human Immunodeficiency virus in dental practice. Annals Internal Medicine 116: 798–805

Coates E A, Gaffney A 1996 Infection control in practice. Annals of Royal Australasian College of Dental Surgery, April 13, 115–118

Department of Health 1997 Guidance on post exposure prophylaxis for health care workers occupationally exposed to HIV. PL/CO (97) 1, 27 June (Letter). Department of Health, London

Fayle S, Pollard M A 1996 Decontamination of dental unit water systems: a review of current recommendations. British Dental Journal 181(10): 369–372

Fuller A 1998 An Investigation to Identify if the General Dental Practitioner Complies with The Principles of Infection Control. Unpublished.

Garrett S J, Robinson J K 1993 Disposable protective eyewear devices for healthcare providers: how important are they and will available designs be used? Journal of Occupational Medicine 35(10): 1043–1047

Health and Safety Executive 1999 Control of Substances Hazardous to Health Regulations (1999)

Horton R 1995 Handwashing: the fundamental infection control principle. British Journal of Nursing 4(16): 926–933

Infection Control Nurses Association 2002 Glove Usage Guidelines. ICNA, Bathgate

Jensen E T, Giwercman B, Ojeniyi B et al 1997 Epidemiology of *Pseudomonas aeruginosa* in Cystic Fibrosis and the possible role of contamination by dental equipment. Journal of Hospital Infection 36(2): 117–122

Kellet M, Holbrook W P 1980 Bacterial contamination of dental handpieces. Journal of Dentistry 8: 249–253

Lewis D L, Boe R K 1992 Cross infection risks associated with current procedures for using high speed dental handpieces. Journal of Clinical Microbiology 30: 401–406

Marshall K 1998 Rubber dam. British Dental Journal 184(5): 218–220

Martin M V 1998 The air/water syringe: a potential source of microbial contamination. British Dental Journal 184(6): 278–279

Medical Devices Agency 1995a The reuse of medical devices supplied for single use only. DBI 9501. Medical Devices Agency, London

Merchant V A, Molinari J A 1991 A study on the adequacy of sterilization of air/water syringe tips. Clinical Prevention Dentistry 13: 20–22

Miller C H, Palenik C J 1994 Infection Control Management of Hazardous Materials for the Dental Team. Mosby, St. Louis

Molinari J A, Molinari C E 1992 Is mouth rinsing before dental procedures worthwhile? Journal of the American Dental Association 123: 75–80

Samaranayake L 1993 Handpiece and water line decontamination and HIV transmission. A Critique. Dental Update, March: 53–56

UK Health Departments 1998 Guidance for Clinical Health Care Workers: Protection Against Infection with Blood-borne Viruses. Recommendations of the Expert Advisory Group on AIDS and the Advisory Group on Hepatitis

Waggoner M B 1996 The New CDC Surgical Water Recommendations. Why they should be implemented and what they require. Compendium of Continuing Education in Dentistry 17(6): 612–614

Williams J F, Molinari J A, Andrews N 1996 Microbial contamination of dental water lines. Origins and characteristics. Compendium of Continuing Education in Dentistry 17(6): 538–540

Wood P R 1992 Cross Infection in Dentistry. A Practical Illustrated Guide. Wolfe, Aylesbury

12

Pregnancy and childbirth

C. Fry

INTRODUCTION

Midwifery and obstetric care differs from other forms of patient care, in that it concerns two patients – the pregnant women and a fetus and then a mother and her newborn infant. The majority of pregnant and post-partum women are healthy with no underlying medical pathology, and do not have the risk factors that can make other groups of patients susceptible to acquiring infections.

BACKGROUND

The importance of preventing and controlling infection was first recognized almost two centuries ago. Ignaz Semmelweis, a doctor working at the great free Vienna Lying-in Hospital in the nineteenth century, noted that a significant number of women were dying of puerperal infection. Semmelweis undertook an epidemiological study that demonstrated that women cared for by medical students had the highest rates of infection and maternal deaths (Semmelweis 1981). Further investigation revealed that women who had their babies prior to admission had the lowest infection rate. Semmelweis noted that the medical students were attending women in labour directly after post-mortem examinations without decontaminating their hands. The introduction of hand washing with chlorinated lime water after performing a post-mortem dramatically reduced the incidence of puerperal sepsis. At the time, Semmelweis was ostracized by his colleagues, who did not agree with his findings. However, two centuries later, most experts agree that adequate hand decontamination is one of the most important infection control measures for protecting patients and healthcare professionals from acquiring infection. Obstetric infections and maternal mortality remained high until the introduction of the first antibiotics, along with improvements in other aspects of obstetric care.

The effect of pregnancy

Although the majority of pregnant women have no underlying medical pathology, pregnancy can make women more susceptible to infection. For example, increased oestrogen and progesterone production cause ureteric dilatation, which together with the pressure of the uterus on the bladder predisposes to urinary tract infections. Chest infections in later pregnancy may be more severe as the diaphragm becomes elevated. Within the bacterial flora of the female lower reproductive tract, there are some organisms that can cause infection. These include *Staphylococcus aureus, S. epidermidis, Escherichia coli.*

Other risk factors that can increase susceptibility to infection include low socio-economic status, multiple sexual partners, poor personal hygiene, alcohol and drug abuse, smoking and poor nutrition. Underlying medical conditions, such as diabetes mellitus and corticosteroid therapy, can also increase this risk. There are also factors that protect a woman and her fetus from infection. During pregnancy, the amount and viscosity of cervical mucus increases, forming a 'plug' in the endocervical canal to prevent ascending infection. The amniotic membranes form a protective physical barrier when intact; amniotic fluid has bactericidal and bacteristatic properties, and the ability to inhibit the growth of bacteria increases with advancing pregnancy.

Antenatal screening

When a pregnant woman has her first antenatal appointment, she will be offered and recommended to have a range of screening tests for communicable infections, including **Hepatitis B** (NHS Executive 1998), **HIV** (DoH 1994, 1996a),

rubella and **syphilis**. Congenital infections acquired during pregnancy can be the cause of multi-system fetal disease, resulting in permanent damage. Early treatment or prophylaxis of infections acquired during delivery or in the postnatal period affords the opportunity to minimize the effects of these infections.

Information should be provided to women so that they can make an informed choice about these screening tests. There are a number of leaflets available as a source of information. Many of these materials are translated into other languages and media such as audiotapes.

INFECTIONS ACQUIRED DURING PREGNANCY, DELIVERY OR THE POSTNATAL PERIOD

Exposure of the fetus and neonate can occur:

- in pregnancy via the placenta
- during delivery
  — exposure to maternal blood due to trauma or placental separation
  — exposure to pathogenic organisms present in the genital tract
  — exposure to pathogenic organisms that may have infected the amniotic fluid or membranes. This is most likely to occur when there is a long interval between membrane rupture and delivery
- in the neonatal period because of the very close contact between mother and baby and via breastfeeding.

Cytomegalovirus (CMV)

Cytomegalovirus is a common cause of congenital infection. Infection in pregnancy is not usually apparent, and there is no specific treatment available. Neonatal CMV occurs in 0.3–1% of births, but 90–95% of these infections are clinically inapparent. Fetal death can occur and infected infants can develop neurological impairment and deafness. CMV is excreted in urine, saliva, breast milk and cervical secretions. CMV can be transmitted by a mother to her baby in utero, during delivery and the postnatal period.

- *Incubation period*: infection acquired during birth can be identified 3–12 weeks after delivery.
- *Period of communicability*: CMV can be excreted in saliva and urine for several years following infection.
- *Prevention and control*: avoiding contact with the urine and saliva of young children has not been proven in preventing infection in susceptible pregnant women. However, it is important to maintain a high standard of personal hygiene, for example by hand washing after exposure to body fluids. Occupational exposure to young children has not been shown to carry additional risk of CMV infection.

Gonococcal infection

Neisseria gonorrhoeae can cause ophthalmia neonatorum, which results in the newborn infant developing acute redness and swelling of the conjunctiva in one or both eyes, with a purulent discharge. Permanent damage to the eyes can occur if specific treatment is not given promptly. Gonococcal infection is acquired almost exclusively through unprotected sexual intercourse, and seen most commonly in those with multiple sexual partners. The infant becomes infected during delivery.

- *Incubation period*: usually 1–5 days in affected infants.
- *Period of communicability*: while discharge persists if untreated, and for the first 24 hours of antibiotic treatment.
- *Prevention and control*: the infant and mother should be cared for in a single room. The infant will require chloramphenicol eye drops or ointment for 7 days and regular eye care. The mother and her partner should be offered investigation and treatment for gonorrhoea and other sexually-transmitted infections. Ophthalmia neonatorum is a notifiable infection.

Hepatitis B (HBV)

Hepatitis B is a viral infection which can be transmitted from mother to baby during labour and delivery, and in the postnatal period. In some inner-city areas, up to 1:100 women are carriers of HBV. HBV is also transmitted sexually and parenterally, for instance by needle sharing by intravenous drug users. Sexual partners of infected individuals and healthcare workers who have direct contact with blood and blood-stained body fluids of infected individuals are also at risk of infection.

The severity of illnesses in individuals infected with Hepatitis B varies from clinically inapparent cases to fulminating, fatal cases of acute hepatic necrosis. The onset of disease is usually insidious. Of those that become infected as adults, 2–10% will become chronic carriers of HBV and 20–25% of HBV carriers worldwide develop some form of progressive liver disease. HBV in developed countries is more common in injecting drug users, heterosexuals with multiple partners, homosexual men and patients in institutions.

- *Incubation period*: variable, from 3–6 months.
- *Period of communicability*: patients who are **'e' antigen positive** (HbeAg) are highly infectious.
- *Prevention and control*: HBV is the only sexually-transmitted infection which may be prevented by **immunization**. Two forms of vaccination are used to protect individuals from infection. HBV vaccine is effective in preventing infection in those at risk. Of HBV immunized individuals, 80–90% will develop immunity to infection, although this may take up to 6 months. HBV vaccine should not be withheld from at-risk pregnant women. As soon as possible after delivery, babies born to mothers who are carriers of HBV should be immunized with HBV vaccine. Further doses of the vaccine are required at one, two and twelve months of age (NHSE 1998).

HBV immunoglobulin provides passive immunity to give immediate temporary protection. This is indicated in babies born to mothers who have had active HBV infection during pregnancy, or who are known to be HBV antigen-positive.

All healthcare workers who may be exposed to blood and body fluids should be vaccinated against HBV (UK Health Departments 1998).

Additional guidance has recently been issued on HBV surface antigen-positive healthcare workers undertaking exposure-prone procedures (NHS Executive 2000a).

Herpes simplex (HSV)

Herpes simplex infection can be transmitted in pregnancy via the placenta and can result in still-birth or severe neonatal disease. Congenital infection in affected infants is associated with a high mortality. Neurological damage and pneumonitis are also common sequelae in infected infants. HSV 1 is transmitted by direct contact with the saliva of infected individuals. HSV 2 is usually acquired via sexual contact. Infection during delivery can occur if a mother has active HSV 2 infection of the cervix or vulva.

- *Incubation period*: 2–12 days.
- *Period of communicability*: persons with primary genital infection are infective for 7–12 days.
- *Prevention and control*: elective caesarean section is often performed on women with active genital herpes because of the high risk of neonatal infection. Infected infants will require intravenous antiviral treatment, e.g. acyclovir. Healthcare workers should wear gloves if direct contact with lesions is anticipated. Occupational health advice should be sought by any healthcare worker with an herpetic whitlow on their hand.

Human immunodeficiency virus (HIV)

It was estimated in 1998 that there were over 300 births to HIV-infected women, of which 220 occurred in London, principally in African communities (Intercollegiate Working Party 1998). Yet it has been shown that by the end of pregnancy, only 25% of these HIV infections were diagnosed. This means that approximately 60 babies will have acquired HIV infection as a consequence of their mother being unaware of their own infection. Of children infected with HIV, 20% develop Acquired Immunodeficiency

Syndrome (AIDS) or die in the first year of life (Intercollegiate Working Party 1998). In the UK the highest incidence of HIV infection has been recorded in men who have sex with men, and intravenous drug users (DoH 2000a).

Mode of transmission

- Sexual exposure and exposure to blood and some body fluids, i.e. semen, vaginal secretions.
- Vertical transmission from mother to baby during pregnancy, delivery and breastfeeding.
- Occupational exposure principally through sharps injuries.

Incubation period

Variable, although the time from infection to the development of detectable antibodies is usually 1–3 months. The time from HIV infection to a diagnosis of AIDS has an observed range of less than one year to more than ten years. Anti-retroviral therapy has been demonstrated to prolong the interval between confirmation of HIV infection and the development of AIDS.

Period of communicability

Infectiousness is higher during the initial period after infection and as individuals become more immunocompromised.

Prevention and control

It is recommended that all women be offered an HIV test during pregnancy (NHS Executive 1999, DoH 1996a). Identification of HIV infection during pregnancy means that women can be offered a range of interventions that can reduce the rate of vertical transmission to less than 5%. Interventions include anti-retroviral therapy, careful obstetric management, delivery by caesarean section and the avoidance of breastfeeding (UK Departments of Health 1999). This advice on breastfeeding is consistent with the 1997 Collaborative statement from the World Health Organization, UNICEF and UNAIDS which states:

When children born to women living with HIV can be ensured uninterrupted access to nutritionally adequate breast milk substitutes that are adequately prepared and fed to them, they are at less risk of illness and death if they are not breastfed. However, when these conditions are not fulfilled, in particular in an environment where infectious diseases and malnutrition are primary causes of death during infancy, artificial feeding substantially increases children's risk of illness and death.

Other important measures to reduce HIV transmission include:

- Effective health promotion and education, for example giving information on how to avoid acquiring sexually-transmitted infections.
- Informing injecting intravenous drug users how to minimize the risk of transmission of infection, i.e. avoiding the use of shared needles, instructing on needle and equipment decontamination, needle exchange programmes.
- Minimizing the risk to healthcare workers of occupational HIV transmission through the safe handling and disposal of sharps and the appropriate use of protective clothing (UK Departments of Health 1999).

Listeria

Listeria monocytogenes can be transmitted from mother to baby in utero or during delivery. This can result in spontaneous abortion or stillbirth. Infected infants can be born with septicaemia or may develop meningitis. The case fatality rate approaches 50% when onset of disease occurs in the first 4 days of life. Neonates, pregnant women and immunocompromised individuals are most at risk of acquiring listeria. Mothers may acquire listeria via the ingestion of contaminated milk, soft cheeses, contaminated vegetables, and ready-to-eat meals, such as pâté.

- *Incubation period*: variable. 3 weeks incubation on average.
- *Period of communicability*: mothers of infected new-born infants may shed listeria in vaginal secretions and urine for 7–10 days.
- *Prevention and control*: *Listeria monocytogenes* is found principally in soil, water, mud and

silage; infected domestic and wild animals. Soft cheese and pâté have been implicated in transmission of listeria. Pregnant women should be advised to eat only properly cooked meats and diary products, avoid diary non-pasteurized products and thoroughly wash raw vegetables before eating.

Group B streptococcal (GBS) disease

Of pregnant women, 10–30% are colonized with group B streptococci in the vaginal and rectal area, although this varies by age, ethnic group and geographical location. Early onset GBS disease is the commonest cause of severe infection in new-born infants in developed countries (Centers for Disease Control 1996). Recent studies in England suggest that at least 400 cases of early-onset GBS disease (in infants less than 7 days old) occur annually (Communicable Disease Surveillance Centre/PHLS 2000), although opinion is divided whether active screening for GBS is indicated (Isaacs 1998). Maternal GBS infection can result in late miscarriage, preterm labour or stillbirth. Early-onset GBS disease in the newborn usually presents as septicaemia, pneumonia or meningitis. GBS can be transmitted vertically, during labour and the post-partum period.

- *Incubation period*: usually 1–3 days.
- *Period of communicability*: with adequate antibiotic therapy, transmissibility is generally reduced in 24 hours.
- *Prevention and control*: infected infants will require intravenous antibiotics. Screening mothers for GBS in late pregnancy or labour is not common practice in the UK. In the USA mothers are screened for GBS and are given antibiotics prophylactically to prevent early onset GBS (Centers for Disease Control 1996).

Parvovirus B19 (slapped cheek syndrome)

Infection may manifest as a sporadic rash, with noticeable redness of the cheeks (slapped cheek appearance). The rash is less commonly seen in adults. When maternal infection occurs during pregnancy, subsequent fetal infection develops in about half of these cases and the majority of infected individuals will recover with no long-term sequelae. Infection in the first half of pregnancy can lead to fetal death. Parvovirus is transmitted via contact with infected respiratory secretions and from mother to fetus in utero.

- *Incubation period*: 4–20 days.
- *Period of communicability*: probably greatest before the onset of the rash.
- *Prevention and control*: susceptible women who are pregnant should avoid contact with infected individuals.

Rubella (German measles)

The acquisition of rubella during pregnancy can lead to congenital disease in the fetus, the severity of which depends on the stage of pregnancy when infection occurs. When infection occurs in the first trimester, 80–90% of babies will develop congenital disease, such as severe brain damage, deafness and cataracts. By the third trimester the risk to the fetus is greatly reduced. Rubella is transmitted via droplet spread or direct contact with nasopharyngeal secretions of infected people.

- *Incubation period*: 14–21 days.
- *Period of communicability*: from one week before to four days after the onset of the rash.
- *Prevention and control*: since the introduction of rubella vaccination, the incidence of Congenital Rubella Syndrome has been extremely low. However, it is important to note that women from countries without a rubella vaccination programme may not have immunity to infection.
- Immunity to rubella should be ascertained antenatally. Women who are susceptible to rubella should be immunized after delivery and before discharge. If a susceptible woman is exposed to rubella during pregnancy, serological confirmation is necessary because clinical diagnosis of rubella is not reliable. If infection is confirmed in early pregnancy, termination of pregnancy can be offered.

All healthcare workers should be screened for rubella and if found to be non-immune should be immunized to avoid transmitting rubella to pregnant women. For most individuals, immunization confers lifelong immunity.

Syphilis

Syphilis (caused by *Treponema pallidum*) is principally a sexually-transmitted infection, and if untreated can be transmitted vertically or during delivery. Untreated infection can result in spontaneous abortion and stillbirth. Congenital infection may be asymptomatic, but can result in intrauterine growth retardation, preterm delivery or stillbirth. The effects of infection associated with *T. pallidum* may become apparent 5–20 years later, for example, central nervous system involvement.

- *Incubation period*: 10 days to 3 months, usually in the region of three weeks.
- *Period of communicability*: congenital transmission is most probable during early maternal infection.
- *Prevention and control*: penicillin is the treatment of choice. Sexual contacts of the mother will need to be followed up. Effective health promotion and education, for example, giving information on how to avoid acquiring sexually-transmitted infections.

Toxoplasmosis

Toxoplasmosis infection occurs in about 1.5/1000 pregnancies, and the majority of these infections are subclinical. Transplacental infection occurs in about one third of affected pregnancies. Infection acquired between the second and sixth month of pregnancy is most likely to cause significant fetal disease, including cerebral palsy, epilepsy and stillbirth.

- *Incubation period*: 10–23 days.
- *Period of communicability*: toxoplasmosis is not directly transmitted from person to person, except in utero. Cats are the definite host of *Toxoplasma gondii*, and harbour the parasite in

their gastrointestinal tract. Playing in sandpits or playgrounds in which cats have defecated can infect children. Intermediate hosts of *T. gondii* include cattle, chicken and sheep.

- *Prevention and control*: it is important that pregnant women avoid cleaning cat litter trays and wear gloves for gardening. Hands should be thoroughly washed after handling raw meat. Women who are infected between the second and sixth month of pregnancy may be offered a termination of pregnancy. Treatment of pregnant women is problematic as the available treatment does not cross the placenta and cannot cure an already infected infant.

Varicella (chickenpox)

Chickenpox is a common, highly infectious disease, transmitted directly by personal contact or droplet spread, or indirectly via fomites (such as medical equipment). Of the UK indigenous population, 90% are immune to chickenpox. Varicella infection during pregnancy, particularly during the second trimester, can result in the development of fetal abnormality. Disease can be more serious in adults, particularly pregnant women who are at greater risk of developing fulminating varicella pneumonia. The risks to the fetus depend on the stage of acquisition of maternal infection. In the first 20 weeks of pregnancy there is a 1–2% risk of congenital varicella syndrome, which has a high associated mortality. Maternal infection, a week before to a week after delivery, can also lead to severe, fatal disease in the neonate.

- *Incubation period*: 13–17 days.
- *Period of communicability*: 1–2 days before the rash appears, until the vesicles are dry.
- *Prevention and control*: Varicella zoster immunoglobulin (VZIG) prophylaxis is recommended:
  — for infants whose mothers develop chickenpox 7 days before and up to 28 days after delivery
  — susceptible neonates exposed to chickenpox or herpes zoster in the first 28 days of life
  — varicella zoster-negative pregnant contacts of infected individuals.

- VZIG does not necessarily prevent infection in susceptible individuals, but will attenuate disease. Treatment with **acylovir** (an anti-viral agent) may also be indicated as about half of neonates exposed to maternal chickenpox will become infected despite VZIG. Non-immune women should avoid contact with infected individuals during pregnancy.

Further information on vaccination can be found in 'Immunisation Against Infectious Disease' (DoH 1996c).

Factsheets on some of the above infections can be found at <www.amm.co.uk>.

INFECTION CONTROL

The majority of pregnant women, wherever they choose to deliver their baby, are fit and healthy. Those mothers who have their babies in hospital usually have a short length of stay. This can vary from a few hours after delivery for those who have an uncomplicated vaginal delivery, to 4–7 days for those who have a caesarean section.

It is recognized that short hospital stays minimize patients' risk of exposure to pathogenic organisms. Many mothers post-delivery will be mostly self-caring, requiring limited hands-on care from healthcare workers. Those that have invasive devices such as urinary catheters and intravenous cannulae will generally have these in situ only for the short term. These factors mean that rates of infections acquired in hospitals are lower than among other patient groups. Minimizing interventions such as urinary catherization, vaginal examinations and the use of fetal scalp electrodes reduces the risk of a mother and her baby acquiring an infection. There is limited surveillance data on infections acquired in hospital by maternity patients due to their short length of stay, as collecting data from patients in the community is less reliable and more resource-intensive (Holbrook et al 1991).

Some of the infections below are more likely to be hospital-acquired, as mothers requiring obstetric and medical interventions will be cared for in hospital. Some infections relate to the management of labour and can therefore be acquired in any delivery setting.

Caesarean sections

Wound infection is the most common complication of caesarean section, and the incidence varies from 5 to 85%, with the highest infection rates being observed in patients with multiple risk factors undergoing emergency caesarean section. Patient risk factors include:

* long duration of labour
* prolonged rupture of membranes
* previous caesarean section.

Other risk factors include:

* frequent vaginal examinations
* the operation being performed in the second stage of labour
* the skill of the operator.

Current evidence on the use of antibiotic prophylaxis at caesarean section does not conclusively support routine use, although this may be indicated in patients at high risk of infection (Nice et al 1996). *Staphylococcus aureus* accounts for about 25% of wound infections associated with caesarean section. This can be caused by the mother's own skin flora, or can be introduced during surgery.

Chorioamnionitis (amniotic infection)

Chorioamnionitis is a major predisposing factor to premature labour, and is caused by ascending infection usually associated with ruptured membranes. Predisposing factors for infection include prolonged premature rupture of membranes, frequent vaginal examinations, retained intrauterine contraceptive devices, amniocentesis, fetal blood sampling and cervical incompetence.

Symptoms may include maternal fever and tachycardia, fetal tachycardia, uterine tenderness and offensive vaginal discharge. If infection is apparent in a woman with ruptured membranes and there is a strong suspicion of chorioamnionitis, delivery of the baby should be expedited. Both mother and infant will require antimicrobial therapy.

Post-partum endometrial infection (infection of the lining of the uterus)

Risk factors for post-partum infection include those that increase the entry of vaginal flora, for example prolonged rupture of membranes, frequent vaginal and rectal examinations, intrauterine monitoring such as insertion of a fetal scalp electrode, tissue damage, for example associated with a forceps delivery, and poor infection control practice. Symptoms include abdominal pain, pyrexia, uterine tenderness and offensive lochia (vaginal discharge).

Episiotomy

Infection following episiotomy is uncommon and not usually serious: approximately 0.09–0.3% infections per 100 deliveries (Association of Practitioners in Infection Control 1996), although this is likely to be an underestimate, as the majority of these infections will manifest after discharge from hospital. Shaving of perineal (pubic) hair does not reduce the risk of infection.

Urinary tract infection

Urinary tract infections are common in pregnancy and the post-partum period. Asymptomatic bacteriuria (the presence of bacteria in the urine) occurs in 2–10% of both pregnant and non-pregnant women, and 20–30% of these will go on to develop a symptomatic urinary tract infection. Urinary tract infections predispose to the onset of premature labour. Risk factors include a history of urinary tract infection, operative delivery (caesarean section, forceps or vacuum extraction), epidural anaesthesia and urinary catheterization. Urinary retention is common during labour, especially in women who have an epidural anaesthetic.

Breast infection

Breast infection manifests as either mastitis, that is, inflammation of the breast, or an abscess. Few breast infections are seen during hospitalization, as mastitis and breast abscesses usually occur several weeks into the post-partum period. A slight fever can develop with breast engorgement on day 2–4 post delivery. Poor personal hygiene and poor feeding technique with inadequate emptying of the breast can predispose to infection. Symptoms include pyrexia and erythema. Breast firmness and pain are usually experienced in one breast. *Staphylococcus aureus* is the most common cause of breast infection and will require antimicrobial therapy. The mother can continue breastfeeding from the affected side. A breast abscess will require surgical drainage.

USE OF ANTIBIOTICS IN PREGNANCY

Antimicrobial agents should be selected with care when administered to pregnant women, as with all drugs used in pregnancy. This is necessary because of the potential effects on the fetus, the expanded maternal blood volume, increased glomerular filtration rate and increased hepatic metabolism. All antibiotics cross the placenta and enter the fetal circulation to some degree. Vomiting, which is common in early pregnancy, may mean that drugs are not well absorbed. Placental transfer of antimicrobials increases as pregnancy progresses. However, certain agents, such as sulfonamides, may be potentially toxic to the fetus and should be avoided in pregnancy (ACOG Educational Bulletin 1998). Additionally, all antibiotics are excreted into breast milk in various amounts, although this is usually relatively small. The neonatal intestinal tract only absorbs a small amount of the ingested drug, and adverse effects in the infant are rarely seen.

PREVENTION AND CONTROL OF INFECTION

The same principles of infection control apply in the care of pregnant women, in maternity care settings and the home, as for all other groups of patients. Universal infection control precautions (UICP) are infection control precautions to be applied in the care of **all patients at all times**

Box 12.1   Universal infection control precautions

- Hand hygiene
- Appropriate use of protective clothing
- Covering cuts and abrasions on hands and forearms
- Safe handling and disposal of sharps
- Safe disposal of clinical waste
- Segregation of linen contaminated with blood and body fluids
- Treatment of spillages
- Decontamination of reusable devices and equipment

(Box 12.1), including home deliveries. The aim of UICP is:

- to protect patients from acquiring infections
- to protect healthcare workers from acquiring infections occupationally.

UICP are based on the principle that communicable infections may not be clinically apparent, for example HIV infection or MRSA colonization, and if precautions are applied in the care of all patients, the risk of transmission of infection is minimized.

Studies (Panililio et al 1992, Popejoy and Fry 1991) have shown that at least one occupational exposure with blood or amniotic fluid occurs in about 39% of vaginal deliveries and in 50% of caesarean sections. Midwives sustained the greatest number of exposures, followed by obstetricians. The researchers have concluded that half of these contacts were potentially preventable with the use of additional barrier precautions. Sharps injuries were most common during repair of episiotomy or perineal laceration.

Hand hygiene

Patients are put at potential risk of developing a hospital-acquired infection when the healthcare worker caring for them has contaminated hands. Effective hand hygiene minimizes the transmission of transient pathogenic organisms. Routine hand hygiene will remove most transient organisms, which can easily be removed either by the use of hand washing agents, such as liquid soap or antiseptic solutions, or agents that can be used instead of soap and water, for example, alcohol hand rub. Hands must be decontaminated immediately before and after every episode of patient care and when visibly soiled (Pratt et al 2001).

Liquid soap and water is adequate for hand hygiene in most care settings. If the correct technique is used the majority of transient organisms will be removed. Liquid soap is preferable to bar soap, which can easily become contaminated with bacteria when left sitting in a pool of water. The effectiveness of alcohol-based hand rubs is well documented (Rotter 1997) and they appear to be more attractive to healthcare workers as their use is less time-consuming than washing with soap and water (Voss and Widmer 1997). Promoting the use of alcohol hand rubs has recently been shown to be associated with a reduction in the rate of hospital-acquired infection (Pittet et al 2000).

Compliance with hand hygiene by healthcare workers remains problematic. Doctors and those working in areas where there is a high risk of cross infection have the lowest levels of hand hygiene compliance (Pittet et al 2000). There is a perception amongst healthcare professionals that they wash their hands more often than they do in practice, and education has only a transitory effect (Dubbert et al 1990).

Patient empowerment programmes to improve hand hygiene could work well in maternity units, as the mothers are naturally very protective towards their babies (McGuckin et al 2000).

Protective clothing

Protective clothing should be selected according to the likely risk of a healthcare worker becoming exposed to blood and body fluids (Table 12.1), and the possible risk of acquiring an infection (Pratt et al 2001). All blood and body fluids (with the exception of sweat) should be regarded as potentially infectious (UK Departments of Health 1998). Universal infection control precautions (UICP) should be used with mothers known to be infected with a blood-borne virus. If UICP are rigorously adhered to, no additional precautions are necessary.

Detailed guidance on reducing occupational exposure to blood and body fluids during exposure-prone procedures can be found in Guidance for Clinical HealthCare Workers: Protection against infection with blood-borne viruses: Recommendations of the Expert Advisory Group on AIDS and the Advisory Group on Hepatitis, March 1998.

Gloves

Disposable gloves provide a barrier against contact with blood and body fluids, although it should be noted that hand washing after removal is still necessary as neither latex nor vinyl gloves are completely impermeable. Gloves should be made available in different sizes, as poorly-fitting gloves can interfere with dexterity and cause loss of tactile sensation. Damaged gloves should be changed immediately. Gloves should not be washed, as water may penetrate through any holes in them, and detergents can damage the glove material. Contaminated gloves should be disposed of as clinical waste. Comprehensive information on the use of gloves is available (ICNA 1999): Table 12.2 is an adaptation from ICNA 1999 and Pratt et al 2001.

Gloves should be worn when contact with the following is anticipated:

- blood/body fluids
- mucous membranes
- non-intact skin
- contaminated surfaces or items.

Table 12.1 Risk assessment for use of protective clothing

No contact with blood and body fluids anticipated	Contact with blood and body fluid anticipated, low risk of splashing	Contact with blood and body fluid, high risk of splashing
No protective clothing required	Gloves and/or disposable apron	Gloves, face protection (mask, protective spectacles, shield), fluid resistant/ repellent gown, protective footwear

Sterile gloves should be worn for invasive procedures and for contact with sterile body sites.

Gloves should be worn as single use items and put on immediately before an episode of patient care and removed when that activity is completed. It is necessary to change gloves when moving from a contaminated procedure to a clean procedure on a patient, and to change gloves between different patients. As other chapters have stressed, gloves should not be used as a substitute for hand washing. Poor use of gloves can facilitate cross infection between patients, in the same way as poor hand hygiene. Unnecessary and inappropriate use of gloves should be avoided, as this can create a barrier between a healthcare worker and their patient.

Other protective clothing

There is a wide range of protective clothing available, which needs to be selected according to the anticipated risk of exposure. During delivery, for example, there is a high risk of splashing of the face with blood or amniotic fluid (Panililio et al 1992); therefore facial protection (mask and protective spectacles) should be worn. However, it is not necessary to wear sterile gowns for most interventions during labour and vaginal deliveries. Fluid-repellent gowns and foot protection should be worn by the scrub team during caesarean section. Face-masks have limited efficacy in protecting patients from infection, but do act as a physical protective barrier for healthcare workers.

Employers have a duty to ensure that their staff are provided with protective clothing fit for their work, and that they are trained to use this clothing correctly. Additional information on risk assessment and personal protective equipment can be found in the following Health and Safety Executive publications:

- Control of Substances Hazardous to Health Regulations (1999)
- Management of Health and Safety at Work Regulations (1992)
- Personal Protective Equipment at Work Regulations (1992).

Table 12.2 Glove selection. Sources: ICNA 1999, Pratt et al 2001

	Advantages	Disadvantages
Latex gloves[*]	Close fitting Do not impair dexterity Not prone to splitting Lower leakage rates Offer better protection against viruses Comfortable to wear	Latex sensitization[†]
Vinyl gloves	Useful for activities such as routine cleaning Suitable for use in areas where there is a low biohazard risk Inexpensive	Lower tensile strength than latex gloves, therefore more prone to splitting Increased permeability to blood-borne viruses Inflexible with increased leakage rates
Nitrile gloves	Acceptable alternative to latex Good biological barrier Effective for handling some disinfectants, e.g. glutaraldehyde	Allergic reactions have been reported Cyanide is released when incinerated
Polythene gloves	Not suitable for use in clinical settings	Provide limited protection as seams have a tendency to split, therefore do not protect against exposure to blood and body fluids Usually ill-fitting

[*]Powdered gloves should no longer be used, as the powder has been shown to have undesirable side effects, e.g. adhesion formation, adverse effect on wound healing.
[†]See Medical Devices Agency 1996a.

Cuts and abrasions

Cuts and abrasions on the hands and forearms should be covered with a waterproof dressing when working in a clinical area or carrying out clinical procedures in the home or other settings, to prevent possible contamination with pathogenic organisms. If a healthcare worker develops an excoriating skin condition like dermatitis, advice should be sought from an Occupational Health Department (NHS Executive 1998).

Safe handling and disposal of sharps

Healthcare workers are potentially at risk of acquiring a blood-borne virus via a percutaneous (sharps) injury. The most effective way of minimizing this risk is by avoiding injury through the safe handling and disposal of sharps. As other chapters have set out, this includes:

- never resheathing needles
- avoidance of passing sharps directly from hand to hand, and keeping handling to a minimum
- disposal of needle and syringe directly into a sharps disposal bin without dismantling
- never allowing sharps bins to become more than three-quarters full
- taking sharps bins to the point of use, including homecare settings
- keeping sharps disposal bins off the floor, and placing them on a shelf, in trolley bracket, etc. This is particularly important in maternity and neonatal units, where there is a risk that visiting children may put their hands into a sharps disposal bin. Sharps disposal bins should conform to BS 7320 and UN 3291, and be disposed of by incineration (Health Services Advisory Committee 1999).

Waste

Clinical waste should be placed into a yellow waste bag and disposed of by incineration. Clinical waste includes blood and other body tissues, contaminated swabs and dressings, and syringes, needles and other sharp instruments (HSAC 1999). In home care settings, collection of clinical waste (including sharps bins) can be arranged with the local authority. Double bagging of waste is required if there is a risk of leakage. **Placentae should be placed in a yellow waste bag and an approved rigid disposal container**, which complies to UN standard 3291, prior to incineration (HSAC 1999). Waste not contaminated with blood or body fluids can be disposed of into a black bag or the domestic waste stream. Sanitary towels and disposable nappies generated in the home, where the source population is generally healthy, are not considered to be clinical waste, and can be disposed of as domestic waste. Always ensure adherence to local waste policies and guidance.

Linen

Current Department of Health guidance on linen recommends that linen infected (contaminated, from patients diagnosed with a communicable infection) and fouled (contaminated by faeces) should be segregated and laundered separately from soiled linen. Some maternity units have elected to treat any linen contaminated with blood and body fluids as 'infected', as patients with blood-borne viruses may not be known to staff, and it is viewed that this is the most pragmatic approach (NHS Executive 1995). In a patient's home, it is usually sufficient to rinse contaminated linen in cold water and then wash in a hot wash cycle of a domestic washing machine.

Equipment

All reusable equipment should be cleaned between patients. All visible soiling should be removed with neutral detergent and hot water. This applies to low-risk equipment (items that come into contact with intact skin or do not come into contact with the patient) and intermediate and high-risk equipment (items that require high level disinfection or sterilization) (Medical Devices Agency 1996b). All single use equipment must be disposed of after use, and should never be reused (MDA 2000a). It is necessary for healthcare workers to be trained in the use of and deconta- mination of medical devices (MDA 2000b, NHSE 2000b). Refer to local policies as required. See also Chapter 5 on Cleaning, disinfection and sterilization.

Spillages

As Chapter 5 illustrates, the accepted treatment of spillages of blood and blood-stained body fluids is either to sprinkle sodium dichloroiso- cyanurate granules (NaDCC) over the spillage or to cover the spillage with paper towels and pour sodium hypochlorite 10 000 ppm over the towels. After two minutes, wearing appropriate protect- ive clothing, the healthcare worker should scoop up the towels or granules with paper towels, dispose of them into a yellow bag, and the area should be washed thoroughly with neutral deter- gent and water. NaDCC should not be used on spillages of urine, as this chemical reacts with the urea in the urine.

This response is considered by many to be impractical on a labour ward, where substantial spillages of blood and amniotic fluid are com- monplace (Fraise 1999). In this setting the spill- age should be absorbed with paper towels and disposed of as clinical waste. The area should then be wiped over with sodium hypochlorite 10 000 ppm, and then washed thoroughly with neutral detergent and water.

Both NaDCC and sodium hypochlorite are cor- rosive to metal and both are bleaches, and they need to be used with care in a patient's home. If a spillage of blood and body fluids is anticipated, carpets and furnishings can be protected with a fluid-repellent, disposable covering. Should a spillage occur, the area should be cleaned using neutral detergent and water.

OTHER INFECTION CONTROL CONSIDERATIONS
Labour ward and delivery

It is not necessary for fathers or other support persons attending vaginal delivery to wear the- atre scrubsuits. Those accompanying a mother during a caesarean section will need to wear theatre scrubsuits and be given information on where they may sit, and what they should avoid touching. Shaving the perineum (pubic hair) prior to vaginal delivery does not reduce the risk of infection. At delivery, mechanical suc- tion should be used on infants requiring airway clearance.

Birthing pools

The use of a birthing pool for labour and/or delivery is an option widely available in mater- nity units and also for home birth. Although only a small proportion of women give birth in a pool, it is likely that many more use pools during labour for relaxation and pain relief. A survey conducted during 1994–96 concluded that 0.6% of all deliveries occurred in birthing pools, and 9% of these were at home (Gilbert and Tookey 1999). Theoretical infection risks include infec- tion with *Pseudomonas aeruginosa*, *Legionella* and other water-borne organisms. There is limited evidence on infection rates associated with water births, although one small study (Hawkins 1995) indicated that infants delivered in birthing pools have a higher infection rate. Women with compli- cated pregnancies should be excluded.

Clear protocols and procedures for pool cleaning and maintenance are needed. After use, any debris should be removed and discarded as clinical waste. The pool should then be thoroughly cleaned with neutral detergent and hot water, followed by sodium hypochlorite (10 000 ppm). The pool should then be rinsed and dried. Always seek infection control advice if in doubt.

Fetal monitoring

Fetal infections can develop from the use of a fetal scalp electrode or as a result of fetal blood sampling. Associated infections range from zero to 4.5%, but most of these are not serious. Fetal scalp electrodes should be avoided in mothers who are known to have active genital herpes sim- plex infection, Hepatitis B or HIV.

Box 12.2 Infection control checklist for home delivery

- Hand hygiene materials – liquid soap, paper towels, alcohol hand rub
- Protective clothing
- Fluid-repellent disposable sheeting to prevent contamination of the environment with body fluids
- Sharps box
- Clinical waste bags and rigid container for disposal of the placenta. Arrangements should be made for the collection of clinical waste

---

Home deliveries

The principles of universal infection control precautions apply equally to a home delivery, that is, hand hygiene, appropriate use of protective clothing, safe handling and disposal of sharps, etc. (Box 12.2) To facilitate this, it is helpful to ensure that the necessary equipment is available prior to the expected date of delivery.

Postnatal period

Education on hygiene for mothers should include advice on the care of the perineal area, breasts and nipples. Mothers should be encouraged to report symptoms that may be indicative of infection, such as offensive lochia (vaginal discharge), or symptoms that may put them or their baby at increased risk of infection, such as cracked nipples. The use of a shower is preferable to a bath.

New-born infants have little natural immunity to infection, therefore it is helpful if mothers and their partners are given advice on basic hygiene, for example how to give eyecare, and the need to wash their hands after nappy changing. Healthcare workers need to be vigilant about decontaminating their hands before and after any contact with newborn infants. A review of the literature has shown that keeping the umbilical cord clean, is as effective and as safe as using antiseptics and antibiotics for cord care (Zupan and Garner 2000).

There is no need to prevent siblings from visiting a mother and her newborn infant. However, anyone with an infection, including siblings and healthcare workers, should be excluded.

INFANT FEEDING
Breastfeeding

Health benefits associated with breastfeeding include protection against gastro-enteritis, respiratory infection, otitis media and urinary tract infections (Heinig and Dewey 1996). Breast milk provides passive immunity and also enhances the benefits from immunization through an increased active immune response (Pabst and Spady 1990). Yet the number of women initiating breastfeeding in the UK remains low at around 40–60%, with women in social class V having the lowest uptake rates (NHS Centre for Reviews and Dissemination, York 2000).

Artificial feeding

Milk can become contaminated with bacteria as a result of inadequate decontamination of teats, bottles and preparation equipment. Contamination can also occur during feed preparation. Therefore, it is essential that mothers who choose this method of feeding understand how to decontaminate all feeding equipment and the need to refrigerate reconstituted milk.

The UK Baby Friendly Hospital Initiative was launched in 1994, with the aim of helping all parents to make informed decisions about feeding their babies and then supporting them in their chosen method. Best practice is represented by the 'Ten Steps to Successful Breastfeeding' (UNICEF UK 1998).

RISK ASSESSMENT

Risk assessment should be undertaken in order to determine if exposure to blood and body fluids could be minimized. Where it is not possible to eliminate a potential hazard, the next step is to assess how exposure can be minimized, for example, by introducing engineering controls such as needleless devices. An ever-increasing number of safety devices are being manufactured for venepuncture, and their use has now become mandatory in the USA (Occupational Safety and Health Administration 1999). These devices should be evaluated before introduction, as some safety intravenous devices have been associated with a higher infection rate (Do et al 1999). The most effective safety devices are those that are simple to use.

Work practice also needs to be evaluated to assess if there is a safer way of conducting a procedure and so minimizing the risk of exposure, such as eliminating hand-to-hand instrument passing in the operating theatre, no-hands procedures for handling contaminated sharps.

SHARPS INJURIES

The risk of acquiring a blood-borne virus via percutaneous exposure is higher than that following mucocutaneous exposure (such as to eyes) or contamination of non-intact skin (Communicable Disease Surveillance Centre 2000). All sharps injuries relating to waste disposal are preventable, and many relating to clinical practice are avoidable. It is helpful to collect sharps injury data within an institution or organization to identify unsafe practice and high risk areas, to target interventions and education. The more sharps injuries sustained, the greater likelihood that healthcare workers will acquire blood-borne viruses: therefore it is important that safer practices are adopted.

This is the responsibility of every healthcare worker who uses sharps.

It is important that all healthcare professionals, whatever their work environment, are educated in the management of sharps injuries and exposure to blood and body fluids. All staff must be able to access services for post-exposure prophylaxis, usually via occupational health or accident and emergency departments, for risk assessment following a sharps injury (UK Departments of Health 2000). Follow local policies and advice.

CONCLUSION

Good practice in infection control remains as important today as it was when Semmelweis discovered the link between poor hand hygiene and puerperal sepsis. Whether a mother chooses to have her baby in hospital or at home, the basic principles of infection control apply and healthcare professionals must adhere to universal infection control precautions at all times.

It is also important that all pregnant women and new mothers are provided with accessible and culturally sensitive information to be able to make informed decisions about their pregnancy, for example antenatal screening, and the care of their baby, such as infant feeding.

REFERENCES

ACOG Educational Bulletin 1998 Antimicrobial therapy for obstetric patients. International Journal of Gynaecology and Obstetrics 61: 299–308

Association of Practitioners in Infection Control 1996 Infection Control and Applied Epidemiology: Principles and Practice. Association of Practitioners in Infection Control. Mosby, St. Louis

Centers for Disease Control 1996 Prevention of group B streptococcal disease: a public health perspective. Morbidity and Mortality Weekly Report 1996; 45(RR-7). CDC, Atlanta

Centers for Disease Control 2000 Hospital-based policies for the prevention of perinatal Group B streptococcal disease – United States, 1999. Morbidity and Mortality Weekly Report 2000; 49(41): 936–940

Communicable Disease Surveillance Centre: PHLS Group B Streptococcus Working Party 2000 Enhanced surveillance of invasive group B streptococcal disease in infants. Communicable Disease Report 2000; 10: 21

Communicable Disease Surveillance Centre 2000 Surveillance of healthcare workers exposed to

blood-borne viruses at work: July 1997 to June 2000. Communicable Disease Report 2000; 10: 293

Department of Health 1994 Guidelines for offering voluntary named HIV antibody testing to women receiving antenatal care. DoH, London

Department of Health 1996a Guidelines for pre-test discussion on HIV testing. DoH, London

Department of Health 1996b Protecting healthcare workers and patients from Hepatitis B: recommendations of the Advisory Group on Hepatitis. HSG (93)40. Addendum was issued under cover of EL(96)77. DoH, London

Department of Health 1996c Immunisation Against Infectious Disease. HMSO, London

Department of Health 2000a Prevalence of HIV and hepatitis infections in the United Kingdom 1999. Report of the Unlinked Anonymous Surveys Steering Group. DoH, London

Department of Health 2000b Hepatitis B infected healthcare workers. HSC 2000/20. DoH, London

Do A N, Ray B J, Banerjee S N, Illian A F et al 1999 Bloodstream infections associated with needleless device use and the importance of infection control practices in the home health care setting. Journal of Infectious Disease 179: 442–448

Dubbert P M, Dolce J, Richter W, Miller M et al 1990 Increasing ICU staff handwashing: effects of education and group feedback. Infection Control and Hospital Epidemiology 11: 191–193.

Fraise A P 1999 Choosing disinfectants. Journal of Hospital Infection 43: 255–264

Gilbert R E, Tookey P A 1999 Perinatal mortality and morbidity among babies delivered in water: surveillance study and postal survey. British Medical Journal 319: 483–487

Hawkins S 1995 Water vs conventional births: infection rates compared. Nursing Times 91(11): 38–40

Health Services Advisory Committee 1999 Safe Disposal of Clinical Waste. Health and Safety Commission, London

Heinig M J, Dewey K G 1996 Health advantages of breastfeeding for infants: a critical review. Nutrition Research Reviews 9: 89–110

Holbrook K F, Nottebart V F, Hameed S R, Platt R 1991 Automated postdischarge surveillance for postpartum and neonatal nosocomial infections. American Journal of Medicine 91(Suppl 3B): 125S–130S

Infection Control Nurses Association 1998 Guidelines for hand hygiene. Infection Control Nurses Association, Bathgate

Infection Control Nurses Association 1999 Glove usage guidelines. Infection Control Nurses Association, Bathgate

Intercollegiate Working Party for enhancing voluntary confidential HIV testing in pregnancy 1998 Recommendations for reducing mother to child transmission of HIV infection in the United Kingdom. Royal College of Paediatrics and Child Health, London

Isaacs D 1998 Prevention of early onset group B streptococcal infection: screen, treat or observe? Archives of Disease in Childhood Fetal Neonatal Edition 79: F81–F82

McGuckin M, Storr J, Bowler I 2000 Hand hygiene practices in Oxford: changing behaviour by empowerment. Proceedings of 4th Decennial International Conference on Nosocomial and Healthcare Associated Infections, P-S1-65

Medical Devices Agency 1996a Latex sensitisation in the HealthCare Setting (use of latex gloves). MDA DB 9601. MDA, London

Medical Devices Agency 1996b Sterilisation, Disinfection and Cleaning of Medical Equipment: Guidance on Decontamination from the Microbiology Advisory Committee to the Medical Devices Agency. Medical Devices Agency, London

Medical Devices Agency 2000a Single-use Medical Devices: Implications and Consequences of Reuse. MDA DB2000(04). MDA, London

Medical Devices Agency 2000b Equipped to care. Medical Devices Agency, London

NHS Centre for Reviews and Dissemination, University of York 2000 Promoting the initiation of breastfeeding. Effective Healthcare July 2000: 6(2): 1–12.

NHS Executive 1995 Hospital laundry arrangements for used and infected linen. HSG (95)18. DoH, London

NHS Executive 1998 The Management of Health, Safety and Welfare Issues for NHS Staff. HSC 1998/064. DoH, London

NHS Executive 1998 Screening of pregnant women for Hepatitis B and immunisation of babies at risk. HSC 1998/127. DoH, London

NHS Executive 1999 Reducing mother to baby transmission of HIV. HSC 1999/183. DoH, London

NHS Executive 2000a Hepatitis B infected healthcare workers. HSC 2000/20. DoH, London

NHS Executive 2000b Decontamination of medical devices. HSC 2000/32. DoH, London

Nice C, Feeney A, Godwin P et al 1996 A prospective audit of wound infection rates after caesarean section in five West Yorkshire hospitals. Journal of Hospital Infection 33: 55–61

Occupational Safety and Health Administration 1999 Enforcement procedures for the occupational exposure to blood-borne pathogens. Directive CPL2-2.44D. OSHA, Washington DC

Pabst H F, Spady D W 1990 Effect of breastfeeding on antibody response to conjugate vaccine. Lancet 336: 269–270

Panililio A L, Welch B A, Bell D M et al 1992 Blood and amniotic fluid contact sustained by obstetric personnel during deliveries. American Journal of Obstetrics 167: 703–708

Pittet D, Hugonnet S, Harbarth S, Mourouga P et al 2000 Effectiveness of a hospital-wide programme to improve compliance with hand hygiene. Lancet 356: 1307–1312

Popejoy S L, Fry D E 1991 Blood contact and exposure in the operating room. Surgery, Gynecology and Obstetrics 172: 480–483

Pratt R J, Pellowe C, Loveday H P, Robinson N et al 2001 The *epic* Project: Developing national evidence-based guidelines for preventing healthcare associated infections. Phase 1: Guidelines for preventing hospital acquired infections. Journal of Hospital Infection 47: S1–82

Rotter M L 1997 Handwashing, hand disinfection and skin disinfection. In: Wenzel R P (ed.) Prevention and Control of Nosocomial Infections, 3rd edn. Williams & Wilkins, Baltimore, 1287–1294

Semmelweis I P 1981 Classics in infectious diseases. Childbed fever by Ignaz Philipp Semmelweis. Reviews of Infectious Diseases 3(4): 808–811

UK Health Departments 1998 Guidance for Clinical HealthCare Workers: Protection against infection with blood-borne viruses. Recommendations of the Expert Advisory Group on AIDS and the Advisory Group on Hepatitis. HSC 1998/063. DoH, London

UK Health Departments 1999 HIV and infant feeding: Guidance from the UK Chief Medical Officers' Expert Advisory Group on AIDS. PL/CO (99)2. DoH, London

UK Health Departments 2000 HIV post-exposure prophylaxis: Guidance from the UK Chief Medical Officers' Expert Advisory Group on AIDS. PL/CO (2000)4. DoH, London

UNICEF 1998 Implementing the 'Ten Steps to Successful Breastfeeding'. UNICEF UK, London

Voss A, Widmer A F 1997 No time for handwashing!? Handwashing versus alcoholic rub: can we afford 100% compliance? Infection Control and Hospital Epidemiology 18: 205–208

Zupan J, Garner P 2000 Topical umbilical cord care at birth (Cochrane Review). The Cochrane Library, Issue 3, Oxford

FURTHER READING

Ayliffe G A J, Fraise A P, Geddes A M, Mitchell K (eds) 2000 Control of Hospital Infection: A Practical Handbook, 4th edn. Arnold, London

Bannister B A, Begg N T, Gillespie S H 1996 Infectious Disease. Blackwell Science, Oxford

Chin J (ed.) 2000 Control of Communicable Disease Manual, 17th edn. American Public Health Association, Washington DC

Department of Health 1996 Immunisation Against Infectious Disease. HMSO, London

Horton R, Parker L 1997 Informed Infection Control Practice. Churchill Livingstone, London

Mayhall C G (ed.) 1999 Hospital Epidemiology and Infection Control, 2nd edn. Lippincott Williams & Wilkins, Philadelphia

McCulloch J (ed.) 2000 Infection Control: Science, Management and Practice. Whurr, London

Wenzel R P (ed.) 1997 Prevention and Control of Nosocomial Infection, 3rd edn. Williams & Wilkins, Baltimore

13

Ectoparasitic infections

G. Xavier

INTRODUCTION

This chapter describes the common parasites which infect man. Human parasites range from the advanced arthropods such as lice and mites, through to worms and the primitive single-celled protozoa. An ectoparasite is an organism that lives on or in the skin of its host and derives sustenance from the host. This term can include those organisms that live on the host only long enough to obtain a blood meal, as well as those that burrow into the superficial layers of the skin and remain there for weeks to months or even years if left untreated.

Infection with lice carries a strong social stigma due to a long-standing association with dirt and poverty. Human lice feed solely by sucking blood, and lice are only transmitted by close contact with an infested person. Human lice have a worldwide distribution, and three species of lice infect humans, producing three different conditions; pediculosis pubis, also known as phthiriasis, caused by the crab or pubic louse, pediculosis corporis caused by the body or clothing louse, and pediculosis capitis caused by the head louse. Scabies infection caused by *Sarcoptes scabiei* and its management are also discussed within this chapter.

THE HEAD LOUSE – *PEDICULUS CAPITIS*

Head lice are not a serious health problem in the United Kingdom. Infection with head lice is most

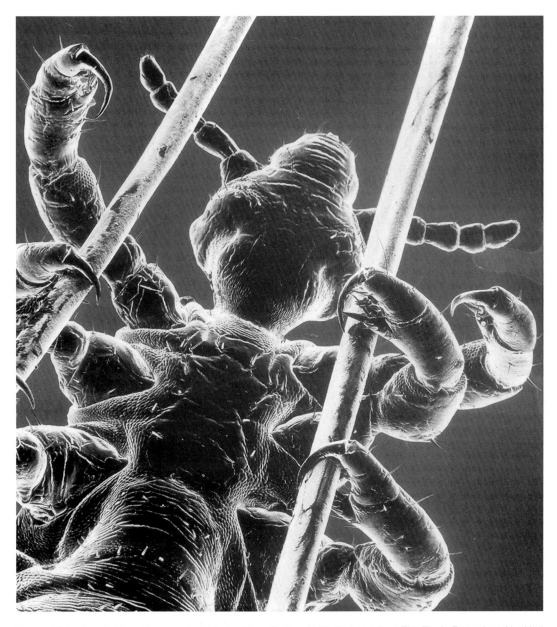

Figure 13.1 An adult head louse on hair shafts. Magnification: ×40. Photographer: Tim Flach. Reproduced by kind permission of Leeds Community and Mental Health Services NHS Trust.

common in children aged 6–11 years, but can affect anybody. It rarely affects general health but can cause much anxiety.

The head louse is a wingless, parasitic insect (Fig. 13.1), which spends its whole life cycle on human hair. It can be difficult to see as it can blend in with the host hair colour. The adult head louse is about 3 mm long. Its mouth is like a very small needle, which it sticks into the scalp to feed on human blood. Head lice cannot live free of the head, and will dehydrate and die if they leave it. The female can lay up to 10 eggs a day. The eggs are not necessarily laid near the root of the hair shaft. The female chooses a position on the hair,

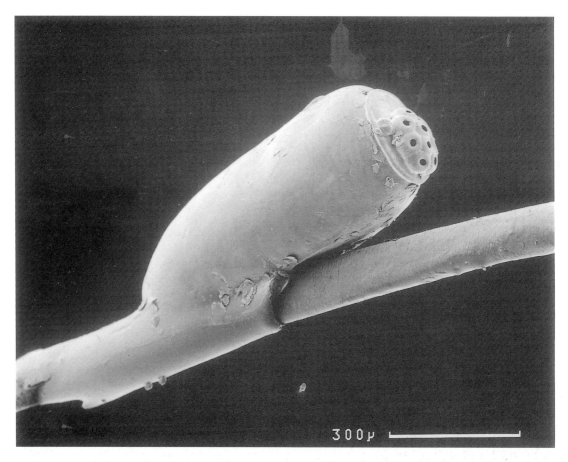

Figure 13.2 An egg attached to a hair shaft, showing typical 'pepper-pot' holes. Magnification: ×40. Photographer: Tim Flach. Reproduced by kind permission of Leeds Community and Mental Health Services NHS Trust.

which is warm enough to incubate the egg at the time of laying.

The live egg (Fig. 13.2) is flesh coloured and not easily seen. The eggs take 7–10 days to hatch; once the egg has hatched, the empty shell, which is called a nit, is white and can be seen easily. Head lice become fully mature after 10 days and can live on the scalp for up to 4 weeks. Before becoming an adult, they shed their skin three times, usually at night.

Signs and symptoms

Itching is often the only symptom of the disease, but, misleadingly, may appear weeks or months after the onset of the infections, particularly in people with a first infection. The louse bite produces an erythematous, itchy papule. Head lice do not bite below the hairline. However, a pruritic rash on the back of the neck caused by an allergic reaction to louse faeces is a fairly common sign of severe infection.

Transmission

Head lice are only spread by prolonged direct head-to-head contact. The contact must be sufficiently close and long to allow a warm zone to develop between the heads. The lice go across this warm zone to spread evenly over the warm scalp area available to them. Clean hair is not protection against head lice, as they do not need unhygienic conditions to survive. Short-haired people get and give lice more easily, and long-haired people who are infected tend to have more lice, as they do not transmit them to others as easily. Because of the mode of spread, transmission tends to occur in settings and groups where there is opportunity for prolonged head-to-head contact. Transmission is more likely to occur amongst families and close friends than within schools.

Diagnosis

Infections are usually asymptomatic, with only 15–35% of people who experience itching. Head lice and live eggs are difficult to see. Diagnosis cannot be based on the presence of nits alone, because these remain firmly stuck to hairs long after an infection has been eradicated. Nits may also be confused with hair muffs (sheaths of keratin around hair shafts) which, unlike nits, will slide along hair shafts. The outermost nit is not an accurate indicator of the duration of the infection, because even though the egg or the nit is carried out on the growing hair at the pace of about one centimetre a month, there is no certainty that the egg was laid at root level.

The only definitive sign of head lice infection is the presence of a living, moving head louse. In longer-term cases, live lice may be seen on the scalp. But, in general, head lice can be more easily found using a detection comb. This is a specially-designed comb available from pharmacies. Ideally, detection combing should be done over a pale piece of paper or sheet. The hair should be damp. It should be combed in small sections starting with the teeth of the comb touching the scalp at the top of the head and drawing the comb carefully towards the end of the hair. If head lice are present they will then be found between the teeth of the comb or on the paper/sheet.

A warning sign of heavy head lice infection is black powder or cast skins on the pillow in the morning or when combing.

Treatment and management

Before starting any treatment it is essential to ensure the correct diagnosis. The best way to confirm an infection is either to find live, moving lice or to see the physical evidence of a louse brought in by the patient. Treatment is only required for those who are infected; there is no need to automatically treat all members of the household. However, it is important to check all people who may have had head-to-head contact with infected members of the family.

Insecticides

Insecticides (Burgess et al 1992) are the only treatments for which there is clear evidence of effectiveness. There are three types of head lice insecticides available: **malathion**, **pyrethroids** and **carbaryl**. In previous years some regions in the United Kingdom have operated a policy of rotating insecticides. However, rotational policies have not been effective in limiting the development of resistance. It is now recommended that if one course of insecticide has failed or re-infection has occurred, a different insecticide be tried. This is known as a 'mosaic strategy' and it prevents the repeated use of a single product. The insecticide should kill live lice and eggs in a single application. However, as very young eggs are difficult to kill, a routine second application is recommended, 7 days after the first, to kill any young lice emerging from eggs missed in the first treatment.

Insecticide treatment for head lice is as follows:

- The manufacturer's instructions should always be followed.
- The insecticide should be applied all over the scalp in a systematic way.
- The hair should be allowed to dry naturally as heat inactivates the insecticide.
- After treatment, the hair can be washed and dried as normal.
- It can take up to 24 hours for the lice to die. Any nits left in the hair may be unsightly but are harmless.

Chlorine in swimming pool water can weaken the effect of insecticides. If the person has been swimming in the pool in the 3 days before treatment, it is recommended that the hair is shampooed and dried before applying the insecticide.

Safety of insecticides

All of the available insecticide preparations are well within safety limits when used correctly. It is important not to overuse insecticides. Most of the insecticide products contain ingredients that can cause skin irritation if used repeatedly. Formulations containing alcohol should be avoided in small children and people with asthma or eczema. Insecticide treatments should not be used in infants under 6 months old. In 1995, carbaryl was restricted to prescription-only use because of data suggesting that it could cause cancers in rodents. A formal rotation policy of insecticides in the treatment of head lice is no longer logical. Prolonged use of one insecticide has also resulted in resistance in some areas. However, this evidence is unpublished and many experts consider that there is no real risk because exposure of the body to the drug through topical application is so small.

Treatment failures

Head lice treatments will fail if used incorrectly. If a treatment fails, the reason for failure should be thoroughly investigated before re-treating. Common reasons for apparent treatment failure include:

- misdiagnosis
- psychogenic itch
- incorrect application of product
- re-infection
- irritation caused by product ingredients
- resistance to insecticides.

Other treatments

Mechanical methods

Mechanical methods of removing lice from the hair such as 'bug busting' are gaining popularity because they do not involve the application of insecticides. The efficacy of these treatments has not been scientifically proven, but there are anecdotal reports of success.

The 'bug busting' technique involves washing the hair with ordinary shampoo, applying conditioner thoroughly and combing the hair with a plastic detector comb. The hair is combed until no more lice are found. Each treatment session takes about 30 minutes and has to be repeated every 3–4 days for a minimum of two weeks. At least three combing sessions are needed after the last adult louse is found. This technique needs to be shown to people and requires a high degree of commitment from them. This is an alternative for well-motivated people who do not wish to use insecticides, or when resistance is a problem.

Alternative remedies for head lice infection

Following concerns over the safety of conventional insecticides, a number of cosmetic shampoo preparations containing herbs or aromatic oils are being promoted as effective ways to prevent or treat head louse infections. They do not have product licences and there are no efficacy or safety data to support their use; these 'natural' products are often perceived as being totally safe, but concentrated oils such as tea tree oil or lavender oil can be toxic.

Electric combs kill lice by electrocution or burning. They do not kill eggs. They seem to work best on hair which is dry, fine and straight, but again evidence is only anecdotal and their general use cannot be recommended. These combs are also relatively expensive.

Management of contacts in the community

As part of a regular health education programme, families should be instructed in contact tracing, that is, listing people likely to have had head-to-head contact with infected members of the family during the 4 weeks prior to the detection of a case. Close contacts may either have given the head lice to the infected members of the family or vice versa. They include family members, partners and close friends. All close contacts should be informed so that they can check themselves for head lice by detection combing and be treated if necessary. Health practitioners should make every effort to support parents/carers in carrying out a good contact tracing exercise, for example by providing them with sufficient information, in the form of factsheets for distribution to contacts, and the practitioners should be aware of local policy and procedures.

Management of head lice in schools

Head lice are not primarily a problem of schools, but of the wider community. Although most common in schoolchildren, about 20% of cases are amongst people over 16 or under 4 years old. Routine head inspections as a screening measure are without value and are not recommended. Head lice cannot be accurately detected by head inspection alone, and the school nurse has limited access to other members of the family who also need to be checked. Schools should work in partnership with their named school nurses in providing educational information to parents and children about head lice. This should not be a special separate topic but integrated with the management of other health problems. If children are found to have head lice, they need not be sent home from school. This practice is unnecessary, as the child has probably had the infection for some time. Alert letters should not be sent routinely to parents when only one case of head lice has been identified. Instead, information about head lice and the school's approach to the management of head lice should be sent out on a regular basis as part of a package dealing with other issues. Parents/carers have the responsibility to deal with cases of head lice within their family. Families with continuing, recurring infection should be assisted and supported, as with any other health problem, by the community (including the school) and health professionals.

THE CRAB LOUSE/PUBIC LOUSE – *PHTHIRUS PUBIS*

Phthirus pubis, the crab louse (Fig. 13.3), acquired its common name because it strongly resembles a miniature crab. *P. pubis* is the most sedentary human louse and dies quickly when separated from its host. It lays several eggs on a single hair.

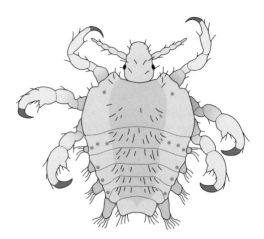

Figure 13.3 The pubic louse, *Phthirus pubis*.

The egg takes 6–8 days to incubate and the life cycle from egg to egg is about 3 weeks. Although infestation with *P. pubis* is a common condition in the United Kingdom amongst adults, its exact frequency is unknown. Person to person contact transmits it. Clothing, bed linen and toilet seats do not play a role in transmission.

Although it is often considered to be sexually-transmitted, as the pubic and peri-anal areas are the most frequently affected, *P. pubis* can infest all coarse body hair. Its claws are large and it has a wide leg span, enabling it to cling to thicker, sparsely distributed hairs including axillary hair, beard, eyebrows and eyelashes. Children often pick up crab lice on the eyelashes through natural family contact, such as with a hairy arm or chest, or a beard.

Signs and symptoms

Itching, often intense, is the main symptom, but may begin some months after onset of infestation.

Diagnosis

All hairy parts of the body must be examined to make the diagnosis. Crab lice are even more difficult to see on the hair than head lice are; they move little between hairs. The presence of 'grit' in the undergarments, possibly crab louse faeces, should lead to further investigation. In the eyelashes, the lice may be unnoticeable whereas the nits are more easily visible. Diagnosis can be made by detection combing on all hairy parts of the body, with the exception of the eyelashes.

Treatment and management

All hairy parts of the body must be treated in adults. In children scalp treatment may be needed in conjunction with eyelashes and eyebrows. The effective management also requires examination and simultaneous treatment, as found necessary, of all family members and sexual contacts.

All head louse formulations can be used to treat crab lice, but aqueous lotions are most effective. For treatment of eyelashes, removal of the hatched lice has been recommended, but this is a difficult procedure as this involves the risk of harming the eye. Smoothing petroleum jelly among the closed lashes twice a day for 10 days kills the nymphs as they hatch. No attempt should be made to remove the eggs or nits, which will be eliminated fairly quickly as the lashes they are attached to fall and regrow. Any lice on the eyebrows also can be treated this way.

THE CLOTHING/BODY LOUSE – *PEDICULUS HUMANUS*

Pediculosis corporis (infestation with body lice) is seen primarily where there is overcrowding and poor sanitation. In the United Kingdom pediculosis corporis is a condition almost entirely restricted to street dwellers and vagrants who are not able to change their clothes regularly: their bedding can become infested.

The body louse (Fig. 13.4) lays its eggs and resides in the seams of the clothing rather than on the skin of its host. The body louse leaves the clothing only to obtain a blood meal from its host. Nits present in the clothing are viable for up to one month. When mature lice have no access to the body they die of starvation in 5 days at low temperatures and more quickly at high temperatures. Adult lice live 13–30 days.

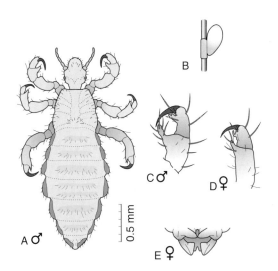

Figure 13.4   The clothing or body louse, *Pediculus humanus*. (A) Male viewed from above; (B) the egg attached to a fibre; (C, D) claw (anterior leg) of male and female; (E) female terminalia.

Transmission

The social isolation of carriers in the United Kingdom restricts the risk amongst the general population. Most transmission occurs during contact between fully clothed persons.

Signs and symptoms

Symptoms can take weeks to develop in a first infestation. However, dermal hypersensitivity to louse bites can develop in 10 days of continuous exposure, so there is a wide variation in reaction to infestation. There are two reactions to the bite, a purpuric papule caused by the bite itself, and/or a pruritic inflammatory wheal, caused by the host immune response.

Diagnosis

The diagnosis must be confirmed by finding the lice or their eggs in clothing or bedding. The bite pattern characteristically follows the seamlines of the underwear. In long-term cases the skin may have thickened due to continuous scratching. Presence of these symptoms should prompt examination of the clothing.

Treatment and management

In the United Kingdom treatment does not usually require pesticides. There are several alternatives:

- Dry clothes turned inside out can be tumble dried at approximately 50 degrees centigrade for 30 minutes; this can kill lice and eggs and the clothes are then washed in the usual way.
- Dry cleaning is effective against lice and eggs but expensive. Infested clothes should not be cleaned together with unaffected clothing.
- Clothes washed on a hot cycle should kill eggs and lice.

Affected individuals should brush, shower or bathe to remove any lice left on the body after removing infested clothing.

SCABIES: *SARCOPTES SCABIEI* VAR *HOMINIS*

Scabies is a condition caused by infestation of the skin by *Sarcoptes scabiei* (Fig. 13.5). The main symptoms of the disease are due to an allergic reaction to the presence of mites and their products in the skin. Symptoms develop in response to certain water-soluble glycopeptide allergens leaching out of the faeces of the mite, which are glued to the floor of the tunnels the mite makes in the skin (Maunder 1992). Scabies is a common public health problem in poor communities, and is widespread in many developing countries.

While infestation with the scabies is not a life-threatening condition, the severe, persistent itch debilitates and depresses people (Green 1989). The level of infection in communities varies, and is influenced by changes in social attitudes, population movements, wars, misdiagnosis, inadequate treatment and changes in people's immune system (Van Neste 1986). Epidemic cycles are said to occur every **seven to 15 years** and these are partly a reflection of population immune status. Meinking and Taplin (1995) note:

… the most practical guide to the epidemiology of scabies, and one that is often of value in family or community management, is to estimate the degree and frequency of close body contact. The rise and fall of scabies incidence in developed countries is due in part to the intervention of health professionals by treating cases when the incidence reaches clearly recognisable levels…

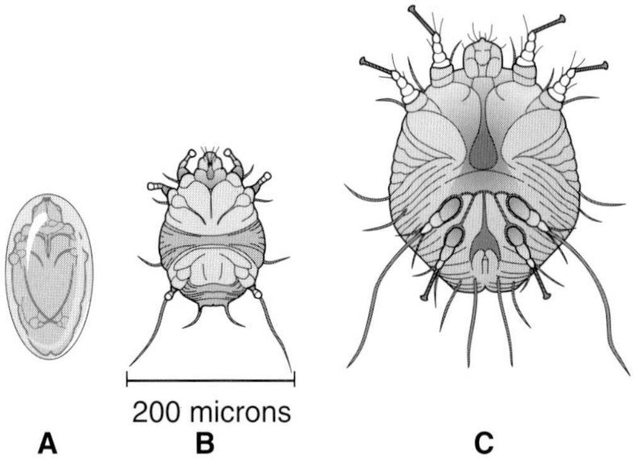

Transmission

Man is the main reservoir for *Sarcoptes scabiei*. Spread is person-to-person via direct skin contact including sexual contact. Transfer from undergarments and bedclothes occurs only if these have been contaminated by infectious persons immediately beforehand. The microscopic mites penetrate the epidermis causing tiny, characteristic, linear burrows that may be seen in the skin. Eggs are laid in the epidermis, and hatch after 3–4 days. The emerging larvae then appear on the surface of the skin before excavating new tunnels. The life-cycle of *S. scabiei* begins with the pregnant female laying two to three eggs a day in burrows several millimetres to several centimetres in length in the skin. After about 50–72 hours larvae emerge, and wander to make new burrows.

They mature, mate and repeat this cycle, which takes 10–17 days. Mites usually live 30–60 days. Animal scabies (mange) can transiently infect people. Sarcoptes in animals is not completely host-specific, and those which are parasitic on domestic animals, including dogs, cats, horses and pigs, may rarely infect humans (Fain 1978).

200 microns

A B C

Figure 13.5 *Sarcoptes scabiei*: the life stages; (A) Egg; (B) 6-legged larva; (C) 8-legged adult male.

Signs and symptoms

Classical scabies

The clinical picture in healthy individuals is the appearance of raised burrows, or small, red, slightly elevated papules or vesicles, particularly on the **wrists, back of the hands and between the fingers**. Further spread is usually confined to the elbows, armpits, beneath the breasts, waist, groin, genitalia, buttocks, knees and ankles (Fig. 13.6). The incubation period is 2–6 weeks before the onset of itching in those infected for the first time, but symptoms may occur 1–4 days after re-exposure. Symptoms are due to an allergic reaction to toxins released by mite faeces, and include itching, particularly at night. Itching is most intense when the patient is in a warm bed or when the body is warm.

The distribution of the rash is unrelated to the location of the mites and burrows, so the whole body of the infected person must be treated (Pankhania 1996).

Atypical and crusted scabies

Immunocompromised people (that is, those with immunosuppressive illness and patients receiving immunosuppressive therapy) and the very young or elderly may present with an atypical form with minimum signs, or rarely a severe, crusted form. When the immune response is impaired, thousands and even millions of mites may be present compared with only a few (10–20) when healthy people become infected. Patients with these atypical forms are highly infectious

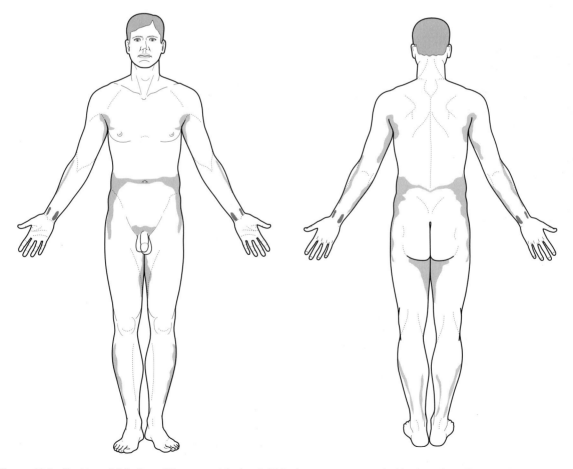

Figure 13.6 Scabies: distribution of the symmetrical rash. This does not correspond with sites of predilection of the mites.

but may not itch, and mites may be present anywhere on the body, including the head. Delay in diagnosis may lead to widespread dissemination including all that have close contact with them.

Diagnosis

The diagnosis of classical scabies is usually based on the history and clinical appearance, but may be confirmed by identification of the mites or their faecal pellets, in skin scrapings of burrows or papules. The eggs are usually present in the deeper parts of the burrows (Barrett and Morse 1993). The diagnosis can be confirmed by following this simple procedure:

- Apply a drop of mineral oil to the skin where there is evidence of a burrow.
- Gently scrape the horny layer using a sterile needle or scalpel blade. The mite (dead or alive) will adhere to the needle point and can sometimes just be seen with the naked eye.
- Apply the skin scrapings directly to a microscope slide.
- Place a cover-slip over the scrapings and examine under a low-power microscope or send the slide to the local microbiology department for examination.
- If the lesions are mite burrows, distinctive eggs, mites and larvae should all be seen.

Treatment and management

A thorough single application of scabicide is usually adequate. For particularly heavy infestations a second application is useful after an interval of 5–6 days; this is long enough for eggs to give rise to larvae but not for adult mites to develop. Transmission ceases after the first treatment has been applied; however, itching may persist for several weeks after the infection has cleared.

Treatment should be applied on cool, dry skin over the entire body and allowed to work between 8 and 24 hours depending on the manufacturer's instructions. **Taking a hot bath or shower before scabies treatment is not recommended** since this facilitates the absorption of the agent from the horny layer into the bloodstream, reducing efficacy and increasing the risk of systemic toxicity. Treatment is best in the evening prior to bedtime.

When there is an outbreak of scabies in the community, some people may be asymptomatic incubators of infection. All close contacts of infected people, bed partners and members of the household of the index case, even if asymptomatic, must be treated simultaneously, even in the absence of signs and symptoms.

The success of any outbreak in the community depends on the expertise of the outbreak team, good communication skills and a well-planned strategy to deal with queries. Forward planning is also important for successful containment of infection (Xavier 1998).

CONCLUSION

A prevention strategy for the common ectoparasitic infections in humans is impossible. A further problem arises when there is not a co-ordinated policy in the community to deal with outbreaks. The value of managing such infections emphasizes the need for infection control teams in the community to adopt an educational role in offering primary healthcare teams help in the early diagnosis and prompt treatment of ectoparasitic infections. This approach enables the life-cycle of most ectoparasites to be broken by the application of relevant treatment, and the adoption of routine infection control measures to prevent further spread. This is the most cost-effective approach to control.

REFERENCES

Barrett N J, Morse D L 1993 The resurgence of scabies. Communicable Diseases Report: CDR Review 3, R32–34
Burgess I F, Veal L, Sindl T 1992 The efficacy of d-phenothrin and permethrin formulations against head lice, a comparison. Pharmaceutical Journal 249: 692–693

Fain A 1978 Epidemiological problems of scabies. International Journal of Dermatology 17: 20–30
Figueroa J, Hall S, Ibarra J 1998 Primary Health Care Guide to Common UK Parasitic Diseases. Community Hygiene Concern, London

Green M 1989 Epidemiology of scabies. Epidemiological Reviews 11: 126–150

Maunder J W 1992 Treating the twenty-year itch. Practice Nurse Jan. 469–473

Meinking T L, Taplin D 1995 Infestations. In: Schachner L A, Hansen R C (eds) Paediatric Dermatology. Churchill Livingstone, New York: 1347–1392

Pankhania B 1996 Management of scabies. Dermatology Update 53: 268–276

Van Neste D J J 1986 Immunology of scabies. Parasitology Today 12: 194

Xavier G 1998 Public relations. Nursing Times 94: 44

FURTHER READING

Aston R, Duggal H, Simpson J 1998 Head Lice, for the Public Health Medicine Environmental Group Executive Committee

Chandler A C, Read C P 1971 Introduction to Parasitology with Special Reference to the Parasites of Man, 10th edn. John Wiley, London

Public Health Laboratory Service 2000 Lice and Scabies: A Health Professional's Guide to Epidemiology and Treatment. PHLS, London

Zaman V, Keong L A 1990 Handbook of Medical Parasitology, 2nd edn. Churchill Livingstone, Singapore

14

Wound care

E. Scanlon

INTRODUCTION

Wound management techniques have been cited as areas of ritualistic nursing practice for many years (Walsh and Ford 1989). A lot of the rituals such as the 'aseptic technique' have been performed with the intention of preventing infection. Unfortunately these procedures were not evidence-based, and through the challenges presented to us by authors such as Walsh and Ford, nurses have moved towards a more rational approach to care. As the extent of available research increases, nursing practice becomes more varied. There has been an expectation for many years that nurses should practice evidence-based healthcare. This message is being emphasized by the current government through the guidance on Clinical Governance, a concept introduced in the White Paper *The New NHS: Modern, Dependable* (DoH 1997) and described in detail in *A First Class service: Quality in the new NHS* (DoH 1998) which strongly links evidence-based practice with quality care. Unfortunately, assimilating all the evidence and transferring it to practice is not easy.

Some areas of wound care have been well researched, and the guidance is clear: for example, compression bandaging for venous leg ulcer management. Other areas remain highly controversial, like the use of EUSOL solution, and despite a huge body of research there is still insufficient evidence to say what its overall effect is in wound healing. Nurses have to be aware of trends in wound management practice. Dressing manufacturers are quick to disseminate these trends if they help to sell their products. Although these are usually based on current research, new evidence is continually coming to light and we have a responsibility to keep our practice up to date.

This chapter will assimilate the body of evidence currently available on the management of infected wounds in the community. The reader is advised that even as they are reading, new papers are being published. It is hoped that they will use this chapter as an essential starting block for current practice and build on it with new information to ensure they maintain 'best practice' over the coming years.

WOUND CLASSIFICATION AND THE HEALING PROCESS

Wounds can be classified according to cause and stage of the healing process:

- **Acute wounds** include traumatic injuries such as burns, scalds, lacerations, abrasions (grazes), cuts and bites. Surgical wounds are intentional acute wounds.
- **Chronic wounds** occur when acute wounds fail to heal within the expected time, and are usually associated with underlying pathologies which delay the healing process such as leg ulcers, pressure sores and malignant tumours.

An understanding of the wound healing process and the mechanisms involved in both acute and chronic wounds is essential to the understanding of wound infection. The information is briefly summarized here but readers are advised to consult more specialist texts for a complete grasp of the physiology (see for example Kindlen and Morrison 1997).

Wound healing process

The process of wound healing can be divided into four stages, which begin once haemostasis has been established: these are the acute inflammatory, destructive, proliferative and maturation phases (Fig. 14.1).

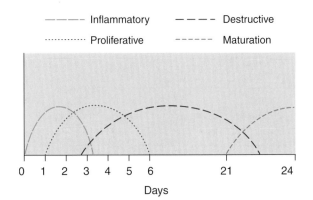

Figure 14.1 The phases of wound healing.

Acute inflammatory phase

Signified by the release of histamine and other mediators from damaged cells and the migration of white blood cells (polymorphonuclear leucocytes and macrophages) to the damaged site, this phase presents at the wound site as the classic signs and symptoms of inflammation, that is, heat, redness, swelling and pain.

Destructive phase

Signified by the clearance of dead, devitalized tissue and bacteria by polymorphs and macrophages, this may be visualized in an open wound bed as debridement, but will also occur in sutured wounds.

Proliferative phase

This phase is signified by the infiltration of the wound by new blood vessels, supported by connective tissue. It is seen at the wound surface as an increase in the granulation tissue; the wound appears red due to the angiogenesis. A sutured wound will continue to appear red due to the new blood vessels.

Maturation phase

The maturation phase occurs when re-epithelialization, wound contraction and connective tissue re-organization take place. This is recognized when new skin grows over the granulation tissue, and contraction causes a reduction in the wound size. Connective tissue re-organization can be seen as changes in the size and shape of scar tissue. The wound is still very fragile at this stage (Kindlen and Morrison 1997).

These phases do not occur in isolation, as there is considerable overlap. The duration of each phase may also vary with the physiology of the individual wound. Most healthcare interventions for wounds are aimed at optimizing the healing time.

Healing by primary intention

We know that if a clean surgical wound or recent laceration has the wound edges opposed, in other words the wound is sutured, taped or glued, then rapid healing will take place. The inflammatory phase commences within a few minutes, following haemostasis. Within hours, neutrophils and macrophages migrate to the wound and begin the removal of debris and bacteria. The wound site will appear hot, red, swollen and painful. This phase usually lasts up to 3 days.

The destructive phase in this type of acute wound is very sensitive to bacterial levels, wound temperature and oxygen levels, each of which may cause wound breakdown or delay healing. If the wound heals within 10–14 days having had the skin edges opposed, this is known as primary intention.

Healing by secondary intention

If a new wound exhibits significant tissue loss or is known to have high bacterial levels, for instance in drainage of an abscess, then it is inappropriate to oppose the skin edges and the wound is left open to heal by secondary intention. This process will allow granulation tissue to fill any cavity and the increased levels of neutrophils and macrophages will deal with the bacteria and debris.

Healing by tertiary intention

Wound healing may be delayed in either primary or secondary intention due to intrinsic or extrinsic factors. These factors may include poor circulation, as in leg ulcers and pressure, and sheer or friction as in pressure sores. This healing process is known as tertiary intention. This chapter will not describe in detail all the known factors that delay healing, but the reader is advised to refer to other texts (such as Kindlen and Morrison 1997).

EPIDEMIOLOGY OF WOUNDS IN THE COMMUNITY

There is a general lack of research in community nursing, especially epidemiological studies on wounds and infection. Some surveys have been carried out on specific wound groups such as leg ulcers (for example Lees and Lambert 1992). Pressure-sore incidence and prevalence may be recorded by individual Trusts but there are no known published community audits. Anecdotal evidence and local audits indicate that approximately 60% of District Nursing time is spent on wound management.

The number and type of wounds treated in the community is very different from hospital: Table 14.1 shows the results of local surveys in Leeds 1998–2000.

Many surgical patients are discharged home with dissolvable sutures and never come into

Table 14.1 Wound treatment in the community: results of local surveys in Leeds

Year	Population	Type of wound	No. of patients	Reference
1998	District nursing caseloads patients	Pressure sores	498	Scanlon 1998
1999	Patients seen by District Nurses, Practice Nurses, hospital outpatients and nursing home staff	Leg ulcers	510	Briggs, Scanlon and Hall 1999
2000	Patients seen by District Nurses and Podiatrists	Foot ulcers	130	Scanlon, Briggs and Hall 2000

contact with community nurses. Occasionally, nurses are required to remove sutures or check healed wounds. Wound management is only needed for these patients where there is delayed wound healing, which may be due to infection.

There is, however, an increasing trend for minor surgery in General Practice, such as excision of in-growing toenails or minor skin lesions, where a knowledge of acute wound management and the associated infection risk is required. Minor traumatic and accidental injuries may be dealt with by the practice nurse in a clinic. The management of these wounds will need to take into account the risks of infection (see Assessment of risk section) and the ability to clean the wound suitably (see Wound cleansing section).

Wounds which are deliberately left to heal by secondary intention, such as following the excision of pilonidal sinuses or breast abscesses, require frequent dressing changes in the community and may have a significant impact on the workload of a district nurse or practice nurse.

Chronic wounds which have associated underlying pathology, such as leg and foot ulcers, pressure sores and malignant tumours, are managed predominantly in patients' own homes.

There is very little reliable information about any of the other factors related to wound management, such as duration of the wounds, infection rates, pain, patient's quality of life, and costs, both to the health services and patients. The financial costs of leg ulcer management alone were estimated at £648 000 in Newcastle Community Health District (Lees and Lambert 1992). If financial costs are calculated, these are usually a crude estimate of nursing time and dressing products.

A study by Law et al (1990), who surveyed surgical patients in hospital and then followed them up after discharge into the community, found that of the patients whose wounds became infected, 41% of cases were diagnosed in hospital and 59% were diagnosed in the community. A survey by Elliston et al (1994) suggested that the extra nursing time required per patient with a wound infection in the community, compared to normal post-surgical nursing care, was on average 6 hours over a 4-week period. These papers suggest that surgical wound infection is probably managed mostly in the community, incurring extra time and resources costs for the health services.

The number of infected wounds in hospital populations has been identified in some areas, with one of the most extensive studies which highlighted the problem being carried out by Cruse and Foord (1980). In their conclusion, they identify that feedback to surgeons about their own patients was an important factor in reducing infection rates. This gave a valuable message about the audit process being used in a cyclical manner so that feedback and dissemination change practice. It is apparent from this section that there is very little formal evaluation or audit of practices in community. For nurses to know whether their practices are good or bad and whether they are improving, there must be better arrangements for surveillance of wound management and infection rates in the community setting.

WHAT IS AN INFECTED WOUND?

Over the years this subject has been hotly debated. Various experts have proposed definitions, most of which are very subjective. Infection is associated with the presence of pathogenic micro-organisms which have a detrimental effect on the health of the host.

Cruse and Foord (1980) used the National Research Council's classification system and definitions from 1964. 'Infection' was identified by them when a wound discharged pus, and 'possible infection' when there were signs of inflammation or a serous discharge.

The presence of micro-organisms in a wound is not unusual, but not all wounds support the same range and number of species (Cooper and Lawrence 1996). Chronic wounds in particular, such as leg ulcers and pressure ulcers, are usually colonized with a mixture of species, many of which can be potential pathogens.

Ayton (1985) categorized different levels of bacterial involvement in wounds:

- Contamination: the presence of bacteria with no multiplication
- Colonization: the presence of multiplying bacteria with no host reaction

- Infection: the presence and multiplication of bacteria in tissue, with an associated host reaction.

Kingsley (2001) proposes the notion of a wound infection continuum where the wound can extend from sterility to infection. Table 14.2 summarizes the continuum with brief definitions of each stage, when this is likely to occur and the recommended action to be taken. More detailed explanations of the information contained in Table 14.2 are given in the text, in particular the actions to be taken.

Criteria used to identify infection may often be restricted to the presence of pus, or pus with inflammation, but these criteria are not very useful when assessing chronic wounds for infection. It must also be remembered that the elderly or immunosuppressed patient (including those on anti-inflammatory drugs) may not present with the classic signs. Cutting and Harding (1994) suggested traditional criteria and identified a list of additional criteria to assist the practitioner in the identification of infection in a wound (Table 14.3).

If the aforementioned 'additional criteria' only are present, this may be an indication of critical colonization which could be managed with topical antiseptics.

For many years the presence of any bacteria was thought to be detrimental to wound healing. It is now known that certain types of wounds in particular patients can heal despite the presence of micro-organisms. It is known that all chronic wounds contain bacteria. However, Gilchrist and Reed (1989) found that this colonization did not necessarily delay wound healing. Trengrove et al (1996) also found that the presence of any specific

Table 14.3 Signs and symptoms of infection. Source: Cutting and Harding 1994

Traditional criteria	Additional criteria
Abscess	Delayed healing
Cellulitis (heat, pain, oedema and erythema)	Discoloration (usually appears dull and dark red)
Increased discharge – serous, seropurulent, haemopurulent, pus	Fragile tissue which bleeds easily
	Unexpected pain or tenderness
	Bridging of soft tissue
	Pocketing at wound base
	Abnormal smell
	Wound breakdown
	Necrotic/sloughy tissue (not explained by pressure damage)

Table 14.2 The infection continuum (Kingsley 2001)

Severity ⟶				
Sterility	**Contamination**	**Colonization**	**Critical colonization**	**Infection**
Acute wounds	Acute wounds	Acute and chronic wounds	Acute and chronic wounds	Acute and chronic wounds
Absence of microbes	Presence of microbes but little active growth	Balanced growth and death of microbes	Host defences unable to maintain healthy balance	Host defences overwhelmed, local spread of cellulitis (may lead to bacteraemia, septicaemia and death)
Very brief period following initial surgical incision or thermal trauma	Present soon after wounding, progresses quickly to colonization	**Situation normal**	Delay in healing	Exacerbation of wound
No action	**Action**	**Action**	**Action**	**Action**
Situation will not persist in wound healing by secondary infection	No need to artificially prevent colonization. Wound healing by secondary intention (with the possible exception of burns)	Do not disturb balance (with the possible exception of diabetic foot ulcers)	Consider using antiseptic dressings to return wound to colonization	Systemic antibiotics +/− antiseptic dressings

bacteria in leg ulcers did not delay healing, but where four or more different bacteria groups were present, healing was delayed. Wounds colonized by non-pathogenic bacteria (that is, with no host reaction) may more readily acquire pathogenic bacteria (producing a host reaction), therefore attention to routes of infection, including self-contamination, airborne contamination and cross infection, is important (Lawrence 1993). Kriezek and Robson (1975) found that wound infection occurred only if more than 100 000 bacteria per gram of tissue were present during wound closure. The work of Robson (1999) over many years has led to the belief that acute or chronic wound infection exists when the microbial load is $>10^5$ Colony Forming Units (CFU)/gram of tissue.

There are several factors which may influence the bacterial effect and determine whether it will lead to the development of an infection. These include:

- the type of pathogen (some bacteria, e.g. *Streptococcus pyogenes*, are known to be particularly virulent)
- the prevalence of the pathogen (the higher the bacterial count, the more likely the wound is to become infected)
- the local wound environment (if the wound does not have the correct moisture balance, i.e. is too wet or too dry, or has pH imbalance, or too little oxygen or nutrients, the bacteria are more likely to become pathogenic)
- the immune response of the host (if the patient has a compromised immune system due to systemic disease, concurrent illness/infection or suppression by medication, then the local wound environment is unable to deal with the bacterial levels)
- the treatments used (if the treatments used have an adverse effect on the local wound environment, as above, or have a specific toxicity for one particular type of bacterium resulting in over-proliferation of other pathogenic bacteria)
- the presence of other disease processes, e.g. concurrent diseases such as diabetes; auto-immune diseases such as rheumatoid arthritis as well as concurrent infections which compromise the immune system

- the presence of devitalized tissue and other foreign bodies (these are known to act as a focus for infection).

MICROBIOLOGY OF INFECTED WOUNDS

Staphylococcus aureus is a major pathogen and the most common micro-organism to cause wound infections. In the national survey of infections in UK hospitals (Emmerson et al 1996), *S. aureus* was found to be responsible for 33% of post-operative wound infections and 33% of skin infections. It can colonize the skin and often the anterior nares of many people. It is transmitted by both contact and air-borne routes via skin squames. It is responsible for a broad spectrum of infections ranging from trivial pyodermas to life-threatening septicaemia, endocarditis and toxic shock syndrome. It is very resistant to desiccation (drying out) and maintains its viability for long periods on work surfaces and in dust particles.

In recent years there has been great concern over the spread of antibiotic-resistant *S. aureus* (for example MRSA). Currently, there is no clinical evidence to say that MRSA is any more virulent in wounds or causes more morbidity or mortality than antibiotic-sensitive strains. Problems have occurred, however, when cellulitis develops and the patient does not respond to systemic antibiotics. This late recognition of resistance has led to delay in appropriate antibiotics being used. This delay may lead to the patient developing septicaemia. Some experts argue that MRSA colonization should be treated, although it may not be a problem to the patient at the time, because if it does become a problem there is a limited range of antibiotics available for treating infection. If infection occurs, the routes of administration (most are given intravenously) and the costs of these treatments, both to the patient in terms of morbidity and side-effects and to the health service financially, are significant. The opposing view, however, is that most patients with a reasonable immune system will cope with colonization, particularly in chronic wounds in the community, and the overuse of antibiotics specific to MRSA will only lead to more resistance. Further guidance on management is given in the section on MRSA-colonized wounds (p. 247).

Streptococci are normally found in the nasopharynx, gastrointestinal tract and female genital tract. They are transferred by hands or are airborne from the throat and are also resistant to desiccation. Although certain strains of Strep. may not become pathogenic in wounds, many experts would actively treat a Group A colonization as the risks of cellulitis, toxicity and even death are very real.

Gram-negative aerobes such as *Pseudomonas aeruginosa*, Proteus species and *Escherichia coli* and other coliforms are all normal flora of the gastrointestinal tract and thrive in warm, moist environments. They are transferred by hands and via contaminated equipment such as commodes. These micro-organisms may commonly be found on chronic wounds with no delay in healing, but in the appropriate environment, such as an excess of moist, sloughy material, they may cause infections.

Anaerobic organisms such as Bacteroides and Peptococcus which naturally grow in the gastrointestinal tract do not present a cross-infection risk as they die quickly on contact with the air. They are, however, frequently found in dead tissue and slough and cause malodour in wounds. They may be a problem in wounds which are ischaemic.

ASSESSMENT

Assessment of risk

It has been established that infection in wounds delays healing. David et al (1983) carried out a multi-centre study of established pressure sores. They observed that only a small proportion of those in the infected category gave any indication of healing.

We know that all wounds are contaminated and many wounds will be colonized with bacteria. Thus an assessment of risk needs to take place. The risk is twofold:

- the possibility of the colonization becoming an infection

- the risk that the number or virulence of the bacteria exceeds the individual's ability to heal the wound.

Consideration needs to be given to the following factors and an individualized plan of care devised.

Site of the wound

Certain areas of the body are known to pose a higher risk of infection than others, for example the groin, axillae and skinfolds. These are sites where the natural skin colonization with bacteria is high. The nurse should be aware of the risk and monitor wounds at these sites carefully.

The patient's immune status

The patient's immune status is influenced by many factors, some longstanding, for example metabolic disorders such as diabetes, some progressive, such as age, and some transient, like concurrent infections. It is difficult to apply a measurement of risk based on these factors, as they vary considerably with each individual. An accurate history of previous infections may indicate the patient's susceptibility.

Age

Although the studies which link increased age to higher levels of infection are all hospital-based, we can rationalize that this is linked to the known decreased immune response in the elderly, rather than the fact that they are hospitalized. There is no evidence to suggest that very young age is linked with a higher risk of infection.

Nutritional status

Cruse and Foord (1973) found a much higher rate of infection in overweight people. Suggestions as to why this occurs include the fact that areas of adipose tissue have been found to impede haemostasis, with resulting haematomas providing an excellent medium for bacterial growth. Adipose tissue generally does not have a good blood supply, and this in itself may be a risk factor. Other suggestions include the problems obese people may incur with moist skinfolds which harbour bacteria, and reduced mobility which may impede circulation.

Malnourished patients have also been found to have a higher wound infection rate. There is an obvious need for carbohydrates for the metabolism of all cells, including white blood cells. The inflammatory response, immunological processes and tissue repair depend upon a good supply of protein. A negative nitrogen balance will impede healing, increasing the opportunity for bacteria to invade the wound (Gould 1987). Research has suggested other factors that are particularly important; ascorbic acid deficiency is thought to increase the risk of wound infection as it is required for the phagocytic action of white blood cells in dealing with bacteria (Penn and Purkins 1991). Some researchers have recommended vitamin C supplements for 'at risk' surgical patients. It is worth considering the vitamin C intake for patients in the community who have been suffering repeated wound infections and those who are thought to be at high risk of infection.

Metabolic disorders

Metabolic disorders affect the body's ability to withstand infection. Cruse and Foord (1980) found a higher infection rate in diabetic patients. The reasons for this are not fully understood but are thought to relate to the numbers of polymorphs at the wound surface. The implications of this for community practice are significant. Many diabetic patients, particularly the elderly, have wounds such as foot ulcers and leg ulcers which often develop due to circulatory problems or diabetic neuropathy. Rigorous aseptic technique should be used when managing these wounds in order to minimize the risk of cross infection.

Steroids

Steroids suppress the immune response by their effect on white blood cells and inflammation. How much effect this has on the patient's risk of infection is not clear.

Hypovolaemia

Low circulatory blood volume is associated with dehydration. This may lead to increased susceptibility to infection. This may be an important factor in community patients where either a sudden acute illness being managed at home may lead to dehydration, or the process may be an insidious one whereby the patient may consciously or unconsciously restrict their fluid intake.

Malignancy

The reasons why a patient with malignancy is at higher risk of infection are multi-factorial. These factors may include anaemia, malnutrition, side-effects of chemotherapy or other medication, stress, haemorrhaging from the wound site, and many others. The nurse should be aware of these risks and intervene where appropriate to maintain the patient's quality of life.

Presence of concurrent infection

Patients who already have an infection, for example a chest or urinary tract infection, are more likely to develop a wound infection. Although the evidence for this was a hospital study of surgical wounds (Valentine et al 1986) we can rationalize this to patients in the community when we consider the effects of an infection on the immune system. If the immune system is compromised through the demands of one infection the patient will be generally debilitated and have lowered resistance to other infections. It is also possible that bacteria may spread haematogenously from one body site to another.

Assessment of the wound

The holistic assessment of the patient should include an assessment of the risk of infection and a detailed assessment of the wound. The assessment of the wound should include the type of wound, the location and position, the grade and classification, the size dimensions, the condition of the surrounding skin, the appearance of the wound bed, the nature and amount of the wound exudate, the odour, and the amount and type of pain.

Assessment of the wound should specifically include inspection for foreign bodies and haematoma formation. Foreign bodies provide a focus for infection and haematomas are toxic, irrespective of any bacteria present in them. Both these elements need to be removed.

Certain people with wounds may not show a classic immune response, such as the elderly, those on anti-inflammatory drugs including steroids, and those with immune disorders. Close observation of these patients is necessary for signs such as:

- increased exudate due to serous fluid, caused by the inflammatory response allowing excess plasma to leak out of the capillaries
- increased pain or change in description of type of pain, often from a dull ache to a throbbing sensation
- change in the visual appearance of the wound, a change in granulating tissue to a deeper red
- a sudden unexplained increase in slough or necrotic tissue due to the toxic effect of the bacteria
- an offensive odour that may be present; this may be difficult to distinguish from the odour associated with colonization of necrotic tissue or a fungating tumour
- a halt in the wound healing process (Gilchrist and Morrison 1997).

The assessment of the wound should be clearly documented. The ongoing assessment and changes in the presentation of the wound will provide indicators of wound infection. Figure 14.2 is an example of a wound assessment chart. It should be noted that the key indicators for infection have been marked with an asterisk to prompt the assessor.

If a wound is to heal by primary intention it must be deemed at low risk of infection. This method of healing is only suitable for clean surgical wounds or traumatic wounds where debridement and mechanical cleansing have successfully removed all bacteria and contaminated matter. This method may be used for some minor surgery within general practice. If a practice nurse is considering opposing skin edges for healing by primary intention in a traumatic wound then a risk assessment of residual contamination must be made. This should take into account how the injury occurred and the type of contaminants; how thorough the wound cleansing has been; whether there is any devitalized tissue still present, and site of the wound on the body which would indicate the level of self-contamination. The presence of a foreign body greatly decreases the threshold for infection; one silk suture can reduce the threshold for clinical infection by a factor of 10 000 (Gould 1987). Resistance to infection is much better in wounds which have been held together with adhesive tapes rather than sutures (Gould 1987).

Obtaining a bacterial specimen

Within the community this can be interpreted as taking a swab. There are other methods of sampling, such as biopsy, aspiration, curettage, contact plates, velvet pads, etc. However, these are generally unavailable in the community so will not be discussed here.

The value of swabbing wounds remains controversial, with many experts questioning whether there is any value in taking a swab at all (Trengrove et al 1996). As with all investigations the findings must be reviewed alongside the clinical information, and treatments should not be based on the swab result alone.

Taking a swab will give a qualitative (not quantitative) picture of the bacteria present on the wound surface. These may not, however, be the bacteria causing the host reaction. When a cellulitis is present we cannot sample the tissue to identify the pathogenic bacteria. Assumptions may be made that the bacteria on the wound surface are also present in the tissues. If antibiotics are prescribed based on the findings of a swab, then regular reassessment of the wound is important to ensure they are being effective.

How to take a swab

There is no clear evidence to support one particular technique for taking a swab; whether to clean

Generic Wound Assessment Chart

Patient name		DOB	
GP/Consultant		Unit/ID no.	
Relevant medical diagnosis		Allergies	

Type of wound	Leg/foot ulcer		Pressure sore		Surgical		Traumatic	

Other (Please specify and complete specific wound assessment)

Position of wound on body Front Back	Location of wound (in words)	Sketch of wound (showing surrounding body region)

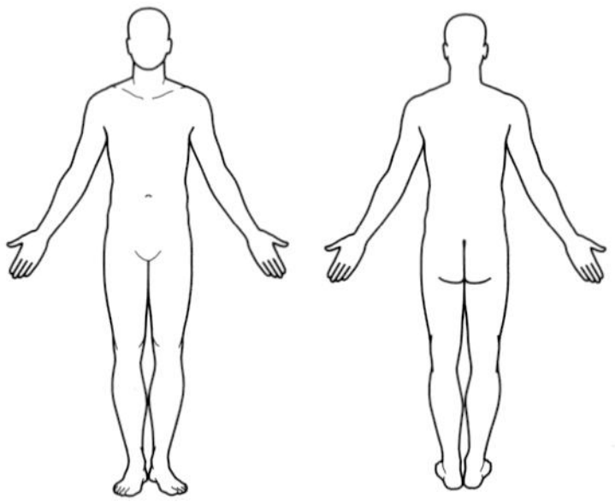

Wound Dimensions

	Date									
Method of measurement (Map/Photo)										
Maximum length (cm/mm)										
Maximum width (cm/mm)										
Superficial skin loss **Grade 1** (Modified Stirling)										
Tissue loss – no cavity **Grade 2**										
Cavity formed **Grade 3**										
Cavity exposing underlying structures, e.g. tendon/bone **Grade 4**										

Are dimensions...

Increasing									
Decreasing									
Static									

Wound Bed Specify Percentage (%)

Necrotic (Black)	%	%	%	%	%	%	%	%	%
Slough (Yellow)	%	%	%	%	%	%	%	%	%
Granulating (Red)	%	%	%	%	%	%	%	%	%
Epithelializing (Pink)	%	%	%	%	%	%	%	%	%

Figure 14.2   Wound assessment chart.

Nutritional Status

Recent weight loss/gain (Please specify) _____

Factors affecting healing (other than infection and nutrition)

Poor blood supply	Poor oxygen supply to wound	Diabetes	Peripheral neuropathy
Elderly	Immunosuppression	Steroids	Chemo/radiotherapy
Smoking	Other (please specify)		

Referrals requested (e.g., clinical nurse specialist, dietician, dermatologist, chiropodist, vascular/plastic surgeon, smoking cessation advisor, pharmacist, pain team, etc.)

Speciality	Name	Contact no.	Date	Brief outcome

N.B.*Where asterisk – may indicate wound infection

Date										

***In addition, suspect wound infection if...**

Granulation tissue bleeds easily										
Fragile bridging of epithelium occurs										
Odour increasing										
Healing is slower than anticipated										
Wound breakdown										

Exudate levels

High*										
Moderate										
Low										
Amount increasing*										
Amount decreasing										

Wound Margin/Surrounding Skin

Macerated*										
Oedematous										
Erythema*										
Eczema										
Fragile*										
Dry/scaling										
Healthy/intact										

Figure 14.2 (*continued*).

Pain (if present, complete a full pain assessment)

Continuous/constant*												
At specific times*												
At dressing change*												
None												
Malodour	On dressing removal											
	When dressing intact											
	On entry to room											

Complete if clinical signs of infection (see guidelines)

Swab taken	Y/N										
Results	+/−										
Action taken	Y/N										

Treatment objective(s)

Debridement											
Absorption											
Hydration											
Other, e.g. odour/pain management											

Signature/initials											

Figure 14.2 (*continued*).

the wound first, use a cotton-tipped or other swab, moisten the swab first, using one or more swabs, wiping with a zig-zag motion, or which medium to use. Until further research is available the reader is advised to use the following technique: if there is pus present a sample obtained by aspiration with a syringe will be the most informative; loose debris on the wound should be removed as this is likely to contain high levels of bacteria, not representative of the infective organism; if the wound is dry and a dry swab is being used then it may be moistened with sterile saline; the swab should be wiped over the wound surface in a zig-zag and rolling motion; the swab should then be placed in the tube and carefully labelled; the nurse must always ensure no contamination from his/her hands or any other part of the patient occurs; the swab should be kept cool and sent to the laboratory as soon as possible; if a serum-tipped swab is available this is preferable to a dry swab as the dry swab may give a false impression of a low bacterial count; if anaerobic bacteria are suspected then a cooked meat broth medium is more likely to sustain the bacteria.

To ensure accurate microscopy and culture it is essential that appropriate clinical details are given with the specimen. Details relating to factors which affect the patient's resistance to infection or the presence of the symptoms of infection (such as an obvious cellulitis) and treatment histories like the current or recent use of antibiotics and/or topical antiseptics will assist the microbiologist in making an accurate diagnosis and appropriate recommendations for management.

Where anaerobic bacteria are considered, for instance if the wound is ischaemic, or if other

Table 14.4 Anti-microbial agents

Term	Definition
Antimicrobial	Substances used to treat infections: include antibiotics, disinfectants and antiseptics
Antibiotic	Substances capable of destroying or inhibiting pathogens, either derived from micro-organisms or synthetically manufactured. Antibiotics are able to selectively target bacteria rather than viable tissue, so can be used in low concentrations and are less toxic than antiseptics
Antiseptics	This is a general term used to describe chemical cleansing solutions used to limit infection in living tissues; they are toxic to viable tissues, unlike antibiotics; they are not able to act selectively. They need to be used in high concentrations in order to destroy invading pathogens

Reference: After Flanagan 1997.

particular pathogens are suspected, it may be useful to contact the microbiologist first for advice. Anaerobic bacteria are often included in the routine cultures but it may be that during the transportation of the swab there is some exposure to air resulting in bacterial death. This could result in an equivocal or negative result.

MANAGEMENT OF WOUNDS

An understanding of definitions of different agents which affect micro-organisms is helpful at this stage: Table 14.4 differentiates between antimicrobial, antibiotic and antiseptic.

Cooper and Lawrence (1996) suggest that the use of topical antibiotics may lead to the formation of resistant bacteria, and therefore advise caution in their use. Whilst bacterial resistance to antiseptics has been less prevalent (Cooper and Lawrence 1996), Harding (1996) advises against their 'wide-spread and indiscriminate use', questioning the effectiveness of these products, due to the lack of research evidence.

It may be appropriate to use prophylactic topical antiseptics for the wound management of immunocompromised patients. It needs to be noted, however, that bacteria can never be completely eradicated from the skin and antiseptics have no healing properties apart from the

antisepsis, so the continual and unselective use of antiseptics is of questionable value.

Wound dressing techniques

From the work by Cruse and Foord (1973) on surgical wounds it has been identified that the development of infection is dependent on the dose of contaminating bacteria. It can be deduced that the longer a wound is exposed, the greater the opportunity there is for bacteria to fall into a wound. A single skin scale from a staphylococcus carrier may transport up to 100 bacterial cells. Staphylococcus may not be pathogenic in a chronic wound on a healthy individual but could present problems in an acute wound or an immunocompromised patient. It would seem prudent, therefore, to keep wound exposure time to a minimum.

The issue of whether an 'aseptic technique' can be carried out in a community environment has always been controversial. Given what we know about ritualistic practice it would seem that whether the procedure achieves its aim, in other words is aseptic, depends more on the individual practitioner rather than the technique itself. It is more appropriate to view the level of asepsis to be a continuum between a safe, clean technique and total asepsis.

The definitions of an aseptic and clean technique are given below.

Aseptic technique

In the context of wound care, an aseptic technique incorporates strategies which prevent the transmission of micro-organisms and involves the use of sterile equipment, fluids and dressings.

Clean technique

A clean technique adopts the same control of infection principles to prevent the transmission of micro-organisms, but clean (rather than sterile) single-use gloves and/or tap water that is safe to drink may be used (Hollingworth et al 1998).

Control of infection principles include hand washing, decontamination and re-processing of instruments and equipment such as bowls used for soaking off dressings; protection of clothing and bedding; and an awareness of the possibility of spreading airborne bacteria.

Given that we know that most chronic wounds are already colonized with bacteria, an aseptic technique may not always be necessary. An individual assessment of risk should be made, taking into account the patient's general well-being, concurrent medical conditions, and current and previous wound history. A flowchart has been designed (Fig. 14.3) to guide the nurse in the decision-making process.

It is important to recognize that wearing gloves to perform wound care procedures is not a substitute for hand washing as a means of infection control. Nurses must still wash their hands before and especially after wearing gloves, as bacterial growth on the hands increases in the moisture which accumulates under gloves and very small tears or holes in the gloves may provide a route of transmission. Hands may also become

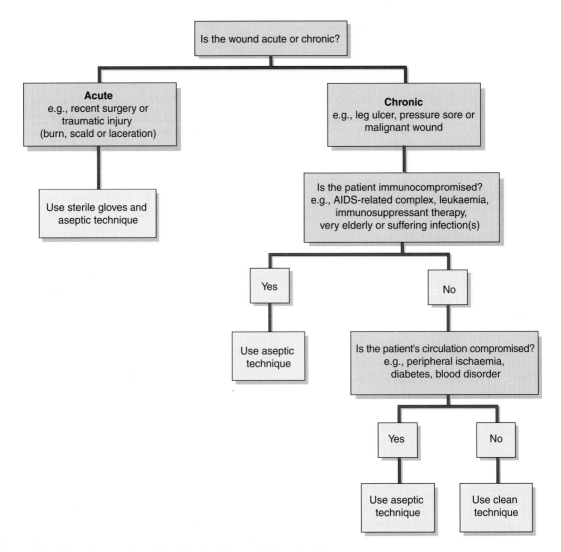

Figure 14.3 Wound management: decision tree for aseptic/clean technique.

contaminated as gloves are removed. The risk of cross infection should be dealt with effectively in every case.

If the patient is being seen in their own home the risk of cross infection by air-borne bacteria is minimal compared to hospital. The nurse must recognize that she/he is the most likely carrier of bacteria, either on the hands or equipment such as scissors or clothes.

In a surgery or clinic setting it is easier to reduce the risk of contamination through contact with surfaces, as these are designed to be decontaminated. It must be remembered, though, even in a busy treatment clinic, that hands and equipment don't clean themselves between patients! If dressings are removed by soaking it is recommended that the bowl or bucket should be lined with a plastic bag which is disposed of after each patient and the bowl washed and dried. Creams and dressing materials must be for individual patient use only.

In the Care Home setting (see Chapter 8), cross infection risks are likely to be similar to hospitals. All nurses working in a Nursing Home should acknowledge the fact that although their residents are not acutely ill they are often frail, elderly and with multiple illnesses. They must also consider the practice of all the staff working with them. It may be that care staff are treating wounds with the best intentions but are lacking knowledge of the risks involved to themselves and other residents. Finally, they must recognize the fact that close contact between residents may lead to an increased risk of cross infection. If dressings are used which allow leakage or 'strikethrough' (the appearance of wound exudate which has soaked through to the outside of the dressing), then contact with the dressing will result in contamination, and bacteria may then easily be passed on to other residents via hands. If occlusive dressings are used and changed before saturation occurs, then the risks of cross infection will be minimized.

Wound cleansing

Wound cleansing has been an area of practice which has been subject to significant change in recent years.

We need to consider when we should cleanse, how, and with what.

The purpose of wound cleansing is to remove 'foreign bodies', excess exudate and bacteria from a wound. This is particularly important in infected wounds or those at risk of infection. Foreign bodies have already been identified as a focus for infection. Excess exudate on healthy skin can cause excoriation and effectively increase the size of the wound, therefore increasing the probability of infection. In addition, the probability of infection is dependent on the number and variety of bacteria present on the wound; thus it would seem advisable to remove them where possible.

Removal of foreign bodies

The choice of wound cleansing technique is not always obvious. It is hoped that any foreign bodies will be removed from a new wound as soon after it has occurred as possible. This may require a pair of forceps, a stitch cutter, a blade or a scrub with a piece of wet gauze depending on the object.

Nurses must be aware of the possibility of introducing new 'foreign bodies' into a wound, for instance leaving a filament of cotton wool or dressing material in a wound. Particular attention needs to be paid to cavities and sinuses where there is a risk of the dressing breaking up on removal. A few fibres of alginate left in the wound, according to the manufacturers, are 'biodegradable' but anecdotal evidence suggests that a piece of alginate being left in a wound is associated with infection and wound breakdown.

Devitalized tissue, for example slough, is considered a foreign body in terms of its effect on wound healing, and therefore requires removal. The removal of devitalized tissue, or debridement, can be classed as wound cleansing. Details of debridement techniques and when to use them will not be given here: the reader is advised to refer to Vowden (1999a, 1999b).

Removing exudates

Exudate is required on the wound surface to maintain phagocyte levels, as well as other wound-healing hormones and chemical stimuli. Wound irrigation will remove these and is therefore best avoided. However, it may be necessary to cleanse the surrounding skin to prevent excoriation from excess exudate. This may be achieved by irrigation or wiping AROUND the wound with a wet swab and then a dry swab. This is not always an easy procedure. It is preferable that a dressing should be used which maintains moist wound healing but absorbs excess exudate and does not allow it to leak onto the surrounding skin. In this case cleansing the wound as a separate procedure is NOT necessary.

Bacterial colonization

Finally, consideration must be given to the prevalence and type of bacteria which may be colonizing a wound. If it is thought that the level of colonization is delaying wound healing, that is, it has reached the point of critical colonization (see Table 14.1) it may be necessary to actively remove some of the bacteria from the wound surface. This is a possibility in debilitated or immunocompromised patients. It is also thought that wound healing in diabetic patients and those with peripheral ischaemia is particularly sensitive to bacterial levels. It may be necessary to be proactive in reducing the number of bacteria at the wound surface. This can be achieved through wound irrigation, the use of topical antiseptics as part of the dressing regime, or systemic antibiotics. Topical antiseptics and antibiotics are considered later in the chapter.

The rationale for different cleansing solutions

If wound irrigation is deemed necessary, a decision will need to be made as to whether the solution needs to be sterile or clean. Nurses are advised to follow the decision pathway found in Figure 14.3. Many nurses are now using non-sterile solutions based on recommendations found in clinical guidelines (RCN 1998).

A decision will then need to be made on the type of solution used. Tap water is not isotonic, that is, water may be drawn into the tissues in an open wound through the cell walls, causing the cells to rupture. Minimal contact time is therefore advocated. Isotonic (normal) 0.9% saline is currently the sterile solution of choice. There are no reported adverse effects and it is relatively inexpensive.

The use of antiseptics for wound cleansing may be considered, but careful consideration should be given to their advantages and disadvantages. In general they should only be used for a specific purpose, as an adjunct to antibiotic therapy, and for a limited period. Their effect is short acting while they are in contact with the wound.

Wound management products

It has been acknowledged previously in this chapter that wound management constitutes a significant proportion of the community nurse's workload. An assumption has been made that the reader will be familiar with the general principles of wound management and will be consulting this text for the specifics of the prevention and management of wound infection.

In recent years the range of wound management products available in the community has significantly increased. With the advent of Nurse Prescribing, many nurses now take full responsibility for their treatment decisions. However, it is well known that many dressings are prescribed by doctors on the recommendation of a nurse. The nurse must remember that he/she is accountable for her own actions and must be fully aware of the indications, methods of administration and contraindications for any dressing they are 'administering' to a patient.

Wound management should be addressed from an holistic perspective and must include maximizing the patient's general physical and psychological well-being. The primary aim should be to maximize their immune function. The management of pain should also be a key priority; if not properly managed the pain of infection may lead to further complications such as immobility, loss of appetite and rest, and stress, which will further delay wound healing.

The choice of dressing must reflect the patient's risk of infection, the management of identified infection, and the risk of cross infection. Where heavy contamination is present the autolysis, or digestion of the bacteria, leads to a proliferation of slough and exudate. The two main aims of the dressing must be:

- To manage this exudate without it either having prolonged contact with the patient's skin, which would lead to excoriation or maceration.
- To contain the exudate and prevent 'strikethrough'. The strikethrough provides a pathway for the bacteria to the external surface, which may then be transmitted to other areas of the body, or other people the patient comes into contact with including nurses or other carers. It may also allow further contamination of the wound from exogenous sources back into the wound.

Healing will also depend on the local wound environment. Factors which influence this include: humidity, gaseous exchange and pH, and the choice of dressing should take into account these factors.

Humidity

The correct balance of humidity can be achieved under an occlusive dressing. The type of dressing will depend on whether there is a need to absorb exudate to prevent this damaging the surrounding skin causing excoriation and maceration. It has been suggested that the use of an occlusive dressing encourages the multiplication of bacteria (Bennett 1982). It is now known that the exudate trapped under the dressing contains a large number of white cells, hormones and chemical stimulants which digest the bacteria and promote wound healing. An occlusive dressing will prevent the entry of new bacteria to the wound and the transfer of bacteria to other people through contact or airborne distribution from the wound. Gilchrist and Reed (1989) found that occlusive dressings did not increase the risk of infection or encourage the growth of anaerobic bacteria. It has been found that wounds dressed with occlusive dressings are less likely to become clinically infected (Hutchinson and Lawrence 1991).

Gaseous exchange

The importance of gaseous exchange at the wound's healing surface is recognized when the high metabolic demands of the repairing tissue are considered. The effect of varying oxygen and carbon dioxide concentrations around the wound is not fully understood. There is an assumption that low oxygen levels in the presence of anaerobic bacteria, especially with a growth medium such as slough or necrotic tissue, will encourage their proliferation and increase the probability of infection. This is a consideration with occlusive dressings and their 'vapour permeability'. A dressing of low vapour permeability is likely to lead to low oxygen levels under the dressing. If the patient is known to have anaerobic colonization such as bacteroides, or to be at high risk of anaerobic infection (for example a patient with diabetes or a wound site on an ischaemic limb), then a dressing with higher vapour permeability seems a more appropriate choice.

pH

The pH of a wound is important, as cell metabolism can only occur within a narrow range. Changes in pH will affect phagocytosis. Consideration needs to be given to the topical agents used: for instance EUSOL is an alkaline solution and hydrogen peroxide is acidic.

Products

There is currently conflicting evidence on the levels of colonization under occlusive dressings. Experimental studies have shown higher levels of bacteria under occlusive dressings (Mertz and Eaglestein 1984) but clinical studies have shown lower rates of infection in dry wounds (Hutchinson and McGuckin 1990). Other products may also be used, such as aromatherapy oils. There is some evidence to support the antiseptic effects of teatree oil in wound management (Baker 1998) but an in-depth review of the evidence is beyond the scope of this book. Dermatologists would also advise caution with these products as there are concerns about the incidence of sensitivity and allergic reactions.

Some of the more common dressings are discussed here, with particular reference to their use in the management of infected wounds.

Absorbent pads These are designed to absorb moisture from highly exuding wounds. They can be used as secondary dressings. Most of them do not have a waterproof backing and the risk of strikethrough leading to cross infection is high, especially with infected wounds. They are relatively low in price and may be considered appropriate if a wound needs frequent dressing changes or assessment.

Alginates These can be used on infected wounds but advice from the manufacturers suggests they need daily changing. Some alginates manufacturers have suggested that when the wound exudate is drawn into the dressing the bacteria are taken with it. Alginates may be beneficial in heavily-exuding wounds where exudate management is a priority for the prevention of strikethrough and cross infection. The combined use of alginates with antiseptics is advocated by some practitioners, for instance soaking the alginate in iodine solution, but this practice is contentious as the alginate loses its absorbency and the duration of the antimicrobial effect of the solution over time is unknown.

Bactroban A topical antibiotic, Bactroban is available as a cream or ointment containing mupirocin 2%. The ointment is used for primary skin infections (impetigo). The cream is used for secondary infected traumatic lesions. It is active against *Staphylococcus aureus* including MRSA, other staphylococci, and streptococci. It is also active against Gram-negative organisms such as *Escherichia coli* and *Haemophilus influenzae* (Morgan 2000). Its use has become widespread for the treatment of wounds thought to be infected with MRSA; unfortunately there have been reports of spreading resistance to mupirocin among *S. aureus* (Morgan 2000). It is important, therefore, to consider alternative topical treatments such as antiseptics, so that over-use of the mupirocin does not lead to more resistance.

Bandages Bandages range from a light retention bandage, used to hold dressings in place when adhesion to the skin is contraindicated, to high compression bandages for the management of oedema associated with chronic venous disease.

The main consideration over bandage choice occurs when high compression bandaging is

being used. If a wound is infected, then it is likely to be painful, and applying a tight bandage will increase the pain experienced by the patient. Also, multi-layer bandaging is cost-effective if left in place for a week at a time. Infected wounds need to be regularly re-assessed, for example daily, and this bandage regime therefore would not be appropriate.

Deodorizing dressings These dressings usually contain charcoal or carbon to absorb wound odour that is often associated with infection. They are used to manage the symptoms of infection and should be used as an adjunct to systemic or topical management. Some deodorizing dressings also contain an antiseptic that helps to control bacterial levels.

EUSOL EUSOL is an antiseptic. Its use in wound management remains controversial. Most of the research carried out is in the form of in vitro or animal studies. The most reputable piece of work was actually performed on acute, clean, granulating wounds in rabbits (Brennan and Leaper 1985). Human studies have been carried out with very small numbers, and very few have used healing rate as an outcome measure. No studies have been found which include economic analysis; although the cost of the product is low, the cost of nursing time is high. No studies have addressed the patient perspective, although some have mentioned pain. It is unlikely that a nurse would initiate a wound treatment with EUSOL in the community but if it was being considered for an infected wound the advantages and disadvantages should be taken into account: see Table 14.5.

A problem-solving approach can be used which will ensure the safest, most effective use of the product: see Table 14.6.

Film dressings Although these dressings on their own are only suitable for minimally-exuding wounds, they are useful as a waterproof secondary dressing to prevent strikethrough with infected wounds. They also allow visible examination of the wound without disturbing the dressing.

Foam dressings Foam dressings may be used in their sheet form or as cavity dressings in the management of infected or colonized wounds. These enable the wound to be occluded (with some of the sheet foams) to facilitate healing and

Table 14.5   Advantages and disadvantages of EUSOL

Advantages	Disadvantages
Cheap	Chemical instability and short shelf-life
Easy to use	Rapidly inactivated in the presence of necrotic tissue and slough
Effective disinfectant of a wide range of micro-organisms and viruses	May lead to production of excessive granulation tissue
Effective at debriding sloughy wounds	May cause pain and skin irritation
No reported resistance by microbial agents	Does not absorb any wound exudate
	Cytotoxic effect on various types of cells involved in the wound healing process

prevent cross infection. They are also highly absorbent. They do not have an active role in the management of infection and should be used as an adjunct to systemic or topical management.

Hydrocolloids   These have been used in the management of infected wounds. Current expert guidance recommends the use of occlusive dressings in the management of MRSA-colonized wounds (Combined Working Party 1998). This is in response to rather limited evidence suggesting hydrocolloids prevent penetration of bacteria for up to 7 days and that they facilitate wound healing. Other studies have shown higher levels of bacteria under occlusive dressings (Mertz and Eaglestein 1984). Anecdotal evidence suggests that they may be unsuitable for infected wounds in diabetic patients. The reasons for this are twofold: the

Table 14.6   EUSOL: guidelines for use

Problem	Action	Rationale
Protection of surrounding skin	Apply barrier cream e.g. zinc & castor oil/petroleum jelly	EUSOL can be corrosive/painful to surrounding skin
Carrier medium for EUSOL	Soak EUSOL in gauze/ribbon gauze	Gauze is cost-effective (non-filamented, does not shed fibres). Whole product can be removed complete
Dressing dries out and sticks to the wound	Whole wound is covered with paraffin gauze tulle. Dressing is changed at least daily	Tulle minimizes water evaporation from wound. It prevents adhesion of dressing to wound. Daily dressing minimizes drying out and prevents tulle being granulated into wound
EUSOL is harmful to granulating tissue	EUSOL soaked gauze is isolated to sloughy/necrotic tissue	EUSOL will slow down healing where the antimicrobial/debridement effect is not needed
EUSOL can be unstable, it has a short shelf-life	EUSOL may be provided by the prescribing hospital department; once opened it must be used within 2 weeks; it must be stored in the dark bottle, away from sun and heat	Community pharmacists do not now stock EUSOL and may have difficulty obtaining it
When debriding a wound EUSOL is rapidly deactivated by organic matter	Dressing changes must take place at least daily	Recommended dressing interval is 3 hours. Consideration must be given to the impact on the patient's quality of life and nursing time
EUSOL does not absorb exudate	Wound requires covering with sufficient gauze to absorb exudate	To prevent exudate reaching the surrounding skin and causing excoriation
The wound healing process is affected by EUSOL	The EUSOL should be isolated to the slough or necrotic tissue; when this is absent from the wound the prescriber should be informed and the treatment changed	EUSOL has an adverse effect on fibroblasts, leucocytes and probably all cell proteins

Reference: Moore 1992.

thicker hydrocolloid dressings have a very low vapour permeability and therefore do not allow gaseous exchange through the dressing. This is thought to lead to low oxygen levels and high levels of anaerobic bacteria, which are frequently responsible for wound infections in diabetic patients. In addition, hydrocolloids are designed to be left in place for up to a week at a time. If a wound is infected, it requires frequent observation which cannot be done with an intact hydrocolloid. There is however more visibility and vapour permeability through the thinner hydrocolloids.

Hydrogels These are available as flat sheets or more commonly amorphous gels. The high water content allows them to hydrate dry wounds. They are most commonly used to promote autolytic debridement of non-viable tissue. They require a secondary dressing. They can be used on infected wounds, although most are contraindicated with anaerobic infections. They should be used as an adjunct to systemic antibiotic therapy.

Iodine products Evidence suggests that slow-release iodine and povidone-iodine based products may be useful in treating wound infections. The effects of antiseptics on wound healing is controversial. The debate was initiated by some early work undertaken by Brennan and Leaper (1985) which examined the early stages of wound healing in a rabbit's ear. Unfortunately this experiment did not follow through to the end healing point and only looked at a small number of wounds. A review by Goldenheim (1993) looked at povidone-iodine (PVP-I) and wound healing in various preparations and in vivo and in vitro experiments. This review concluded that there was no difference in healing rates for most forms of povidone-iodine compared to the controls, except where a 'detergent' form (skin cleansers/ surgical scrubs) was used. This paper was not, however, a systematic review of the evidence. It also did not specifically discuss the use of iodine in colonized or infected wounds.

An experiment by Mertz et al (1999) found that cadexomer iodine ointment did not have a detrimental effect on wound healing and resulted in a significant reduction in levels of *Staphylococcus aureus* including MRSA. It did not however have a significant effect on *Pseudomonas aeruginosa*.

Povidone-iodine is found impregnated in viscose dressings which provide a useful topical antiseptic for minimally-exuding superficial wounds. It is used for prophylaxis and treatment of colonized and infected wounds. The dressings should be changed when the colour changes from yellow to white, indicating that the iodine has all been used up. If the level of exudates is too high then the iodine is deactivated very quickly and the dressing is ineffective.

Povidone-iodine is also found as a 10% ointment or cream. This may be useful for very dry, for example necrotic, wounds which are infected or critically colonized where hydration of the devitalized tissue is a priority.

Metronidazole gel An antibiotic gel used topically on wounds, it is active against anaerobic bacteria such as bacteroides, *Clostridium perfringens*, and certain protozoa. It may be used as well as or instead of oral metronidazole, and is shown to be effective at reducing odour. Concerns exist about the possibility of antibiotic resistance developing with topical use, and its use therefore should be restricted.

Silver impregnated dressing These are impregnated films or foam dressings which contain silver that is slowly released from the dressing to give a constant anti-bacterial effect.

Silver sulfadiazine This is prepared as a topical cream and combines antiseptic with antibiotic properties. Its activity is broad spectrum against most pathogenic bacteria and fungi. It is used in the treatment of wound infections and where heavy colonization is delaying wound healing. Although currently there is no reported resistance, caution should be exercised when deciding on treatment to reduce the possibility of any developing resistance. A study found that silver sulfadiazine reduced the number of *Pseudomonas aeruginosa* in burns wounds (Boeckx et al 1985).

Sugar and honey Although sugar and sugar pastes have been used for many years on dirty, infected and malodorous wounds, the evidence to support their use is sparse. Honey is currently subject to research, as it has been found to be effective as a natural antibacterial agent with the ability to debride sloughy wounds. There are anecdotal reports of the applications of sugar and honey being painful for some patients.

Tulle dressings These dressings consist of impregnated paraffin gauze. Those that are impregnated with chlorhexidine are thought to have some effect on superficial infected wounds. Those impregnated with antibiotics are thought to be more likely to lead to antibiotic resistance and should be avoided. A secondary dressing is required.

All infected wounds should frequently be reviewed. The choice of wound management product should take this into account. It may not be cost-effective to use a dressing or bandage designed to stay in place for a week on a low-exuding wound which is being redressed every day.

SPECIFIC TYPES OF WOUNDS

Traumatic wounds (contributed by M. Steen)

Traumatic wounds are caused by either intentional or unintentional injury. The majority of this type of wound will heal by primary intention (see Fig. 14.4). The clinician, however, needs to be aware of risk factors such as age, site and extent of injury, a person's general well-being and social habits, i.e. smoking, that can influence the rate at which the healing of a wound will occur (Desai 1997, Mera 1997, McPhee et al 1998, Dealey 2001, Flanagan 1997). Some traumatic wounds, therefore, are more at risk – for example in an elderly person with a pre-tibial laceration who smokes. In such cases a preventative measure such as occluding the wound by applying a dry sterile dressing and promoting cessation of smoking would be advantageous.

An example of a traumatic wound is a perineal wound following childbirth injury. A perineal wound can be surgically induced by performing an episiotomy, or can spontaneously occur as a tear which is classified by its severity.

Management of perineal wounds

The vast majority of perineal wounds will heal rapidly. Nevertheless, preventive care is advocated to reduce the risk of infection, and health professionals promote good standards of personal hygiene as the urogenital region is not a sterile area. Organisms commonly isolated include: *Streptococcus faecalis, Staphylococcus epidermidis, Staphylococcus aureus, Escherichia coli, Candida albicans, Clostridium perfringens* and *Bacteroides fragilis*. The incidence of perineal wound infections has been reported to be between 2% and 8% (McGuiness et al 1991, Steen and Marchant 2001). There is some evidence that the severity of the perineal injury increases the risk of a wound infection occurring, for example in the combination of an episiotomy and tear (Hulme and Greenshields 1993). Suture material itself can become infected as it is a foreign body in living tissue until it is completely absorbed; some synthetic absorbable sutures can take a minimum of six weeks to absorb and this may also contribute to a delay in healing. Women are advised that warm bathing can help the sutures to absorb by the process of hydrolysis which will minimize tissue reaction and inflammation.

One of the oldest remedies for perineal and other trauma is the addition of salt to the bathwater and this still appears to be popular. Salt is believed to soothe discomfort and speed the healing process but its precise mode of action is unclear. Claims that it has antibacterial or antiseptic properties remain unsubstantiated (Ayliffe et al 1975). There is no consensus as to the type or amount of salt to be used (Sleep 1990). A randomized controlled trial involving 1800 women compared three bathing policies. One group were asked to add salt, another group were asked to add savlon and the final group were asked to use no additives. Few if any differences were reported between the three groups in healing or infection rates (Sleep and Grant 1988). On the basis of these results, there is no case for recommending the use of salt or savlon bath additives.

Burns

Wounds caused by burns are acute wounds healing by secondary intention and are therefore colonized by micro-organisms. When the burns are extensive the patient is at high risk of infection and septicaemia. This is probably due to the systemic effects of the burns, such as hypovolaemia,

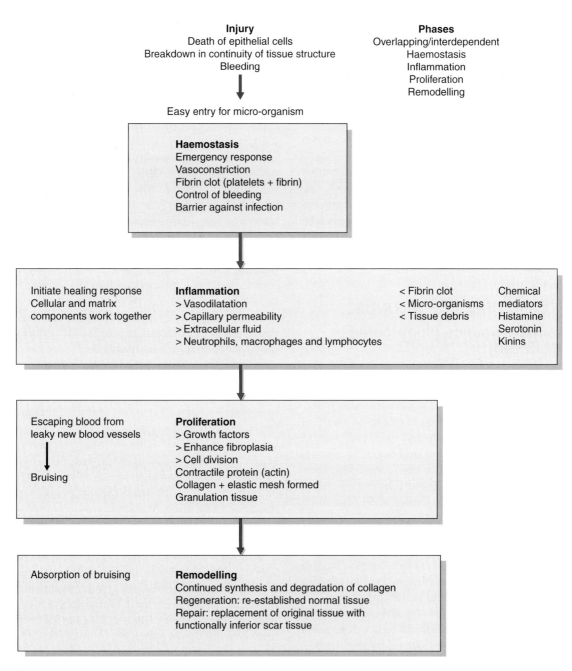

Figure 14.4 Wound healing – primary intention.

and the large wound surface area devoid of skin and containing devitalized tissue which becomes colonized with skin flora.

Burn wounds are often colonized with Pseudomonas, Acinetobacter and Staphylococci. These are particularly resistant to drying out and are easily introduced through air-borne or direct contact routes.

Management should be carried out with an aseptic technique due to the high risk of infection.

Debridement of devitalized tissue may be necessary. Treatments may include topical antimicrobials such as silver sulfadiazine (Flamazine) cream or povidone-iodine (Betadine) cream which may be used to minimize colonization and therefore reduce the risk of infection.

A study carried out in Iraq (Mousa 1997) analysed the type of bacteria in infected burn wounds. It found the dominant organisms to be *Pseudomonas aeruginosa* and *Staphylococcus aureus*. Mousa also carried out cultures for anaerobic bacteria with a rigorous technique and found anaerobes in 55% of the wounds, mostly Bacteroides (several of these patients had septic shock). Anaerobes are often not identified with routine swabbing, and it may be that their virulence leads to more frequent systemic infections. More anaerobic organisms were found in cases where the wound was dressed with an 'open dressing' (70%) compared to 42% in wounds dressed with an 'occlusive dressing'. However, there were no details of the precise dressings and techniques used.

Infected burn wounds should be treated with systemic antibiotics. Topical antibiotics or antiseptics are unlikely to reach organisms in the superficial tissues.

Surgical wounds

The majority of the evidence related to surgical wound infection is derived from the studies by Cruse and Foord (1980). Their conclusions have been supported and developed by other researchers since then. Post-operative wound infection is mainly influenced by the type of surgery and the number of bacteria present at the end of the operation. There are, however, several pre-, peri- and post-operative factors which may also influence its development. These include:

- site of the surgical incision
- length of pre-operative stay
- pre-operative skin preparation and hair removal
- the use of prophylactic antibiotics
- length of operation
- peri-operative skin preparation of the operation site

Table 14.7 Classification of surgical wounds. Source: National Research Council, Ad Hoc Committee on Trauma 1964

Clean	These are operations in which the gastrointestinal, genitourinary or respiratory tracts are not opened. No inflammation is encountered and there is no break in aseptic technique (e.g. varicose vein surgery)
Clean-contaminated	Operations in which a viscus (respiratory, gastrointestinal or urinary tract) is opened but there is minimal spillage (e.g. elective cholecystectomy)
Contaminated	Operations in which acute inflammation without pus is encountered or when there is gross spillage from an opened viscus (e.g. elective colorectal surgery with poor bowel preparation or acute appendicitis)
Dirty	Operations in which pus is encountered or a perforated viscus is found (e.g. perforated sigmoid diverticulitis, abscesses) or the wound is an old traumatic injury

- methods of wound closure
- post-operative care
- wound dressings
- wound drainage
- use of antiseptics
- washing and bathing after surgery (Briggs 1997).

With effective audit and surveillance measures, feedback and education, many of these factors can be minimized.

The types of surgical wounds can be categorized based on the likely degree of intra-operative bacterial contamination, as set out in Table 14.7.

Dressing choice for surgical wounds should follow the same principles as for other infected wounds. The supporting evidence concurs with the view that occlusive and semi-occlusive dressings should be used to prevent the risk of cross infections.

MRSA-colonized wounds

It has already been acknowledged in the Microbiology section that MRSA in itself is not a problem in wound healing. Management decisions will be based on an individual risk assessment. It may be that patients who are deemed at high risk, such as those who are immunocompromised with MRSA colonization of their wounds may have antibacterial therapy as a prophylactic measure, given the difficulty treating an infection due to MRSA.

Wound cleansing has been discussed earlier. These principles need to be applied to wounds with MRSA. It is not uncommon to use antiseptic solutions for cleansing MRSA-colonized wounds. Although the antibacterial effect of the solution is short-acting, the effect of reducing the prevalence of the bacteria may be beneficial.

The use of topical agents in MRSA management will now be discussed.

Mupirocin (Bactroban)

This product has been described in detail on page 242. It is a topical antibiotic with a high level of activity against *Staphylococcus aureus* including MRSA. Its primary use is to de-colonize the nose (anterior nares), which is a common site of MRSA colonization. It is important, therefore, to preserve the useful life of Mupirocin by restricting the frequency and duration of use and avoiding inappropriate usage. It is not licensed for use on wounds, except superficial infected lesions. Although case reports suggest it has been effective, it is not the treatment of choice and its use should be restricted whenever possible.

Chlorhexidine

Chlorhexidine is not generally used in wound management but a 0.05% aqueous solution may be used for wound cleansing in patients where high levels of staphylococcal colonization are thought to be delaying wound healing.

Povidone-iodine (PVP-I)

PVP-I is a potent, rapidly bactericidal antiseptic with high activity against MRSA. It is used for the prophylaxis and treatment of colonized skin and mucosae and wounds. It can sustain an antimicrobial action in between applications, although its activity is neutralized in the presence of organic material like pus.

PVP-I is available in various forms:

- 10% in aqueous and alcoholic solutions (e.g. Betadine). It is used for hand and skin disinfection prior to surgery and invasive procedures. It can be used for cleansing minor wounds but the concentration is too high for body cavity irrigation.
- 7.5% in aqueous surfactant solution for use as a scrub for hands and skin and in seborrhoeic conditions of the scalp and acne vulgaris of the face and neck.
- 4% in surfactant basis for infective skin conditions.
- 2.5% in a dry powder spray for skin and wound disinfection.
- 10% ointment for treatment of superficial septic lesions.

The safety and efficacy of PVP-I has been studied in depth. It has been found to work through a sustained release system whereby the level of free iodine is maintained at 25 ppm (parts per million) in solution. As this iodine is used up, more is released from the compound. This process will continue until all the iodine is used up, thus ensuring safe levels are maintained for a prolonged period of time. It has also been identified that this process is most effective in dilutions of between 1 in 10 and 1 in 100 (using the 10% solution). Therefore where the 10% solution is being used this should be diluted by at least 1:10 (Goldenheim 1993).

Staphylococcal resistance to iodine is currently unknown.

Other wound management products are known to be effective against MRSA, when used topically to reduce colonization. These have been specified above under Wound management products.

Malodorous wounds

It is very important to deal effectively with wounds which are malodorous in the community. An odour in a family home seems to be much more offensive than in hospital. Smells in nursing or residential homes seem to permeate through large areas. If patients are able to go out and mix with the public, a factor which may prevent them doing so may be a self-consciousness about an odour. Assessment of odour should always be included in any wound assessment and documented so that changes can be identified.

Malodours are due to the presence of bacteria and can be related to colonization or infection. It is necessary to make a detailed assessment of the type of wound and wound history to ensure the cause of the odour is correctly identified and an appropriate management plan drawn up.

If the wound has a history of necrotic or sloughy tissue and this is in the process of being hydrated for autolytic debridement, there will naturally be an odour as the colonization of bacteria assists in the breakdown of the non-viable tissue. Products can be used on the wound to absorb the odour, such as charcoal dressings. Manufacturers' instructions need to be followed, as some should be used wet and some dry.

Where there is evidence of cellulitis around the wound or other evidence of infection in an acute wound, systemic antibiotics should be used. Topical antiseptics may be used as an adjunct, such as iodine and/or silver products.

Topical antiseptics may be used in wounds at high risk of infection, as noted in Assessment of risk, above. Where there is uncertainty over assessment or diagnosis, or expected outcomes are not achieved, then an expert opinion should be sought.

Other technologies and regimes may be used in the management or prevention of infection, for example larval therapy, ultrasound, Vacuum Assisted Closure (VAC) therapy, but these are unlikely to be commonly available in the community in the near future so have not been discussed in this chapter.

REFERENCES

Ayliffe G A B, Babb J R, Collins R J, Davies J, Deverill C, Varney J 1975 Disinfection of baths and bathwater. Nursing Times 71(37): 22–23

Ayton M 1985 Wounds that won't heal. Community Outlook Nov. 13: 16–19

Baker J 1998 Essential oils: a complementary therapy in wound management. Journal of Wound Care 7(7): 355–357

Bennett R G 1982 The debatable benefit of occlusive dressings for wounds. Journal of Dermatologic Surgery and Oncology 8(3): 166–167

Boeckx W, Focquet M, Cornelissen M, Nuttin B 1985 Bacteriological effect of cerium-flamazine cream in major burns. Burns, Including Thermal Injury 11(5): 337–342

Brennan S S, Leaper D J 1985 The effects of antiseptics on the healing wound: a study using the rabbit ear chamber. British Journal of Surgery 72: 780–782

Briggs M 1997 Principles of closed surgical wound care. Journal of Wound Care 6(6): 288–292

Briggs M, Scanlon E, Hall T E 1999 The prevalence of open leg ulceration in an area health authority. Abstract from Venous Forum of Royal Society of Medicine Conference 1999

Combined Working Party: British Society for Antimicrobial Chemotherapy, Hospital Infection Society and Infection Control Nurses Association 1998 Revised guidelines for the control of MRSA infections in hospital: combined working party report. Journal of Hospital Infection 39: 253–290

Cooper R, Lawrence J C 1996 Microorganisms and wounds. Journal of Wound Care 5(5): 233–236

Cruse P J E, Foord R 1973 A five year prospective study of 23 649 surgical wounds. Archives of Surgery 107: 206

Cruse P J E, Foord R 1980 The epidemiology of wound infection: a 10-year prospective study of 62 939 wounds. Surgical Clinics of North America 60(1): 27–40

Cutting K F, Harding K G 1994 Criteria for identifying wound infection. Journal of Wound Care 3(4): 198–201

David J A, Chapman J G, Chapman E J et al 1983 An investigation of the current methods used in nursing for the care of patients with established pressure sores. Nursing Research Unit, Northwick Park

Dealey C 2001 The Management of Patients with Wounds: A Guide for Nurses, 2nd edn. Blackwell Science, Oxford, Ch. 2: 20–23

Department of Health 1997 The New NHS: Modern, Dependable. The Stationery Office, London

Department of Health 1998 A First Class Service. Quality in the New NHS. The Stationery Office, London

Desai H 1997 Ageing and wounds. Part 1: foetal and postnatal healing. Journal of Wound Care 6(4): 192–196

Elliston P R, Slack R C, Humphreys H, Emmerson A M 1994 The cost of post operative wound infections (Letter). Journal of Hospital Infection 28(3): 241

Emmerson A M, Enstone J E, Griffin M, Kelsey M C, Smith E T M 1996 The second national prevalence survey of infection in hospitals – overview of the results. Journal of Hospital Infection 32: 175–190

Flanagan M 1997 Wound Management. Churchill Livingstone, London

Gilchrist B, Morrison M 1997 Wound infection. In: A Colour Guide to Nursing Management of Chronic Wounds. Mosby, London, Ch. 3

Gilchrist B, Reed C 1989 The bacteriology of leg ulcers under hydrocolloid dressings. British Journal of Dermatology 121: 337–344

Goldenheim P D 1993 An appraisal of povidone-iodine and wound healing. Postgraduate Medical Journal 69(Suppl. 3): S97–S105

Gould D 1987 Infection and Patient Care: A Guide for Nurses. Heinemann Nursing, London, Ch. 9

Harding K G 1996 Managing wound infection. Journal of Wound Care 5(8): 391–392

Hollingworth H, Kingston J E, Paget J 1998 Using a non-sterile technique in wound care. Professional Nurse 13, 4

Hulme H, Greenshields W 1993 The Perineum in Childbirth: a Survey Conducted by the National Childbirth Trust. National Childbirth Trust, London

Hutchinson J, Lawrence J 1991 Wound infection under occlusive dressings. Journal of Hospital Infection 17: 83–94

Hutchinson J J, McGuckin M 1990 Occlusive dressings: a microbiologic and clinical review. American Journal of Infection Control 18: 257–268

Kindlen S, Morrison M 1997 The physiology of wound healing. In: Morrison M, Moffatt C, Bridel-Nixon J, Bale S (eds) Nursing Management of Chronic Wounds, 2nd edn. Mosby, London, p. 1

Kingsley A 2001 A proactive approach to wound infection. Nursing Standard 15(30): 50–58

Kriezek T J, Robson M C 1975 Biology of surgical infection. Surgical Clinics of North America 55: 1262–1267

Law D J W, Mishriki S F, Jeffery P J 1990 The importance of surveillance after discharge from hospital in the diagnosis of post-operative wound infection. Annals of the Royal College of Surgeons of England 72: 207–209

Lawrence J 1993 Wound infection. Journal of Wound Care 2(5): 227–280

Lees T A, Lambert D 1992 Prevalence of lower limb ulceration in an urban health district. British Journal of Surgery 79: 1032–1034.

McGuiness M, Norr K, Nacion K 1991 Comparison between different perineal outcomes on tissue healing. Journal of Nurse-Midwifery 36(3): 192–198

McPhee I B, Williams R P, Swanson C E 1998 Factors influencing wound healing after surgery for metastatic disease of the spine. Spine 23(6): 726–732

Mera S 1997 Wound Healing. Pathology and Understanding Disease Prevention. Stanley Thomas, Cheltenham, 140–151

Mertz P M, Eaglestein W H 1984 The effect of a semi-occlusive dressing on the microbial population in superficial wounds. Archives of Surgery 119(3): 287–289

Mertz P M, Oliveira-Gandia M F, Davis S C 1999 The evaluation of a cadexomer iodine wound dressing on methicillin resistant *Staphylococcus aureus* (MRSA) in acute wounds. Dermatologic Surgery 25: 89–93

Moore D 1992 Hypochlorites: a review of the evidence. Journal of Wound Care 1(4): 44–53

Morgan D A 2000 Formulary of Wound Management Products: A Guide for Healthcare Staff. Euromed Communications Ltd, Haslemere

Morrison M, Moffatt C, Bridel-Nixon J, Bale S (eds) 1997 Nursing Management of Chronic Wounds, 2nd edn. Mosby, London

Mousa H A L 1997 Aerobic, anaerobic and fungal burn wound infections. Journal of Hospital Infection 37: 317–323

National Research Council Ad Hoc Committee on Trauma 1964 Post-operative wound infections: factors influencing the incidence of wound infections. Annals of Surgery 160(Suppl. 2): 33–75

Penn N, Purkins L 1991 Effects of dietary supplements with vitamins A, C, E on cell-mediated immune function in elderly long stay patients. Age and Aging 20: 169–174

Robson M C 1999 Lessons gleaned from the sport of wound watching. Wound Repair and Regeneration 7: 2–6

Royal College of Nursing 1998 Clinical Practice Guidelines: the Management of Patients with Venous Leg Ulcers. RCN, London

Scanlon E 1998 Audit of pressure sore prevalence. Unpublished internal report.

Scanlon E, Briggs M, Hall T E 2000 Foot ulceration in the community: results of a survey of district nurses and podiatrists. Abstract for EWMA conference, Advances in Wound Management, Sweden

Sleep J 1990 Postnatal perineal care. In: Alexander J, Levy V, Roch S (eds) Midwifery Practice: Postnatal Care: a Research-based Approach. Research based Midwifery Practice 1. MacMillan Press, Basingstoke

Sleep J, Grant A 1988 Routine addition of salt or savlon bath concentrate during bathing in the immediate post-partum period. A randomized controlled trial. Nursing Times 84(21): 55–57

Steen M P, Cooper K J 1998 Cold therapy and perineal wounds: too cool or not too cool? British Journal of Midwifery 6(9): 572–579

Steen M P, Marchant P R 2001 Alleviating perineal trauma: the APT Study. RCM Journal 4(8): 256–259

Trengrove N J et al 1996 Qualitative bacteriology and leg ulcer healing. Journal of Wound Care 5(6): 277–280

Valentine R J, Weigelt J A, Dryer D et al 1986 Effect of remote infection on clean wound infection rates. American Journal of Infection Control 14: 64–67

Vowden K R 1999a Wound debridement, part 1: non-sharp techniques. Journal of Wound Care 8(5): 237–240

Vowden K R 1999b Wound debridement, part 2: sharp techniques. Journal of Wound Care 8(6): 291–294

Walsh M, Ford P 1989 Nursing Rituals: Research and Rational Action. Butterworth-Heinemann, Oxford

15

Immunosuppressive diseases

G. Manojlovic

INTRODUCTION

To protect itself against invasion the human body has developed a complex defence strategy. Using non-specific and specific immune responses the healthy body protects itself against micro-organisms and foreign matter which may cause disease. However, this defence system can become deficient, resulting in an inability of the body to prevent invasion and therefore disease. This chapter intends to arm the community healthcare worker with the necessary knowledge of the immune system, the diseases which affect its function and the subsequent risks faced by those with immunosuppression in order to promote appropriate infection prevention and control practices for this client group.

Why do we need an immune system?

Antigens are the reason the human body has developed an incredibly complex immune system. An antigen is the collective name given to anything able to trigger an immune response; therefore bacteria, viruses, fungi and other micro-organisms are all antigens. Weiner (1986) posed the question 'How are we able to survive in this sea of antigens, this swarm of invaders threatening from without, and within?' The answer is the immune system. The immune system protects the body using several mechanisms, which fit into two categories, either non-specific or specific responses. Non-specific responses are exactly that, non-specific.

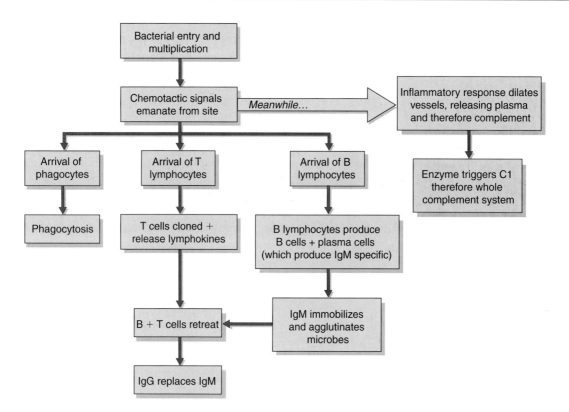

Figure 15.1 Example of immune response following bacterial invasion.

These act against all invading antigens using both internal and external mechanisms. The specific immune response is composed of the humoral and cell-mediated immune systems, which react rapidly to invasion from specific antigens. Figures 15.1 and 15.2 chart the immune process.

THE NON-SPECIFIC RESPONSE

External protection from micro-organisms

The external structures of the body are the first line of defence against micro-organisms, and include the skin and mucous membranes.

Skin

Not only does the skin provide a tough, waterproof barrier from potentially harmful pathogens but the secretions from the sebaceous and sweat glands contain antimicrobial properties to discourage colonization of the skin with organisms such as methicillin-resistant *Staphylococcus aureus* (MRSA). The skin also has its own resident micro-organisms (flora) such as *Staphylococcus epidermidis*, which compete for nutrients with invading pathogens, preventing colonization.

The skin's ability to protect can become compromised as a result of trauma, conditions such as eczema or dermatitis, chronic wounds, surgical procedures, sharps injury or insect bites, and once breached the body can be invaded by micro-organisms through these sites. Those external areas of the body not protected by skin have their own mechanisms of defence.

Mucous membranes

Mucous membranes are found at entry sites to the body like the mouth, the urethra and the female external genitalia, and also internally through the entire gastrointestinal tract and respiratory tract. They are often only one cell thick and can therefore

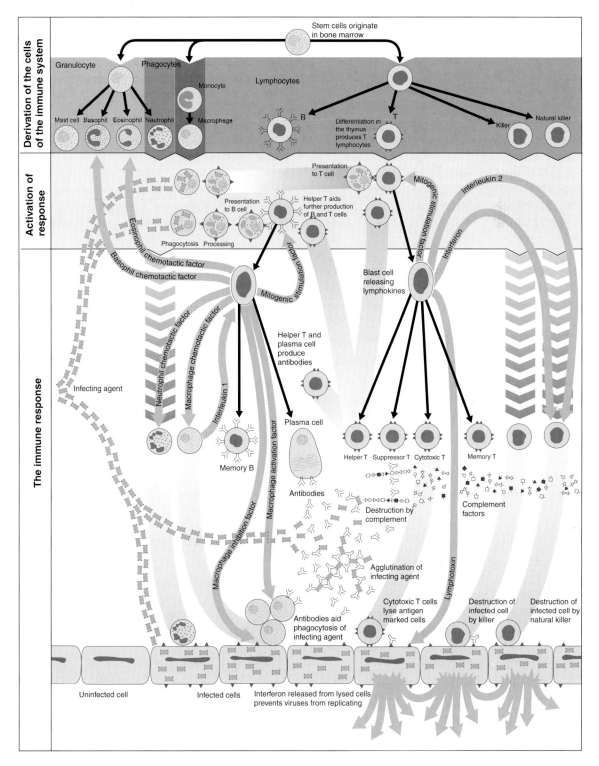

Figure 15.2 Diagrammatic overview of the immune system. Edwin Burgess Ltd., Princes Risborough, Bucks.

be more readily invaded by potential pathogens; however, these membranes contain lysozyme, which is an enzyme capable of destroying the cell walls of micro-organisms.

Areas of the body such as the eyes have other defence mechanisms in addition to the properties of the mucous membranes.

- The eyes are washed with tears, which also contain lysozyme.
- The genitourinary tract is additionally protected through the regular washing through of acidic urine, and the direction of flow of vaginal secretions.
- The respiratory tract protects against invasion with nasal hairs, the cough reflex and the action of mucosal cilia, which move material upward and so away from the lungs. In cystic fibrosis sufferers, the upward movement of mucous is affected, leading to a stasis of secretions, and the lungs are left susceptible to infection (Meers et al 1995).

  So effective are the defences of the urinary and respiratory tracts that other than the external sites like the mouth and urethral entrance, they are deemed bacteriologically sterile areas (Bannister et al 1996) – that is, they have no normal resident flora.

- The gastrointestinal tract is further protected by lysozyme in saliva, gastric acid that destroys many intestinal pathogens, and further down in the small intestine bile inhibits bacterial growth. In the large intestine the resident bacterial flora

compete against invading organisms for nutrients and attachment sites.

As with the skin, a breach in these defences, such as insertion of a urinary catheter or the disruption of the protective resident flora (Box 15.1), offers a route for invasion by pathogens.

Internal protection from micro-organisms

Phagocytosis

The aim of phagocytic cells is to remove substances from the body, whether they are living or dead and of no use to the body. They do this by ingestion, the word phagocyte coming from the Greek 'phagein', meaning to eat.

They are produced continuously in the bone marrow. Polymorphonuclear neutrophils (PMN) are the most abundant of the phagocytic cells, although they only survive a few days. Macrophages are larger and live longer but are less abundant. Many macrophages are attached to sites within the mononuclear phagocyte system (MNPS), mostly in the lymph nodes, bone marrow, liver, lungs, spleen and central nervous system. Phagocytosis by these cells occurs in four stages (Fig. 15.3).

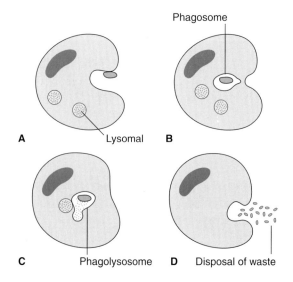

Figure 15.3 Phagocytosis. (A) contact; (B) ingestion; (C) digestion; (D) exocytosis.

Box 15.1 Practice-based example

Mrs Green has developed a chest infection and is prescribed the antibiotic amoxycillin to treat it.
After a week, although her chest infection has improved she has now developed profuse diarrhoea. What could be the cause?

The normal flora of the gut is affected by antibiotic therapy, which can lead to an overgrowth of *Clostridium difficile*, if present. This organism produces toxins, which in turn cause symptoms ranging from mild diarrhoea to pseudo-membranous colitis. If this is the cause of Mrs Green's diarrhoea, discontinuation of her antibiotic may be enough to stop it, but she may require further antibiotic therapy in order to treat the *Clostridium difficile* infection.

Complement

Complement is a complex of enzyme proteins numbered C1–C9 found in plasma. Each component of complement has a function in triggering and enhancing the immune response. Complement (C3 and C5) acts alone or synergistically with antibodies to aid phagocytosis. This action is called opsonization, which comes from the Greek word opsonion, 'to prepare food for'. Complement also plays a vital role in the initiation of the inflammatory response promoting vasodilation and capillary permeability (C3 and C5), attracting phagocytes (C5, C6 and C7) and destroying some bacteria itself (C8 and C9) through the piercing of cell membranes, allowing the entry of fluid and ultimately bursting the organism.

The inflammatory response

The inflammatory response is the body's immediate non-specific response to injury or infection. Signs of this response on the skin and mucous membranes are redness, swelling, heat and pain (caused by adjacent nerves being pressed as the area swells). The sequence is as follows:

- Blood vessels dilate on the release of histamine, complement and other substances released from an injured cell.
- Plasma-containing phagocytes, fibrinogen and lymphocytes converge at the site, passing through the blood vessel wall.
- Fibrin forms a dense mesh wall around the area, preventing the micro-organisms from escaping.
- PMN and macrophages ingest the micro-organisms by phagocytosis with the aid of complement and antibodies.
- Exudate containing fluid and cells collects. This exudate may be fibrinous if there is adequate fibrin to result in clotting, serous if there is more plasma than cells, or purulent if the offending organism is pus-forming such as *Staphylococcus aureus*. Abscesses form where the pus collecting within the wall is not discharged or reabsorbed, and may require surgical intervention.

The aim of this activity is to isolate and kill as many of the invading organisms as possible to avoid further spread; however, some organisms have the ability to survive phagocytosis. Mycobacterium has this ability due to a waxy cell wall and ability to multiply intracellularly, killing the phagocytic cell. Specific defences may destroy the organism if available, or it may survive, developing into a primary tuberculosis lesion (Morello et al 1994).

Other non-specific influences

- Age: children are protected for the first few months of life by maternal antibodies, but are then susceptible to many infections until they produce antibodies of their own. The elderly are more susceptible to infection as a result of a reduction in the cell-mediated immune system, and physical, physiological and nutritional deterioration that often accompanies increasing age.
- Malnutrition and obesity affect healthy tissue function, which affects the body's ability to produce plasma proteins.
- Hormone production from the adrenal gland (corticosteroids) leads to a depression in antibody production and the inflammatory response, for example physical or emotional stress, increases hormone production from the adrenal gland. Puberty, pregnancy and the menopause result in extreme changes in hormone activity which affect healthy tissue function.
- Genetic characteristics in humans provide immunity from many of the infections which affect other species, such as animal and plant infections.

THE SPECIFIC IMMUNE RESPONSE

Lymphocytes are white blood cells that act against specific antigens. They produce the antibodies required for humoral immunity through the B lymphocytes, play a part in cell-mediated immunity through the T lymphocytes, and work in conjunction with phagocytes and the complement system.

Cell-mediated immunity

Cell-mediated immunity is the collective name for the activity of T lymphocytes as they influence, control and mediate the immune response of the body. All T lymphocytes possess surface receptors for specific antigens. Once activated, the T lymphocytes modify and multiply to produce a number of different T cells with specific functions:

- T helper cells are regulatory and assist B-lymphocytes to produce antibodies. They possess the surface molecule CD4. A count of T helper cells is used to measure the severity of Human Immunodeficiency Virus (HIV) infection.
- Natural killer cells are large lymphocytes which are cytotoxic to some viruses, protozoa and to tumour cells.
- T suppressor cells restrain and regulate the activities of helper and killer cells.

The result of T lymphocytes modifying and multiplying is the production of lymphokines. Lymphokines are a collection of chemical mediators that act in different ways to attract phagocytes and promote the inflammatory response:

- Migratory inhibition factor (MIF) prevents further migration of phagocytes.
- Macrophage activation factor (MAF) increases macrophage phagocytic activity.
- Lymphocytic mitogenic factor (LMF) induces cloning of T lymphocytes.
- Lymphotoxin (LT) kills infected cells with antigen on the surface.
- Interferon acts non-specifically against viruses by blocking their replication.

Humoral immunity

The term humoral comes from the Latin for moisture, as in body fluid.

B-lymphocytes are responsible for the production of antibodies (immunoglobulins). Antibodies are proteins shaped like a 'Y'. The two 'arms' attach to specific receptors on the surface of an antigen, different in each antibody. The 'leg' of the antibody binds to phagocytes and complement. Of the thousands of circulating B-lymphocytes, each one has different antibody on the surface, which acts as the specific receptor.

On encountering the matching antigen to its antibody, the B lymphocyte attaches to the antigen

Table 15.1 Immunoglobulin (Ig) activity

Immunoglobulin (antibody)	Activity
IgA	Found in the secretions of the respiratory, gastrointestinal and genitourinary tracts, IgA prevents the attachment of antigens to epithelial receptors.
IgD	Possibly associated with the B-cell receptor activity of IgM, IgD is at its peak during childhood.
IgE	Associated with allergy reactions and the release of histamine, IgE is found mostly in the respiratory and gastrointestinal tract.
IgG	The most abundant of the antibodies, IgG appears after IgM and is involved in opsonization, complement activation. IgG is produced for up to a year after infection, and can cross the placenta.
IgM	The first Ig produced on recognition of an antigen, with 10 attachment sites. A complement activator, IgM also agglutinate (stick together) and coat antigens, to aid phagocytosis.

and divides over and over, creating clones, all carrying the antibody to the encountered antigen. These clones then evolve into plasma cells, which in turn synthesize. This releases the antibodies to opsonize with the phagocytes, while also creating antibody-producing memory cells which remain in the circulating bloodstream for years. The presence of the different types of antibodies is summarized in Table 15.1.

If the same antigen invades the body again it is recognized by the memory cells, inducing a rapid response and thus preventing the establishment of infection: for instance immunity to chickenpox is acquired following initial infection.

IMMUNIZATION

Following successful immunization programmes the global eradication of smallpox was confirmed in 1979 by the World Health Organization. The eradication of polio is also imminent. Immunization can be passive through the administration of immunoglobulin (antibodies) or active through vaccination, defined as 'the administration of inactivated or attenuated live organisms or their products' (DoH 1996).

Passive immunization

Immunoglobulins (Ig) offer protection against some infections, although this protection is short-lived as immunoglobulins do not result in the production of memory cells. They are particularly useful following exposure of a susceptible individual to a potentially dangerous infection, for example a pregnant woman exposed to chickenpox with no history of prior infection.

Derived from plasma, immunoglobulin may be general or specific. Human normal immunoglobulin is obtained from pooled donor plasma and contains the antibodies to those viruses commonly occurring in the community. Specific immunoglobulins are obtained from those donors with high antibody titres or donors who have been recently immunized or infected. *Examples of available specific immunoglobulins include tetanus, rabies, hepatitis B and varicella zoster.*

Active immunization

Immunity to many infections can also be achieved artificially through vaccination. There are a number of identified factors that need to be taken into consideration when those who are to be vaccinated are immunosuppressed (DoH 1996):

- Live vaccines should not be administered to people on high-dose corticosteroid treatment. High-dose treatment is taken as 2 mg prednisolone/kg/day for a child and 40 mg prednisolone daily for more than a week's duration for adults. Live vaccines should also not be administered within 3 months of completion of a course or a reduction in the dose to a non-immunosuppressing level.
- Live vaccines should also be avoided for those being treated for malignant disease, those on immunosuppressive therapy and those with impaired immunological diseases. Following chemotherapy treatment, 6 months needs to elapse prior to administration of live vaccines.

- For clients who have HIV the BCG vaccine should be avoided as this may cause dissemination of tuberculosis, and the Yellow fever vaccine should also be avoided due to the lack of evidence to its safety in this client group.

IMMUNODEFICIENCY

There are many disorders and deficiencies of the immune system and a deficiency of one component can affect the function of others reliant on its presence. Immunodeficiency may be related to dysfunction of immune system components such as B and T lymphocytes, complement system and phagocytes, or be due to the effects of immunosuppressive diseases or treatments.

For people with damaged immune systems, not only are they more susceptible to those infections known to be pathogenic but also micro-organisms which would not normally cause infection in a healthy individual, have the potential to cause severe disease. Infections caused by these micro-organisms are called opportunistic.

Conditions affecting the immune system

The diseases or conditions affecting the immune system may attack one or more components, though in many cases the deficit through disease of one directly affects the activity of another as many components rely on the presence of others in order to function.

Breaks in physical barriers

As discussed at the beginning of this chapter, the external properties of the body provide an excellent barrier to invading pathogens. However, it is sometimes necessary to break those barriers for therapeutic reasons. Indwelling urinary or vascular catheters provide the opportunity for organisms to bypass those barriers. Likewise, therapies that neutralize gastric acid will allow micro-organisms to pass through the stomach into the intestine.

Neutrophil deficiency

Neutropenia is a deficiency in circulating neutrophils, essential in the immune response for their phagocytic activity. The level of neutropenia is measurable by the number of neutrophils present in the blood, the normal level being between 1500 and 2000/mm^3. The risk of infection rises dramatically when the level is below 500/mm^3 (Mandell et al 1990). Neutropenia can be acquired or hereditary. Acquired neutropenia may be as a result of acute leukaemia or drug therapy such as chemotherapy. Antibiotic therapy with penicillins, vancomycin and others has been associated with adverse reactions resulting in neutropenia, though this is rare. Auto-immune diseases can also result in neutropenia. Hereditary neutropenia may be severe, as in *infantile genetic agranulocytosis*, a condition where the phagocytic cells do not mature and which results in severe infection and infant death.

T lymphocyte deficiency

Cell-mediated immunity relies on the activity of T lymphocytes. One condition that affects this activity adversely is HIV. The virus attaches to cells that carry the CD4 protein, including the T helper lymphocytes. By depleting the quantity of circulating T helper cells, the immune system is less able to protect against specific infection. This increases the virulence of micro-organisms which have the ability to survive phagocytosis through intracellular survival, such as *Mycobacterium tuberculosis,* or through the ability to destroy phagocytes by the production of the toxin leukocidin, for example in streptococci and staphylococci (Morello et al 1994).

Immediately before and for some time after organ transplantation, T lymphocyte suppression is essential in order to prevent the rejection by the body of a transplanted organ. This is achieved through drug therapy that severely suppresses the cell-mediated immune response. This therapy leaves the recipient at greater risk of infections. The mortality rate of recipients who contract cytomegalovirus pneumonitis within the first 3 months post transplant is over 50% (Bannister et al 1996).

Bone marrow transplant recipients not only have their underlying disease affecting their immune status but also, prior to transplant, have therapy to cause the near-total suppression of all their immune response systems in order to prevent graft-versus-host disease. Depending on the source of the bone marrow, some recipients may require long-term or even permanent immunosuppression.

Chemotherapy used in the treatment of cancer and high dose corticosteroid treatments can also result in T lymphocyte deficiency.

Gammaglobulin deficit

A decrease in production or an increase in destruction or loss of immunoglobulin may result in *hypogammaglobulinaemia*. Hereditary failure of immunoglobulin production, *agammaglobulinaemia*, may not become apparent until an infant has lost the maternal antibodies and become susceptible to infections and allergies. Disorders of the lymphatic system or bone marrow can result in *hypogammaglobulinaemia*. These conditions can be treated with *gamma globulin (IgG) therapy.*

Complement deficiency

As complement works as a chain reaction, deficiency in one component affects the function of the rest.

Splenectomy

The spleen plays an important role in the immune system in the removal of bacteria from the bloodstream in phagocytes and promoting their destruction. Following splenectomy due to trauma or disease, immunization against *Streptococcus pneumoniae* (pneumococcal vaccine) and *Haemophilus influenzae b* (Hib) influenza and meningococcal meningitis A and C are required (DoH 1996). Lifelong penicillin prophylaxis is also required to protect the individual from pneumococcal infections.

PREVENTION OF INFECTION

The level of susceptibility of a client to infection is as individual as the client is. The environments to which they are exposed also differ greatly, as illustrated in the case study below (Box 15.2). A person with a physical break in their external defences does not have the same risks as one who is immunosuppressed following cytotoxic therapy. Therefore it is important to consider the necessity and practicability of actions and advice. The following sections relate to those clients with a high risk of infection, for example *post transplant, cytotoxic therapy, dialysis and medical conditions such as cystic fibrosis.*

Clinical situations

Basic infection control principles, such as hand hygiene, are central to good clinical practice. However, with the immunosuppressed, further considerations need to be taken into account and practice enhanced especially with regard to the insertion, care and removal of invasive devices.

Intravenous access

For many clients in the community setting, intravenous (IV) access is an essential aspect of their care, for example the administration of chemotherapy, antibiotics or total parenteral nutrition (TPN). Frequent handling of IV devices and clients' own skin flora are accepted as significant sources of infection in relation to IV devices

(Astagneau et al 1999, Maki 1991). For the immunocompromised host, the risk and consequence of infection is far greater, both in the severity of the potential infection but also as a result of the loss of venous access. In addition to standards of care for the immuno-competent client, the following should be considered:

- Sterile gloves should be used for the insertion of peripheral devices (Goodinson 1990).
- Where possible, long-term devices should be inserted prior to immunosuppressive therapy (Risi and Tomascak 1998).

Enteral feeding

Guidance for home enteral feeding is discussed in Chapter 6. The lack of research into the risk of infection as a result of home enteral feeding on the immunocompromised client makes it difficult to offer recommendations. However, there is evidence supporting the inherent problems of re-processing enteral feed equipment (Anderton and Nwoguh 1991), and of the potential for bacterial contamination of feeds in the home (Anderton et al 1993). With this in mind, the highest standard of care should be followed to prevent infection in the immunocompromised patient:

- Client and/or carer needs to be informed of all aspects of administration and equipment care, including hand hygiene and storage of feeds.
- Consider the choice of delivery system for ease of use, to reduce the risk of contamination during use.
- Use pre-packaged sterile feeds, and avoid the use of feeds that require decanting, to reduce the risk of contamination during handling.

Maintaining a safe environment – reducing the risk

Food and water

The avoidance of certain foodstuffs is prudent for the immunocompromised, as many foods such as raw vegetables and salads may be contaminated and have been the cause of a number of outbreaks (Little et al 1997, Bouchier 1998). Advice should

Table 15.2 Food and water: possible infectious agents

Food	Associated infectious agent
Water	*Pseudomonas aeruginosa* *Cryptosporidium parvum*
Uncooked vegetables, salads (including pre-packed)	*Escherichia coli* *Listeria* species *Salmonella* species *Shigella* species
Pepper	*Aspergillus* Other fungi
Soft cheeses	*Listeria* species
Blue cheeses	Fungi
Unpasteurized dairy produce	*Campylobacter* *Listeria* species *E. coli* 0157
Eggs	*Salmonella* species
Seafood	Hepatitis A
Pâté	*Listeria* species

come from the medical team caring for the client, and some clients such as bone marrow transplant patients should have received written guidance on foods to avoid prior to hospital discharge. Table 15.2 shows a list of foodstuffs and their associated infectious agents.

In addition to avoiding certain foods, food hygiene guidelines need to be followed:

- Hand washing, before and after handling food, and between raw and cooked foods.
- Maintain a clean environment for food preparation and storage.
- Storage and preparation for raw food needs to be separate from that of cooked, i.e. store raw meat, fish and eggs at the bottom of the fridge.
- Ensure fridge is maintaining adequate temperatures, i.e. the fridge should be at or below 5°C, the freezer should be at −18°C.
- Avoid re-freezing defrosted foods or re-heating previously cooked foods.
- No produce should be consumed after its 'use by' or expiry date.
- Clean the external surfaces of tin cans prior to opening, to avoid contamination of the contents.

- All foods must be thoroughly cooked: therefore avoid cooking in the microwave unless it is tinned food.

Activities and associated risks

The avoidance of certain activities is prudent for the immunocompromised person. Many activities may expose the individual to potentially pathogenic micro-organisms and result in severe infection. If certain activities are to be avoided, the medical team should provide this information for the client. Some basic considerations include:

- *Gardening* – Digging over compost heaps or dealing with manure would not be advised, but this may need to be explained to the client, as an ardent gardener may not consider compost to be an infection risk.
- *Pets* – Hand washing following contact with pets and avoiding dealing with their excreta where practicable is essential. Some pets carry pathogenic micro-organisms. These include the parrot, who can carry *Chlamydia psittaci*, the terrapin who can carry *Salmonella*, to cats and dogs who can carry *Campylobacter, Salmonella, Toxoplasma* and *Yersinia*. More so, pets with symptoms of an infection should be avoided, such as cats or dogs with diarrhoea. Opportunistic organisms may also be associated with pet care, for example atypical *Mycobacterium marinum* related to the maintenance of fish tanks.
- *DIY* – The demolition of walls, plaster dust, building works, etc. produce large amounts of *Aspergillus* species, fungi that can cause pneumonia in the immunocompromised. Avoidance of such activity would be advisable.

Whatever the advice given to the client and carers, it is important to consider their psychological as well as physical needs. Extreme restrictions on a person's life may result in none of the recommendations being followed; therefore any recommendations made should be practicable in order for them to work.

REFERENCES

Anderton A, Nwoguh C E 1991 Re-use of enteral feeding tubes – a potential hazard to the patient? A study of the efficiency of a representative range of cleaning and disinfection procedures. Journal of Hospital Infection 18: 131–138

Anderton A, Nwoguh C E, McKune I et al 1993 A comparative study of the numbers of bacteria present in enteral feeds prepared and administered in hospital and the home. Journal of Hospital Infection 23: 43–49

Astagneau P, Mauget S, Tran-Minh T et al 1999 Long-term central venous catheter infection in HIV-infected and cancer patients: a multicenter cohort study. Infection Control and Hospital Epidemiology 20: 494–498

Bannister B A, Begg N T, Gillespie S H 1996 Infectious Disease. Blackwell Science, Oxford

Bouchier I 1998 for the Department of the Environment, Transport and the Regions, Department of Health. Cryptosporidium in water supplies: third report of the group of experts. DoH, London

Department of Health 1996 Immunisation Against Infectious Disease. HMSO, London

Goodinson S 1990 Keeping the flora out. Professional Nurse 5(11): 572–575

Little C L, Monsey H A, Nichols G L, deLouvois J 1997 The microbiological quality of refrigerated salads and crudities. PHLS Microbiology Digest 14(3): 142–146

Maki D G 1991 Infection caused by intravascular devices: pathogenesis, strategies for prevention. In: Maki D G (ed.) Improving Catheter Site Care. Royal Society of Medicine Services, London

Mandell G L, Douglas R G, Bennett J E 1990 Principles and Practice of Infectious Diseases, 3rd edn. Churchill Livingstone, New York

Meers P, Sedgwick J, Worsley M 1995 The Microbiology and Epidemiology of Infection for Health Science Students. Chapman and Hall, London

Morello J A, Granato P A, Mizer H E, Wilson M E 1994 Microbiology in Patient Care, 5th edn. McGraw-Hill, New York

Risi G F, Tomascak V 1998 Prevention of infection in the immunocompromised host. American Journal of Infection Control 26(6): 595–604

Watkins E J, Brooksby P, Schweiger M S, Enright S M 2001 Septicaemia in a pig-farm worker. The Lancet 357: 38

Weiner M A 1986 Maximum Immunity. Gateway, Bath

Wilson J 2001 Infection Control in Clinical Practice. Baillière Tindall, Edinburgh

16

Gastrointestinal disease

J. Howard

INTRODUCTION

Infectious gastrointestinal (GI) illnesses are increasing in industrial countries, including the United Kingdom, and remain a major cause of mortality in developing countries (WHO 1998).

Outbreaks are not always linked to food/water consumption and may be due to direct human contact with animals or direct human-to-human contact. Secondary cases occur when spread occurs usually via the faecal–oral route or hand to mouth route. Other cases may be linked to antibiotic administration.

In the community cross infection occurs readily if strict attention to hygiene is not observed. Certain areas and activities will facilitate the spread and large outbreaks which can be linked to a breakdown in infection control precautions, rather than the consumption of offending foodstuffs, are reported quarterly in the Communicable Disease Report published by the Public Health Laboratory Service Communicable Disease Surveillance Centre, London.

Food-related outbreaks when they occur may be localized or diffuse, the latter being linked to the wide and fast distribution networks of the major food production companies (Potter 1992) (see Fig. 16.1).

QUANTIFYING THE PROBLEM

- A national surveillance system in the United Kingdom provides information on trends, incidence and outbreaks of infectious intestinal disease.

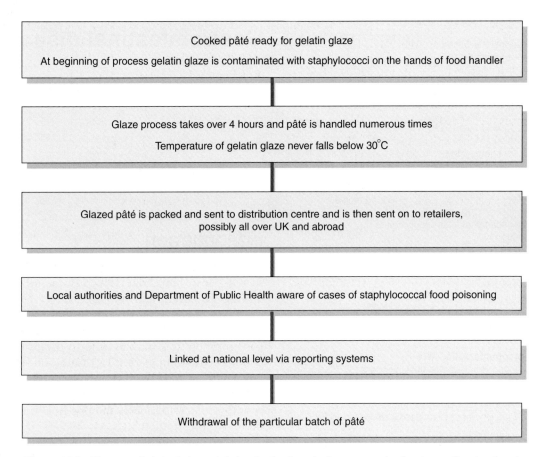

Figure 16.1 The spread of staphylococci during the food production process leading to a national outbreak.

- All doctors are required to notify cases of food poisoning to the Local Authority Proper Officer, usually Consultant in Communicable Disease Control (CCDC), under the provision of the Public Health (Control of Diseases) Act 1984.
- Initially all cases of gastro-enteritis should be regarded as infectious until proven otherwise (PHLS 1995).

It is the duty of the Proper Officer to ensure that all notifications made are then collated and sent on to the Regional Epidemiologist and to the Office for National Statistics (ONS), formerly the Office of Population, Censuses and Survey (OPCS). It is necessary to define food poisoning/food-borne disease for the purposes of notification.

The following definition was formulated by the Advisory Committee on Microbiological Safety of Food and accepted by the Government. All doctors in England and Wales were informed in September 1992,

any disease of an infectious or toxic nature caused by or thought to be caused by the consumption of food or water. This includes all suspected food and waterborne illnesses and does not depend on identification of a causal organism (Chief Medical Officer 1992).

A second source of data is the voluntary reporting of organisms identified by diagnostic microbiology laboratories to the Public Health Laboratory Service (PHLS) Communicable Disease Surveillance Centre (CDSC). These are collected and published quarterly.

The third source are the standardized reports on general outbreaks collected by CDSC and published quarterly.

The fourth source collects data on occupationally-acquired infectious diseases and commenced in 1996 (Ross et al 1998). During 1996–1997 921 new cases of diarrhoeal diseases were reported via this system, the predominant bacterial causes being salmonella, campylobacter, viral causes, and small round structured viruses (SRSV). A total of **531** cases were reported in **healthcare workers**, with rates among healthcare assistants being twice the rate of that amongst nurses. Viral infections predominated among **healthcare workers in residential homes**.

In contrast, within the food industry, **156** cases were reported, the highest number being poultry dressers (campylobacter and salmonella infection). However, it is important to put these figures in perspective by looking at the rates per million workers per year. These are:

- 674 for care assistants
- 308 for nurses
- 4226 for poultry dressers.

Infectious intestinal disease is common, with 9.4 million estimated cases each year in England alone. Of these only 1.5 million cases report to their general practitioner (Wheeler et al 1999).

It is known that official notifications are not representative of the actual level of infection and that of those who do present to their GP, only a fraction are reported to the CDSC; therefore the annual totals compiled by CDSC are only representative of a fraction of actual cases occurring. Nevertheless they provide information on trends and show a year-on-year increase in the number of cases in England and Wales. In addition they provide information on the most serious cases.

A Dutch publication quantifies the loss of information on food-borne infectious disease as follows (Beckers 1987):

- 20% consult doctor
- 15% stool specimens examined
- 10% stool positive
- 5% reported to correct authority.

Thus, there is a 95% loss of reported information about actual cases. The majority of these will be self-limiting illnesses, and there would be no public health gain in encouraging everyone with mild stomach upsets to go to the doctor. The public health gain is to be found in promoting practices and standards of hygiene which prevent GI illnesses, mild or otherwise.

Socioeconomic impact

In general gastrointestinal illness is considered mild, and full recovery occurs. However, there are exceptions amongst the very young and the elderly. Deaths due to intestinal infection in people aged over 65 years accounted for 77% of all deaths attributable to infectious disease for that age group. The causative organisms in order of importance were campylobacter, *Clostridium difficile*, salmonella, other pathogens, rotavirus, SRVS. The total burden of infectious intestinal disease in the elderly is substantial and associated with institutional living, although increasing numbers of elderly people live alone, and without adequate support may be more vulnerable to episodes of intestinal infection due to an inability to prepare food adequately or practise safe hygiene (Djuretic et al 1996, Johnson et al 1998).

For the very young, the risk is rapid dehydration and collapse following the onset of symptoms (Barker and James 1999). The proliferation of day-care nurseries in the community means that outbreaks of infectious intestinal diseases are common, as reported quarterly in the Communicable Disease Report from CDSC.

Infectious intestinal disease costs a lot of money, and is difficult to assess properly. The financial cost to the individual affected should also be considered. These may include prescriptions, extra disposable nappies and the costs involved in disruption to social life, such as cancelled holidays due to illness. In 1988 it was estimated that the total cost per case of human salmonellosis was £789 (Voss 1993) and these costs related to the public sector costs like healthcare, and industrial costs due to loss of production and loss of business (Buzby and Robert 1997). There is often a severe knock-on impact on commercial interests, even if the outlet or institution is blameless.

Historical perspectives

The oldest theory of disease causation was 'The Wrath of God' (Stolley and Laskey 1995). In the Book of Leviticus the laws laid down by Moses for the Israelites address all the issues involved in keeping food safe for consumption.

Accounts of food poisoning recorded in ancient history were generally associated with chemical poisoning, and food poisoning became associated with spoiled, tainted food. It is now known that food contaminated with micro-organisms may be normal in appearance, odour and flavour (Hobbs and Roberts 1987).

Food poisoning organisms were first described by August Gaertner in 1888 (Hobbs and Roberts 1987). They were isolated from the organs of a man who died during an outbreak of gastro-enteritis in Germany. Similar organisms were found on the beef eaten and the original animal carcass. They were later generically named Salmonella. Dr E Salmon isolated the first member of the genus Salmonella in 1885. In 1896 Botulism was described by Van Ermengen in Belgium.

Staphylococci were associated with food poisoning in 1914, and *Clostridium perfringens* was recognized from 1945–1953.

John Snow (1813–1858) made a major contribution to our understanding of epidemics of intestinal infection when he traced the source of a cholera epidemic in London in 1854 to one water pump (Donaldson and Donaldson 1988). Ignaz Semmelweis's conviction that unwashed hands contributed to the spread of infection underpins the infection control message and is of particular importance to GI infections (Stolley and Laskey 1995).

Since World War II the incidence of food-related GI illness has risen. Certain changes in society are thought to have contributed to this:

1. More women working outside the home
2. Changes in eating habits, i.e. grazing effect
3. Increased affluence (microwaves, freezers, eating out, barbecues)
4. Ease of foreign travel
5. Healthy eating (i.e. fewer traditional barriers to organisms, e.g. salt, sugar, preservatives)
6. Membership of European Union with movement of foods
7. Innovation in the food production industry
8. Economics within the food industry.

The love affair between the freezer and the microwave is an example of how the food revolution has liberated us but at the same time deskilled us in terms of culinary expertise (Hardyment 1995).

People see food and health as connected, but there is still a major problem both in improving food hygiene and in reducing the incidence of gastrointestinal illness in the community due to a lack of conceptual understanding about the nature of micro-organisms and their spread (Bloomfield and Scott 1997). It is easy to understand bacterial contamination in the context of visible dirt or smell, but less so when for example a person's hands or the environment appears visibly clean.

WHAT IS INFECTIOUS GI ILLNESS?

Infectious gastrointestinal illness can be viewed as a syndrome. Presenting signs and symptoms may include:

- fever
- abdominal pain and cramps
- nausea and vomiting
- diarrhoea, i.e. a change in bowel habit which differs from the normal for that individual. Stools may be frequent, loose, watery and contain blood or mucus.

Severity may vary from mild, lasting a few hours, to severe purging as in cholera (Chin 2000). Severe dehydration with an accompanied electrolyte imbalance can occur. Hypernatraemia is common in infants.

Non-infectious agents may cause signs and symptoms similar to the above. Figure 16.2 shows a breakdown of infectious and non-infectious causes of gastrointestinal disease.

Non food-related infectious GI illness

The presence of certain organisms in the gut can predispose the individual to GI illness.

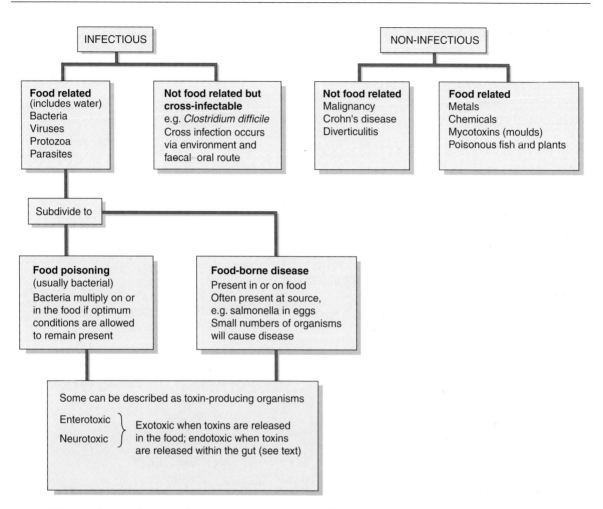

Figure 16.2 Infectious and non-infectious causes of gastrointestinal illness.

Clostridium difficile

Following antibiotic administration an overgrowth of *Clostridium difficile* can occur in the lumen of the gut; this results in a pseudomembranous colitis, and some antibiotics will stimulate toxin formation as well (Finch and Ball 1991). The illness can vary from mild to life-threatening, more commonly seen in the elderly. Outbreaks occur where there is transmission via the faecal–oral route and via contaminated fomites. Between January 1992 and December 1996, *C. difficile* accounted for 109 hospital outbreaks of infectious GI illness (Djuretic et al 1999). Incidence of sporadic cases in the community is not clear but with earlier discharge from hospital and increasing numbers of elderly receiving care in the community either at home or in institutions, the potential for outbreaks is ever-present.

Helicobacter pylori

H. pylori is probably the most common bacterial infection of humans (Williams 1999) and is an important cause of acquired peptic ulceration. It is primarily a human pathogen, and transmission is via the faecal–oral route or the oral route. Those infected are potentially infected for life and infection is more likely if people live in poor conditions (Chin 2000). Cross infection can occur via inadequately decontaminated endoscopes, and studies suggest that medical staff performing endoscopy may be at risk of cross infection (Williams 1999).

Food-related infectious GI illness

It can be seen from Figure 16.2 that food-related infections may be caused by:

- bacteria
- viruses
- protozoa
- helminths.

Food poisoning

Infectious GI illness due to food poisoning occurs as a result of bacteria multiplying in or on the food. The ideal conditions for multiplication are needed, as illustrated in Figure 16.3:

- optimum temperature
- moisture
- nutrients
- either O_2 or CO_2.

Following ingestion of the affected food, symptoms (nausea, vomiting, stomach pain) occur if the number of organisms present is sufficiently high. The incubation period is short: 1–72 hours at the most. The illness is usually of short duration and self-limiting. Table 16.1 sets out the common causative organisms, together with symptoms, vehicles of transmission and routes of transmission. Poor hygiene on the part of the food handlers can be a contributory cause of food poisoning but it is also associated with poor temperature control during preparation, cooking, cooling, storage and reheating processes (Hobbs and Roberts 1987).

Food-borne illnesses

A food-borne illness occurs as a result of ingesting food contaminated by micro-organisms. Relatively small numbers of organisms are required and they do not need to multiply on the food. The food acts solely as a vehicle. Incubation periods tend to be of a longer duration. These illnesses affect body systems other than the gut. Symptoms may or may not include vomiting and diarrhoea. These infections may cross the placental barrier and affect the developing fetus.

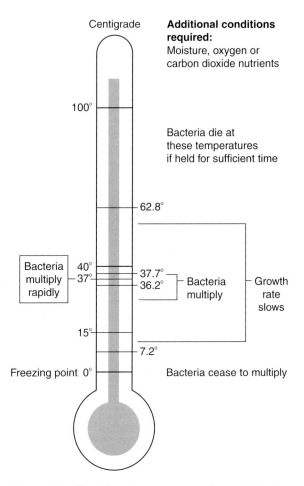

Figure 16.3 The effect of temperature on the multiplication of bacteria.

Table 16.2 sets out the common causative organisms. Poor food hygiene practices and poor hand washing are contributory factors to the secondary spread of these infections. Control methods which trace all the way back to the origins of the raw product or contaminated water supplies are needed.

Control measures for food-borne transmissions (relevant infections are typhoid, paratyphoid, bacillary dysentery, Hepatitis A)

- Ensure safety of all water supplies – chlorinate all water used for food preparation and drinking.
- Ensure satisfactory disposal of sewage.

Table 16.1 Food poisoning

Illness and organism	Source	Incubation period	Symptoms/duration	Vehicles	Transmission routes
Salmonellosis: Salmonella spp. (not enteric fever)	Gastrointestinal tract wild/domestic animals –poultry –terrapins –occasionally humans	12–72 hrs	Diarrhoea Vomiting Fever Septicaemia may develop Carriage may be for years	Undercooked food, particularly poultry, eggs, red meat Contact with infected animals	Raw milk Consumption of under-cooked risk foods Poor kitchen hygiene (1) contaminated surfaces (2) raw meat having contact with cooked products (3) poor standards of personal hygiene
Staphylococcal: Staphylococcus aureus	Grows on meat and bakery products. Food handlers may carry organisms in their noses	1–8 hrs	Intense vomiting Duration 24–48 hrs	Infected lesion on food handler's hand Nostrils or hands	Consuming contaminated foods which have stood at room temperature Unwashed hands
Bacillus aureus	Found in soil, vegetation, cereals, spices	1–8 hrs or 8–16 hrs	Vomiting Diarrhoea 2 clinical syndromes seen associated with exo- and endotoxins Vomiting is the most common	Rice spores survive normal cooking and rapid growth occurs with production of exotoxins	No person-to-person transmission Reheating and consumption of rice Normal reheating will not destroy exotoxins
Clostridium perfringens	Gastrointestinal tract of food animals Soil and dust	8–24 hrs	Vomiting and diarrhoea for 1–4 days Diarrhoea profuse as enterotoxins cause hypersecretion in the gut	Contaminated cooked meats and poultry Food handler's hands	No person-to-person spread Ingestion of inadequately cooked, reheated food or slow cooling of already contaminated foods
Clostridium botulinum type A, B and E	Spores contaminate fruit and vegetables and when inadequately processed produce the toxin in anaerobic conditions	12–24 hrs	Nausea, vomiting, faintness Type E, severe paralysis within 48 hrs Type B, slower onset over a week	Inadequately cooked preserved food Canned food	Consumption of inadequately processed foods Fresh food not a problem to adults as organism does not colonize the gut – it is toxin production which causes illness

(continued)

Table 16.1 *(continued)*

Illness and organism	Source	Incubation period	Symptoms/duration	Vehicles	Transmission routes
Escherichia coli: Enteropathogenic *E. coli* (EPEC) affects under 2 yrs	Human sewage Water Raw meat Human gut	24–72 hrs	Vomiting Diarrhoea Toxin may invade epithelium of gut Toxin causes	Human waste Water Raw meat	Person-to-person faecal/oral route Occasionally contaminated food ETEC via consumption of contaminated food and water
Enterotoxigenic *E. coli* (ETEC, travellers' diarrhoea)	Animals have important role as commonly in gut		hypersecretion in small intestine (presents as Travellers' diarrhoea) Duration 1–3 days		Flies Institutional outbreaks – infection spreads via communal toilets, shared equipment
Enteroinvasive *E. coli* (EIEC)			EIEC – bloodstained diarrhoea	Fruit and vegetable crops irrigated with contaminated water	
Escherichia Coli (*E. coli* 0157-H7) Enterohaemorrhagic *E. coli* (EHEC)			EHEC – mild diarrhoea to severe haemorrhagic colitis. 2–7% develop haemolytic uraemic syndrome with 17% mortality rate	Yoghurts	Very infectious low dose required – especially *E. coli* 0157-H7
Vibrio parahaemolyticus	Aquatic organisms especially in warm climates	6–96 hrs	Fever Vomiting Diarrhoea Duration 1–3 days Recovery complete	Seafood, especially crabs	Consumption of raw seafood
Yersiniosis: *Yersinia enterocolitica*	Wild and domestic animals Birds	3–7 days (under 10 days)	Fever Vomiting Diarrhoea can mimic appendicitis	Pork meat	Contaminated food and water Faecal–oral route Direct contact with animals

Table 16.2 Food-borne infections

Illness and organism	Source	Incubation period	Symptoms	Vehicles	Transmission routes
Tuberculosis: *Mycobacterium bovis* *Mycobacterium tuberculosis*	Cattle Man	4 weeks	Lesions in lungs, bones, kidneys, intestines, skin Chronic illness	Raw milk and dairy foods – low infective dose, so multiplication in food not necessary	(i) Person-to-person spread (sputum) (ii) Consumption of infected food *Control:* Eradication schemes for infected animals Heat treatment of milk Vaccination
Campylobacter enteritis: *Campylobacter jejuni* *Campylobacter coli* (bacteria) (Camps. *need* living host to multiply)	Intestines of animals – especially birds, poultry	2–11 days; usually 3–5 days	Diarrhoea, headache, fever, abdominal pain – organism disappears from stool quite quickly	Water, milk, offal, raw meat – heat-treated milk pecked open by birds has been implicated (especially chicken)	Person-to-person spread unlikely Person to food spread unlikely (i) contact with live *or* dead animal may cause illness (ii) consumption of contaminated food (direct or cross contamination) *Control:* Heat treat milk Educate food handlers
Bacillary dysentery: In UK usually *Shigella sonnei* (bacteria)	Faeces of infected humans	1–7 days, usually less than 4 days	Fever, diarrhoea (may be bloody), stomach pain, vomiting Fatality <1% (dependent on *Shigella* type). Recovery within 1–2 weeks	Organism is very infective so multiplication in food is not of importance Any food type or water	(i) Person-to-person spread by faecal–oral route (ii) Consumption of infected foods and water Problem ir schools/institutions *Control:* Personal hygiene – excretion may be prolonged and intermittent following illness Exclusion of food handlers
Typhoid (enteric fever): *Salmonella typhi* (bacteria)	Faeces of infected humans	1–3 weeks	Fever, malaise, slow pulse, spleen enlargement, constipation or severe diarrhoea	Very infective – very small numbers necessary for illness to result	Transmission is by faecal contamination of food or water – up to 5% of those infected become permanent carriers

(continued)

Table 16.2 (continued)

Illness and organism	Source	Incubation period	Symptoms	Vehicles	Transmission routes
Paratyphoid: *Salmonella paratyphi*	Infected humans	7–10 days	Similar to salmonella food poisoning	Very infective – multiplication in food not necessary so any food type by faecal contamination	As for typhoid
Hepatitis A (infective hepatitis): Virus	Infected humans	15–50 days. Lasts 1 week–several months	Fever, nausea, abdominal pain, jaundice	Water, milk, shellfish – any type of food possible due to low infective dose. Viruses do not multiply in food	(i) Person-to-person spread (often by faecal–oral route) (ii) Consumption of contaminated food (often due to contact with sewage) Virus excreted in faeces during latter half of incubation period
Brucellosis: undulant fever – causative organism *Brucella abortus* *Brucella melitensis*	Cattle Sheep	5–21 days	Intermittent fever, depression, headache, weakness, aching	Raw milk and dairy products Low infective dose	(i) Direct contact with infected animals (ii) Consumption of infected milk and products *Control:* Heat treatment of milk
Listeriosis: *Listeria monocytogenes* (bacteria)	Environment, intestines of domestic and wild animals	1–70 days dependent on dose and health of consumer	Starts with flu-like symptoms; 'weaker' individuals develop full-blown listeriosis – fever, septicaemia, meningitis, abortion/stillbirth Host resistance of importance	Soft ripened cheeses, pâté, cook–chill meats, coleslaw, prepared salads, raw milk	Bacteria of this type can multiply at refrigeration temperatures so if not killed in processed foods, can multiply to dangerous levels – 'danger' depends on host resistance – problem in cook–chill operations *Control:* Ensure processing kills listeria Heat treat milk Ensure no further contamination after processing Observe use-by dates Risk groups should not consume known 'risk' foods

- Ensure heat treatment of milk and milk products.
- Ensure adequate heat treatment/cleansing of shellfish.
- Identify carriers and remove from food preparation environment.
- Train all food handlers about adequate personal hygiene and prevention of cross contamination.
- Maintain high standards at all stages of preparation and distribution.

Toxin production and its relevance to GI illness

All bacteria vary in their ability to cause disease in man; this depends on a combination of two mechanisms (Sleigh and Timbury 1990):

- invasiveness
- toxin production.

There are two toxin types produced by bacteria, exotoxins and endotoxins.

Exotoxins

Classic exotoxins include:

- *Bacillus cereus*
- *Clostridium perfringens*
- Other Gram-positive bacteria.

Enterotoxins include:

- *Staphylococcus aureus*
- *Vibrio cholerae*
- *Escherichia coli*
- Shigella dysentery.

Neurotoxins include:

- *Clostridium botulinum.*

Endotoxins

These are structural elements of the cell wall of Gram-negative bacteria. They are produced by:

- Salmonella spp.
- Campylobacter spp.
- *Vibrio parahaemolyticus.*

Streptococcus and *Escherichia coli* can produce both exotoxins and endotoxins.

Exotoxins are produced whilst the bacteria are multiplying on the food; they leave the intact cell wall of the bacterium and mix with the food. When the food is eaten, the body reacts violently to the toxin, with fever and vomiting. Endotoxins on the other hand are not released on the food but when the bacteria die in the gut; therefore there is usually a delay before onset of signs or symptoms following ingestion.

The significance of toxin production to food safety

Most bacteria can be effectively killed in food if held at 100°C for 1–2 minutes but if exotoxins are released in the food it takes 20–30 minutes at 100°C to kill them; therefore they are much harder to control (Sprenger 1991).

Endotoxins are not released into the food, and therefore it is much easier to kill these bacteria during the cooking process. However, if food is contaminated after cooking and then ingested, illness will follow.

Texts frequently refer to enterotoxic or endotoxic food poisoning or food-related illness, and an understanding of the mechanisms is important when considering infection control measures and the impact the infection has on outcome for the patients (see Further reading).

Viruses

The infective dose for viral infection is low; therefore spread is relatively easy. Food may be contaminated at source by polluted water used for irrigation. Shellfish are known to concentrate the viruses taken up from contaminated water, and cleaning of the shellfish removes bacteria but not viruses (Roberts et al 1986).

Infected food handlers may contaminate food during preparation, particularly items such as sandwiches which require a lot of handling.

Secondary transmission to contacts occurs readily, not only because of poor food hygiene practices but direct spread via the faecal–oral route and the hand to mouth route as surfaces and equipment become contaminated. Outbreaks are common in institutions.

Rotavirus enteritis

Rotaviral infection often causes a severe gastro-enteritis in young children; secondary cases do occur in adults. The virus is of human origin and transmission is via the faecal–oral route, contaminated environmental surfaces to hands and via the respiratory tract. Although viruses present in the tract do not multiply, they can be swallowed along with respiratory secretions (Chin 2000, Ansari et al 1988).

Small round structural viruses

These viruses include Norwalk virus, astro-viruses, caliciviruses, parvoviruses and adeno-viruses. They usually cause a self limiting disease which lasts for 24–48 hours. Sufferers are highly contagious during the acute phase and for up to 48 hours after the diarrhoea has stopped. A short-term immunity develops on recovery (Chin 2000). Ease of spread is similar to rotaviral infections and has implications for infection control and outbreak control in institutions.

Protozoa

Giardia lamblia and Cryptosporidium spp. are common protozoa causing infectious GI illness. They may be transmitted via contaminated water, food, the faecal–oral route and animal to human route.

Cysts which form part of the life cycle of the protozoa are not easily destroyed by conventional use of chlorination, and therefore water filtration methods must be of the highest quality to exclude these organisms. Asymptomatic infections are common. If they do cause illness these are self-limiting infections for people with normal immune systems (Chin 2000).

Large outbreaks of cryptosporidiosis have been associated with drinking water in the UK. Seasonal outbreaks are associated with children visiting farms to feed lambs or see calves (PHLS 1995). With both organisms, person-to-person spread is common in families and spread occurs readily in institutions.

Helminths

In developing countries, helminth infections cause considerable morbidity. The most common intestinal helminths seen in the UK are:

- threadworm (*Enterobius vermicularis*)
- whipworm (*Trichuris trichiura*) which may present as diarrhoeal illness.

Threadworms can be transmitted via the faecal–oral route and food handlers may contaminate food.

Taenia solium (pork tapeworm) is usually imported from abroad but infected persons can spread infection as eggs passed in faeces are infective (PHLS 1995).

PATHOGENS EMERGING AS PUBLIC HEALTH PROBLEMS

The problems associated with these pathogens (see Table 16.3 for list) may be due to a number of factors (Morris & Morris 1997):

- Changes in the micro-organism, e.g. developing resistance to antibiotics
- Changes in its mode of transmission, e.g. *E. coli* is now recognized as an integral part of the food chain rather than a contaminant
- Changes in host susceptibility, e.g. an increased number of immunocompromised persons
- Changes in demography, i.e. increasing elderly population
- Increasing numbers of displaced people, refugees and socially excluded
- Continuing spectre of malnutrition world-wide.

The organisms of concern listed in Table 16.3 share a number of characteristics:

- Most have an animal reservoir.
- There is usually no illness in host animal.
- Contaminated fodder and water are identified as vehicles of cross infection among these animals.
- These organisms spread globally very quickly and the reason is not yet understood.
- Some are becoming resistant to the conventional antibiotics which are also used in veterinary practice.

Table 16.3 Examples of emerging food-borne pathogens and their characteristics

Pathogen	Reservoir	Preparation	Comments
Escherichia coli 0157-H7	Healthy cattle Possible in USA – wild deer	Survives gentle cooking, i.e. rare hamburger Survives in foods with pH below 4.0	Causing illness via consumption of products related to cattle reservoir, e.g. apple juice where contaminated manure used Raw milk Previously *E. coli* seen as relatively benign cause of gastro-enteritis
Salmonella enteritidis	Healthy chickens with lifelong ovarian infection	Contaminated eggs produced and pathogen survives gentle cooking	Serious health problem Utensils used for preparation of egg dishes known to have contaminated other foods. Dried egg products implicated as well
Norwalk-like viruses Small round structures	Human reservoir	Survives usual steaming process Aerosol contamination of surfaces and equipment	Oysters harvested from pristine waters thought to be contaminated by oyster catchers urinating and defecating into water Easy transmission faecal–oral route
Campylobacter jejuni	Cattle, poultry, wild birds	Survives gentle cooking in raw milk	Originally known as rare opportunistic infection until identified as common cause of diarrhoea
Yersinia enterocolitica	Pigs	Survives gentle cooking	
Listeria	Domestic/wild animals	Soft ripe cheeses Survives normal refrigeration temperatures ↓5°C	Fairly recently associated with food-borne transmission. Particularly severe in immunocompromised persons Crosses placental barrier
Salmonella typhimurium DT 104	Healthy cattle herds Widespread contamination of farms – often seen contracted by humans handling sick animals	Survives gentle cooking of sausage and meat pastes	Spreads due to frequent movement of infected calves Drug-resistant strains common High mortality rate in humans, which is unusual for salmonella infections

- Contaminated food usually looks, smells and tastes normal.
- These pathogens usually survive traditional food preparation methods and use of traditional recipes.
- The rate at which new pathogens have been discovered suggests there may be many more awaiting discovery.

The impact of these characteristics is compounded as food vehicles are usually:

- contaminated very early in production rather than just before consumption
- distributed widely very quickly
- made with ingredients from many countries, making identification of a specific source of contamination difficult.

PREVENTION STRATEGIES

From the information so far it can be seen that a broad approach must be taken to prevent and control infectious GI illness. This is now considered as:

- primary prevention
- secondary prevention
- tertiary prevention.

Primary prevention of infectious GI illness

In an ideal world primary prevention would include:

- elimination of infected birds/animals from the breeding stock

- provision of safe, potable water for all, i.e. filtration, chlorination and prevention of slurry run-off from farmland
- high standards of practice to prevent human-to-food transfer of human-source pathogens
- high standards of practice in food processing industry to prevent proliferation of environmental organisms
- adherence of antibiotic policies to prevent overprescribing in medical and veterinary practice
- safe processing of equipment to prevent nosocomial spread of *H. pylori*.

There are a number of agencies and personnel who work together in the community in an attempt to develop strategies for primary prevention. They include:

- Rivers authorities
- Department for Environment, Food and Rural Affairs
- Local veterinarians
- Environment Agency
- Environmental Health Officers of Local Councils
- Trading Standards Officers
- The Meat Inspection Service
- Public Health Laboratory Service
- Public Health Medicine Departments
- Microbiologists
- Food hygienists
- Infection Control doctors and nurses.

In some areas, these personnel meet together on a regular basis to exchange information and education. These meetings provide a basis for ongoing preventative work.

The Food Standards Agency, which was established on April 1 2000 via primary legislation, is described as a force for change and places an emphasis on primary prevention (www.foodstandards.gov.uk).

Secondary prevention

Hazard control approach

Preventative work at this secondary level is vital and aims at:

- destruction of organisms on raw food
- prevention of recontamination of cooked food

- standards of practice which prevent human-to-human spread, either from an index case or from a carrier who is symptomless
- standards of practice which prevent animal-to-human spread.

Within the food processing/catering industry a Hazard Analysis and Critical Control Point system is used (WHO 1995).

It involves the identification of all ingredients, stages in process, environmental features and human factors which can lead to food-borne hazards for the consumer. Critical control points are identified to prevent potential hazards becoming actual hazards (Hotel Catering and Institutional Management Association 1991). They are:

- Inspection and temperature checks on goods at delivery and before use
- Separate storage and handling of ingredients and the finished product
- Correct temperature ranges for fridges and freezers
- Cleaning procedures and correct usage for utensils and equipment
- Prevention of cross contamination of foods
- Personal hygiene and health standards.

These control points have been established for the food industry but apply equally to care institutions (see Practice points, Boxes 16.1–16.4). Environmental Health Officers have an enforcing and educational role, with legal powers to act where standards do not meet the minimum legal

---

Box 16.1   Practice point: Human salmonellosis

Chicken in white wine sauce served at large function. Consumption leads to illness within 24–48 hours. High percentage of guests who ate chicken ill.

Critical points:
Frozen chicken – not all salmonella killed on freezing.
Thawing preparation – hands, surfaces, equipment become contaminated.
Cooking – salmonella survive – cooked too slowly.
Cooked carcasses recontaminate equipment, surfaces and hands.
Inadequate refrigeration allows bacteria to grow and multiply.
Warming meat (e.g. in sauce) encourages growth.

Box 16.2 Practice point: Staphylococci

Nursing home – tongue sandwiches contaminated with food handler's nasal staphylococci.
Poor temperature control on refrigerator.
Half residents consume sandwiches.
Illness 1–8 hours later.
Residents who did not consume sandwiches remain well.

Critical points:
Poor hygiene – food handler.
Poor temperature control – fridge allowed bacteria to multiply.
High risk population – serious implications for home owners' lack of training.
Lack of adherence to food hygiene regulations.

Box 16.3 Practice point: Campylobacter

Family gathering – roast turkey inadequately thawed.
Parts of bird did not reach high enough temperature to kill bacteria.
7 of 10 family members ill.
Child – symptoms resembled appendicitis.
Stool samples submitted.
Meat samples submitted.
Campylobacter jejuni grown.
Campylobacter isolated from other turkeys at same supplier.

Critical points:
Inadequate thawing time.
Inadequate temperature control.
Demonstrates potential for serious outbreaks via domestic setting.

Box 16.4 Practice point: Small round structured virus

Nursery – staff member works with mild diarrhoeal type symptoms.
24–48 hours later 4 children ill.
Over period of two weeks:
5 of 8 staff ill, 25 of 32 children ill, spread via siblings to local junior school.

Critical points:
No staff education about importance of reporting illness.
High infectivity of virus and aerosol spread leads to ease of transmission in nursery and school.
Nursery closed – loss of business.
Exclusion of staff and children until asymptomatic for 48 hours.
Cost of contract cleaners to nursery owner.

---

requirements (see Further reading list and Chapter 8).

A hazard control basis for safe food handling and preparation in the domestic setting is similar.

Education of food handlers and the public

The Food Safety (General Food Hygiene) Regulation 1995 states that all food handlers must receive training. The Pennington Group (Ellison and Williams 1998) recommends food hygiene training for the following groups:

- all those involved in food handling
- school children
- local authorities, to ensure those involved in non-registered catering, i.e. private catering for parties, are aware of safe food handling practices.

This group also recommends that those working with vulnerable groups should be trained to at least a basic level in food hygiene, and the implications for nurses are obvious. Food hygiene is included in the P2000 curriculum and its importance to nursing care needs to be stressed. Nurses need an understanding of the hazard analysis as outlined above, and in addition an awareness of the vulnerability of the patient groups. Infection control audits addressing areas such as kitchen hygiene, hand washing practices and facilities, decontamination procedures and environmental cleaning are key preventative measures in infectious GI illness. They should be combined with regular training sessions. Community infection control nurses have a key role in promoting this, and they should form part of quality care delivery in institutions. (Other chapters address this issue in more detail and relate it to specific institutions, such as nursing homes, nurseries.) Public participation is an important element in secondary preventative strategies, and nurses have a role in education and helping them choose safe foods, prepare food safely and understand the rationale behind personal and environmental hygiene.

Appendix 1 at the end of this chapter is a quiz, and as such provides the basic information for inclusion in educational sessions.

> **Box 16.5** The nurse's role in prevention
>
> • To ensure recognition of an outbreak and inform relevant others
> • To arrange isolation or cohort facilities
> • To ensure maintenance of patients' fluid balance
> • To take all steps to prevent transmission of infection (enteric precautions)
> • To educate others, including patients, carers and relatives
> • To ensure specimens are obtained as requested

Tertiary prevention of infectious GI illnesses

There are three key elements to tertiary prevention:

• provision of nursing care if illness occurs
• prevention of cross infection by implementation of enteric precautions
• outbreak control procedures and investigations.

The latter are discussed in Chapter 4. Responsibilities of the outbreak team are:

• To ensure that it is possible to implement the above points.
• To provide information about the causative organism so that infection control measures specific to that organism can be implemented, such as the need to consider heavy environmental contamination during viral outbreaks or *Clostridium difficile* outbreaks.
• To advise on decisions about exclusion of staff or children.
• To advise on admission and discharge policies during the outbreak.
• To advise on closure of day care centres, schools, hotels, nurseries, etc.

Box 16.5 outlines the nurse's role in preventing the spread of an outbreak.

ENTERIC PRECAUTIONS

The basic enteric precautions outlined below are common to all incidents of infectious GI illness.

Hand washing

Thorough hand washing with soap under running water is essential. Hands should be washed:

• after handling patient
• after handling bedding
• after handling their clothing or other equipment in the vicinity of ill person
• after assisting the patient to the toilet
• prior to preparation and serving of food
• after defecation and urination – carers must also ensure the patient or any children wash their hands.
• It is important in institutions to ensure that adequate soap is available, together with paper towels. Cloth or roller towels should not be used.
• In the home, towels must not be shared.

Disposal of excretions and soiled materials

In the home, patients will normally use a flush toilet. If bedpans, commodes or urinals are used, gloves and plastic aprons should be worn by carers when disposing of contents. Toilets, handles, rails and commode chairs should be cleaned after use. Hands must be washed – both patient and carer.

Soiled clothing and bed linen should be washed in the home using a pre-wash and 'hot main wash', i.e. 65°C or more; this eliminates the need for soaking or use of disinfectant. Any solid matter can be disposed of into the toilet bowl. Sluicing of soiled linen or clothing is to be discouraged as it can place the carer at further risk of cross infection.

In a residential setting, soiled linen and clothing should be washed separately, and in all settings it is essential to ensure the washing machine is not overloaded as this prevents the clothing or linen having adequate contact with the water; therefore cleaning and disinfection will not take place.

Cleaning and disinfection

Thorough cleaning with detergent and water is essential prior to the use of disinfectant. Particular attention should be given to cleaning door handles, taps, flush handles, toilet seats, safety rails, and any surface the infected person may have touched with contaminated hands. The spread of some organisms via an aerosol has already been described: therefore surface cleaning in the vicinity of the patient becomes even more important.

After cleaning, a disinfectant solution containing 1000 ppm hypochlorite may be used.

In the home a bleach-based household cleaner is adequate. Neat bleach should not be used. The dilution is 1 part bleach to 10 parts water.

In the community the various agencies and organizations use a wide variety of cleaning and disinfecting agents. It is therefore essential to check that what they are using and how they are using it is appropriate.

Alcohol-based wipes or sprays may be used, and provide effective disinfection provided the area has been thoroughly cleaned first.

Implementation of these basic enteric precautions depends on a number of factors:

- Everyone understanding the basics of personal hygiene and hand washing
- Good communication by the outbreak team in terms of supplying relevant support and advice quickly
- In isolated cases nursed at home, provision by the GP and/or primary care team of advice and support to the patient and carers
- In a residential home, school or nursery setting, it may be necessary for the outbreak team or infection control team to support management in a request for funding for extra domestic cleaning and laundry staff during an outbreak. This is particularly so where very restrictive domestic cleaning contracts are in place.

Nurses and carers working in the community have a key public health role to play by promoting high standards of personal hygiene, that is hand washing, at all times.

Prevention and control of infectious GI illness in the community is dependent on:

- Good working relationships between all the relevant agencies
- Ongoing education programmes on food hygiene and infection control
- Ongoing audit and monitoring of standards
- The understanding and willingness of community nurses and care workers to play a key role in promoting good personal and environmental hygiene standards
- The provision of a good diagnostic microbiology service
- The support and co-ordinating function of Environmental Health Officers and the Department of Public Health Medicine
- The provision of adequate acute nursing and medical care facilities to ensure prompt treatment of any infection
- Ongoing surveillance systems to pinpoint potential community outbreaks early.

Nurses have a key public health role to play in promoting the good practices which prevent the development and spread of infectious GI illnesses. Nurses work with some of the most vulnerable groups in the community and will understand how best to tailor the basic health promotion messages for the client groups they work with. Eradication of infection at source is not yet achievable; therefore secondary and tertiary preventative methods are essential and education of all concerned, including the public, lies at their heart.

REFERENCES

Ansari S A, Syed A, Sattar V et al 1988 Rotavirus survival on human hands and transfer of infectious virus to animate and non porous inanimate surfaces. Journal of Clinical Microbiology 26: 1513–1518

Barker J, James F 1999 Managing gastroenteritis in early childhood. Community Practitioner 72(5): 131–133

Beckers H J 1987 Public health aspects of microbial contaminants in food. The Veterinary Quarterly 9(4): 342–347

Bloomfield S F, Scott E 1997 Cross contamination and infection in the domestic environment and the role of chemical disinfectants (review). Journal of Applied Microbiology 83: 1–9

Buzby J, Robert T 1997 Economic costs and trade impacts of microbial foodborne illness. World Health Statistics Quarterly 50, part 1–2: 57–66

Chief Medical Officer 1992 Definition of food poisoning. (PL/CMO(92)14). DoH, London

Chin J (ed.) 2000 Control of Communicable Disease Manual, 17th edn. An official Report of the American Public Health Association, Washington DC

Djuretic J, Ryan M, Fleming D, Wall P 1996 Infectious intestinal disease in elderly people. Communicable Disease Report (review) 6(8) July. PHLS, London

Djuretic T, Wall P, Brazier J 1999 *Clostridium difficile:* An update on its epidemiology and role in hospital outbreaks in England and Wales. Journal of Hospital Infection 41: 213–218

Donaldson R J, Donaldson L J 1988 Essential Community Medicine. MTP Press, Lancaster, 115–117

Ellison J, Williams P 1998 Coping with the Pennington Report. Environmental Health 106(11): 331–332

Finch R G, Ball P 1991 Infection. Blackwell Scientific, London, ch. 10

Hardyment C 1995 Slice of Life – The British way of eating since 1945. BBC Publications, London

Hobbs B, Roberts D 1987 Food poisoning and food hygiene, 5th edn. Edward Arnold, London

Hotel Catering and Institutional Management Association (HCIMA) 1991. Technical briefing sheet no. 5. HCIMA, London

Johnson A E, Donkin A J M, Morgan K 1998 Food safety knowledge and practice among elderly people living at home. Journal of Epidemiology and Community Health 52(11): 745–748

Morris J G, Morris R 1997 Emergence of new pathogens as a function of change in host susceptibility. Emerging Infectious Diseases 3(4), Oct–Dec

Potter M E 1992 The changing face of foodborne disease. Journal of Veterinary and Medical Association 201(2): 250–253

Public Health Laboratory Service 1995 The prevention of human transmission of gastrointestinal infection, infestations and bacterial intoxications. A working party of PHLS Salmonella Committee. CDR Review 5(11), October

Roberts D, Hooper W, Greenwood M 1986 Practical food microbiology. Public Health Laboratory Service, London

Ross D J, Cherry N M, McDonald J C 1998 Occupationally acquired infectious disease in the UK 1996–1997. Communicable Disease and Public Health 1(2). PHLS, London

Shanson D C 1989 Microbiology in Clinical Practice, 2nd edn. Wright, London, ch. 14

Sleigh J, Timbury M 1990 Medical Bacteriology, 3rd edn. Churchill Livingstone, Edinburgh

Sprenger R 1991 Hygiene for Management – A text for food hygiene courses, 5th edn. Garnett Dickinson print, London

Stolley P, Laskey T 1995 Investigating disease patterns – the science of epidemiology. Scientific American Library

Voss S 1993 Cost to affected individuals following an outbreak of food poisoning. A pilot study. Public Health 107: 337–341

Wheeler J, Sethi D, Cowden J et al 1999 Study of infectious intestinal disease in England: rates in the community, presenting to general practice and reported to national surveillance. British Medical Journal 318, 17 April: 1046–1050

Williams C 1999 *Helicobacter pylori* and endoscopy. Journal of Hospital Infection 41: 263–268

World Health Organization 1995 Hazard analysis critical control point system concept application. WHO/FNU/FOS/957. WHO, Geneva

World Health Organization 1998 Life in the 21st Century – a Vision for All. The 1998 World Health Report. WHO, Geneva

FURTHER READING

Bignardi G E 1998 Risk factors for *clostridium difficile* infection (a review). Journal of Hospital Infection 40(1): 1–15

Bouchier I (Chair) 1998 Cryptosporidium in water supplies. Third report of the group of experts to Department of Environment, Transport and the Regions and Department of Public Health. DoH, London

Caddow P (ed.) 1989 Applied Microbiology. Scutari Press, London

Chin J (ed.) 2000 Control of Communicable Disease Manual, 17th edn. An official Report of the American Public Health Association, Washington DC

Department of Health 1995 A Guide to Food Hazards and your Business. DoH, London

Domestos Advisory Service. Your guide to home hygiene – Wise up to food – What is bleach? Domestos, London

Food and Drink Federation. The A–Z of food safety. Food Link, London

Green J, Wright P A, Gallimore C et al 1998 The role of environmental contamination with small round structured viruses in a hospital outbreak investigated by reverse transcriptase polymerase chain reaction assay. Journal of Hospital Infection 39(1): 39–45

Gould D 1996 Hygienic practices. Journal of Infection Control Nursing 23(5)

HMSO 1995 Report on Verocytotoxin producing E. coli. Advisory Committee on Microbiological Safety of Food. HMSO, London

International Scientific Forum on Home Hygiene 1998 Guidelines for Prevention of Infection and Cross Infection in the Domestic Environment. http: www-ifh-homehygiene.org/2library/2lbr00.htm/

International Scientific Forum on Home Hygiene 2000 Recommendations for selection of Suitable Hygiene Procedures for Use in the Domestic Environment. A Consensus Document. http: www.ifh-homehygiene.org/2library/2lbr00.htm

National Centre for Infectious Diseases 1997 Emerging infectious diseases – an overview of key issues in food safety 3(4). (Entire journal devoted to subject.)

Pennington Group 1997 Report on the circumstances leading to 1996 outbreak of infection with *E. coli* 0157 in central Scotland, the implications for food safety and lessons to be learned. Stationery Office, Edinburgh

Public Health Laboratory Service (PHLS) 1993 Outbreak of gastroenteritis associated with small round structured viruses. Viral Gastroenteritis Sub Committee of PHLS Virology Committee. PHLS Microbiology Digest 10(1): 2–8

PHLS 1993 Surveillance and control of *Shigella sonnei* infection. Communicable Disease Report Review (5): 23 April

PHLS 1994 *Clostridium difficile* infection, prevention and management. DoH/PHLS Joint Working Group, London

PHLS 1998 Editorial and original reports. Communicable Disease and Public Health 1(3): 144–196

Shanson D C 1989 Microbiology in Clinical Practice, 2nd edn. Butterworth, Oxford

World Health Organization 1998 Prevention and control of enterohaemorrhagic *Escherichia coli* (EHEC) infections. Memorandum from WHO meeting by A Reilly. WHO Bulletin 76(3): 245–255

APPENDIX 1

Tick one answer only for each question. Answers appear at the end of the quiz.

1) If food is kept hot before serving, what is the lowest temperature it must be kept above?
a) 37°C   c) 63°C
b) 53°C   d) 83°C

2) When food is put in a fridge, bacteria:
a) stop growing   c) grow fairly fast
b) grow very fast   d) are all killed

3) You're cooking a piece of meat that will be served cold with salad tomorrow. How should you cool it?
a) put it into the fridge straight away
b) leave it on a work surface in the kitchen for up to 1½ hours
c) put it in a well-ventilated food store for up to 1½ hours
d) turn the oven off and take the meat out after 1½ hours

4) You have been making a pudding and have half a tin of peach slices left over. Should you put them into the fridge in:
a) the open tin?
b) the tin with a cover on it?
c) an open bowl?
d) a covered bowl?

5) Which one of the following is not a physical contaminant of food?
a) paint   c) screws
b) bacteria   d) earrings

6) At what temperature should frozen food be stored?
a) 4°C   c) − 10°C
b) −4°C   d) − 18°C

7) There are four containers of cream in the fridge. You should use the one where the 'best by' date is:
a) last week   c) next week
b) tomorrow   d) next month

8) The main reason why jewellery shouldn't be worn in the kitchen is:
a) it gets in the way
b) it might be broken
c) it might be stolen
d) it harbours dirt and bacteria

9) Overclothes worn by people who handle food must be:
a) white   c) linen
b) clean   d) ironed

10) You are off work with an upset stomach. You can go back to work:
a) as soon as you are better
b) a week after you feel better
c) ten days after you feel better
d) as soon as you get medical clearance and have discussed this with your employer

11) You come back from your mid-morning break (1)
Then you wash and cut up some salad vegetables (2)
Then you empty the waste bin (3)

Then you put some sausage rolls on to cook (4)
When should you wash your hands?
a) after points 1, 2, 3
b) after points 2, 3, 4
c) after points 1, 3, 4
d) after points 1, 2, 4

12) Which one of the following pairs of items should be disinfected frequently?
a) fridge handles and ovens
b) fridge handles and food preparation surfaces
c) food preparation surfaces and floors
d) fridge handles and floors

13) Which one of the following is important when cleaning floors?
a) clean exposed areas
b) always leave them wet
c) disinfect them every day
d) removing dirt with hot water and detergent

14) Disinfectants are used for:
a) reducing germs to a safe level
b) removing stains
c) removing grease and dirt
d) removing germs completely

15) Disinfectants should be:
a) kept regularly topped up
b) made up each time they are needed
c) made up as strong as possible
d) kept in clear glass containers

16) What is the best temperature for the growth of food poisoning bacteria?
a) 10°C   c) 37°C
b) 27°C   d) 63°C

17) One of the four things bacteria need in order to grow is:
a) darkness   c) moisture
b) light   d) dry atmosphere

18) The most common cause of food poisoning is:
a) water   c) chemicals
b) bacteria   d) poisonous plants

19) A common symptom of food poisoning is:
a) cough   c) sore throat
b) diarrhoea   d) kidney pain

20) High-risk foods are:
a) high in fat
b) likely to have bacteria on them
c) where bacteria will grow easily
d) the most difficult to cook satisfactorily

21) How do food poisoning bacteria get into food premises?
a) people   c) raw food
b) insects   d) all of these

22) Dangerous bacteria are called:
a) poisoners
b) pathogens
c) saprophytes
d) spoilage bacteria

23) Which one of the following materials is not suitable for worktops in a kitchen?
a) wood   c) formica
b) marble   d) stainless steel

24) The main reason why food pests should be controlled is that they:
a) spread disease
b) upset customers
c) make food taste unpleasant
d) increase the amount of cleaning

25) Which one of the following is the best way of keeping rats and mice out of food premises?
a) keeping a cat
b) putting poison down
c) keeping everything clean
d) leaving a light on at night

26) Which one of the following must be provided in food premises by law?
a) shower   c) fridge
b) cooker   d) wash hand basin

27) Which of the following foods should you never store close together:
a) liver pâté and cheese
b) fried bacon and salami
c) ham and uncooked mince beef
d) raw chicken and uncooked sausages

28) Hair must be controlled and covered because:
a) long hair gets in your eyes
b) hair and dandruff can contaminate food
c) hats are smarter than bare heads

29) Hands quickly become contaminated by contact with:
a) raw foods
b) dirty surfaces
c) cleaning equipment
d) your face
e) your hair
f) all of these

Answers:

1) c	**2)** a	**3)** a	**4)** d
5) b	**6)** d	**7)** b	**8)** d
9) b	**10)** d	**11)** a	**12)** b
13) d	**14)** a	**15)** b	**16)** c
17) c	**18)** b	**19)** b	**20)** c
21) d	**22)** b	**23)** a	**24)** a
25) c	**26)** d	**27)** c	**28)** b
29) e			

17

Prisoners, travellers, the homeless and refugees

S. Lowe

INTRODUCTION

There are sections of the community that have become marginalized. This chapter aims to look at these client groups and identify their infection control risks and how these can be reduced.

Many of the health problems of these client groups require social as well as medical intervention and therefore they require a multidisciplinary approach. It is often the social problems that give rise to the infection control and communicable disease risks. Understanding the impact that some of these social problems can have on the community is important.

Social exclusion is a process that does not happen alone. Healthcare alone cannot rectify this.

THE PRISON ENVIRONMENT

It is estimated that prisons in the United Kingdom have a throughput of around 150 000 annually. Of this number, the prison population at any given time is over 45 000, of whom 2500 are serving life sentences (Mason and Adams 1992). Some of these prisoners are only on remand, and so will be in the system for only a short period of time; the remainder are living in conditions which are conducive to the spread of infection. Prisoners are housed in large numbers in close proximity to each other, with many communal and shared facilities. It is important therefore that guidance is in place to assist staff in prisons to minimize the risk of infection to themselves and prisoners.

A recent consultation document on the 'Future organisation and delivery of prison healthcare' (NHS Executive 1999), reviewed prison health services and the National Health Service working much closer together to provide a better service for prisoners. It also highlighted the need for prisoners to have access to all areas of the health service, from mental health through to the prevention of infectious diseases, equal to those in the community outside prison.

Prison healthcare may be the first real chance that a prisoner has of medical care in an otherwise disordered life (Levy 1997).

Earlier chapters have looked at general infection control matters which all need to be taken into account on a day-to-day basis. However, there are certain factors which may be more problematic or harder to deal with in the prison setting. One of these areas is dealing with blood or body fluids.

Blood and body fluids

Contact with these substances can be frequent and unexpected and so must be considered a potential risk at all times. There are however particular situations in which the risk of contact with these body fluids may be increased.

One particular situation is 'dirty protests' where prisoners smear body fluids such as blood, urine and faeces over walls, clothing and other surfaces. This increases the risk of others coming into contact with these body fluids. The risk, whilst not always avoidable, can be minimized.

Where applicable, inmates should be encouraged to clean up their own mess. When this is not possible, staff or those who undertake the cleaning must wear personal protective clothing (Box 17.1). The protective clothing should consist of a plastic apron and gloves. If there is a risk of splashes to the eyes, then eye protection must be worn (Department of Health Expert Advisory Group 1998).

Spillages

Spillages of blood or any other body fluids should be cleaned up as soon as safely or reasonably possible. Guidelines on how to deal with spillages

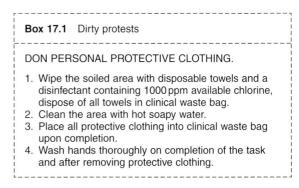

Box 17.1 Dirty protests

DON PERSONAL PROTECTIVE CLOTHING.

1. Wipe the soiled area with disposable towels and a disinfectant containing 1000 ppm available chlorine, dispose of all towels in clinical waste bag.
2. Clean the area with hot soapy water.
3. Place all protective clothing into clinical waste bag upon completion.
4. Wash hands thoroughly on completion of the task and after removing protective clothing.

of blood and body fluids are described and illustrated in Chapter 5.

Blood-borne infections

In order to manage the risk of blood-borne infection safely, all staff should be encouraged to have a course of Hepatitis B vaccination.

A study examined the prevalence of Hepatitis B in prison (Hutchinson et al 1998). But what implications does this have for healthcare workers in the prison setting?

It is known that injecting drug use does occur in prison, but as this is an illicit act the full extent of drug use can only be speculated. The Dinamap study reported by Bolling (1994) looked at the physical health of prisoners. Prisoners were asked if they had used any drugs in the 12 months prior to imprisonment, and 63% declared they had. Each one of these prisoners has the potential to be infected with Hepatitis B or C or Human Immunodeficiency Virus (HIV). Prisoners do not have ready access to clean needles and syringes and there is likely to be more sharing of this equipment by inmates, thus increasing the risk of spread of infections with blood-borne viruses. The equipment used may present a risk to staff at any time, but especially during body or cell searches, and all staff should be aware of these risks and the action to be taken if a sharps injury occurs.

Prison authorities are unlikely to completely stop the traffic of needles and syringes into prisons; they can, however, reduce the flow. By doing this they may in turn increase the risk of disease, through increased needle sharing. Prisoners have

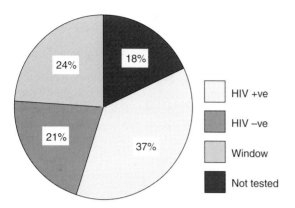

HIV +ve

HIV −ve

Window

Not tested

Figure 17.1 HIV testing results from prison inmates. Window: the window period when the virus may not be present on testing.

anecdotally reported up to 20 people sharing needles and syringes until such time as the needles became blunt and had to be forced through the skin, resulting in tissue damage with a further risk of infection from open wounds. Decontamination using bleach is questionable on biological and behavioural grounds, as drug users underestimate the time needed to sterilize using this method (Dolan et al 1995). In 1993 the first documented outbreak of HIV infection amongst imprisoned drug injectors was reported from a Scottish prison (Taylor et al 1995). They found that of the 378 inmates in the prison, 227 came forward for counselling after the outbreak. A third of these prisoners (76) had injected drugs at some time and 33 admitted to injecting whilst in prison. They were all offered testing for HIV and the results are shown in Figure 17.1.

They also found that all prisoners infected with HIV had injected whilst in prison and the DNA viral sequencing showed that it was highly likely that all of the infections occurred in prison. At this time there were also 11 inmates who presented with Hepatitis B infection, all of whom had contracted the infection within the prison. Interestingly, six of these were also infected with HIV. The intervention of the medical officer authorizing the counselling and testing limited the spread of Hepatitis B and HIV. Recent guidelines (DoH 1996) recommend that all prisoners should be offered immunization against Hepatitis B. A recent study of French prisons showed

that 75% of inmates who participated in the study required immunization against Hepatitis B (Rotily et al 1997).

As yet there has been no reported data about Hepatitis C in prison populations. That is not to say it does not exist, only that it has not yet been reported. As the risk factors for this form of hepatitis are the same as those for Hepatitis B, it is reasonable to expect some transmission to occur in the prison setting.

Accidental inoculations

Accidental inoculation is:

- all penetrating sharps/needle injuries
- contamination of abrasions with blood or body fluids
- scratches or bites involving broken skin (causing bleeding or visible skin puncture)
- splashes of blood/body fluids into the eyes or mouth.

Within the prison environment any of the above accidents can take place. Staff may be injured by a needle from a prisoner or whilst administering drugs to a prisoner. During 'dirty protests' abrasions can become contaminated or blood/body fluids can splash onto the face of others. Biting can also break skin during violent outbursts, causing bleeding, thus creating a high risk of infection.

A policy should be in place outlining the course of action to be followed in the event of such incidents taking place. This should include:

- immediate first aid required
- whom to report incidents to
- identifying source of inoculation
- blood specimens and where to be tested
- possible need for post-exposure prophylaxis and where to seek advice
- checking Hepatitis B status
- documentation
- follow-up of the incident.

Sexual relationships

Any activity that involves the transmission of body fluids from one individual to another increases the risk of further spread of these diseases. This includes unprotected sexual intercourse, whether consenting or not. There is always a great reluctance for male prisoners to discuss the extent of sexual relations within the prison environment. The extent therefore of sexual relationships within prisons can only be estimated, as can the extent of the risk of sexually-transmitted disease. Condoms may be issued by the prison but this remains a local decision by the prison governors.

Staff protection

All staff have a duty to ensure they are aware of the risks of disease transmission from blood and other contaminated body fluids. They must take action to protect both themselves and all prisoners from exposure.

This may be through health education for both prisoners and staff, or through screening programmes. However, a negative result for any disease tested for upon entry to prison does not mean that they will remain negative during their stay.

Further information, support and advice about blood-borne viruses and other sexually-transmitted diseases can be obtained from specialist nurses in the local genitourinary medicine clinic and infection control nurses in the community.

Any guidelines produced for practices within prison healthcare settings should take into account staff protection as well as prisoner protection.

Suggested guidance which should be in place

- Blood and body fluid spillage
- Sharps use and disposal
- Accidental inoculation
- Post-exposure prophylaxis
- Hand hygiene guidance
- Protective clothing
- Clinical waste disposal
- Laundry guidance
- Vaccine programmes
- Screening programmes
- Communicable disease reporting
- Notifiable disease reporting (see Chapter 4)
- Management of specific infections (e.g. scabies, gastrointestinal, tuberculosis)

- Outbreak control
- Record keeping
- Isolation of prisoners for specific infections.

When developing policies/guidelines related to infection control, assistance can be sought through the Consultant for Communicable Disease Control and the Control of Infection Nurse responsible for the community.

Tuberculosis (TB)

Tuberculosis is a bacterial infection which has seen a rise in the number of cases nationally. It should therefore be no surprise that there are cases of TB within prisons. Prisons provide all the factors associated with the spread of TB, namely overcrowding, poverty, drug abuse and concurrent infection with HIV (Drobniewski 1995).

It is recommended that all prison staff know their TB immunity status and, where needed, be offered vaccination.

When a case of TB occurs in a prison, contact tracing will take place by the public health department through the TB nurse specialist. Contacts would include all staff and any other inmates that may have been in close contact with the infected prisoner, particularly those who have shared a cell in the recent past as well as at present. Contacts may also include prisoners at other prisons if the prisoners had been moved around, transport staff, and also any regular family or friends outside the prison. Cases of tuberculosis must be treated promptly to reduce the risk of spread to other prisoners, particularly any HIV-positive individuals. Prompt treatment will also reduce the risk of spread into the community, when prisoners are released.

Prisons that have detainees from other countries, such as illegal immigrants, should ensure that if they have not already had health checks undertaken at the port of entry they should have this done as soon as possible on entry to the prison. This should include testing for tuberculosis.

Diagnosis of tuberculosis should be notified to the Consultant for Communicable Disease Control (CCDC) in the local community. They can ensure that if a prisoner is from another area, liaison with the CCDC for that area takes place, thus ensuring that anyone requiring testing can be contacted and followed up.

Notifiable diseases

Any cases of communicable diseases that are notifiable (see Chapter 4) must be notified to the Consultant for Communicable Disease Control (CCDC) for the area, who will then liaise with the prison, specialist medical staff and the prisoner's home to ensure that the correct advice, contact tracing and treatments are undertaken.

As many prisoners are frequently in prisons many miles from their own home, liaison is also important when a prisoner is released. This allows for continuation of treatment of any disease to be maintained through the person's local health services.

It should be remembered that although prisons have high walls, bacteria and viruses do not respect these boundaries of brick and mortar; they will use the most convenient method of transport to reach the outside world, namely humans.

THE HOMELESS

During the time of Florence Nightingale it was stated, 'The connection between health and the dwellings of the population is one of the most important that exists' (Lowry 1989). A survey by Surrey University found 2307 people living on the street in 1.75 square miles of the city of London (Hudson 1989). The legal responsibility for housing the homeless lies with the local authority housing department. However, individuals need to meet certain criteria to be deemed a priority for the council to be obliged to home them. Emergency housing in bed and breakfast establishments, bed-sits, hostels, old army barracks and old isolation hospitals often has conditions which are as bad as, or in some cases worse than, a life on the streets.

Living on the streets is a precarious existence. Homeless people are often the target of personal attacks, leaving them with wounds, fractures and head injuries that go unreported and untreated.

The basis of all infection control is that of good hygiene, both personal and environmental. Homeless people face a daunting daily task to find somewhere to carry out the basic hygiene needs.

In the past local swimming pools offered private bathroom facilities for a small cost, providing hot water, soap and towels. Many of these have now closed, particularly in the inner cities. The local authority would be able to advise where these facilities are, if any still exist in the local area. Often the only access to clean water is in public toilets, where there is no privacy to wash thoroughly. Often no soap or towels are available, and the attendants may evict them from the facilities.

Evidence on being homeless and the effects on health has already been reported in studies (Davies 1987, Gaze 1997, Mathews 1998). Common infections include skin infections, wound infections, tuberculosis and influenza.

Skin infections and wounds

A study by *Big Issue* magazine (Gaze 1997) found that out of 157 homeless people, most of whom were less than 35 years of age, 17% had chest problems, 12% had abscesses and 19% had foot or dental problems. Many of these infections will go untreated until they become such a problem that admission to hospital is required. It is difficult to know what can be done to prevent and overcome these problems.

In some areas health authorities have established drop-in clinics. These are specifically for the homeless, who can access a range of services in the centres, covering both social and health needs, including basic needs such as bathing and laundry facilities. Once these basic needs are met then specific health issues and the risks of infection facing the homeless can be addressed. Any treatment needed is given in a way which is non-judgmental and supportive of the choices made by the client.

Wounds run the risk of becoming infected. Infected wounds can take a long time to heal and will often become re-infected. Wounds should be cleaned thoroughly and a suitable dressing applied, which will give some protection to the wound from contamination that may be faced from a life on the streets in all weathers. Advice needs to be given about care of the wound which the client is able to carry out, bearing in mind the client's lifestyle. If wounds have been caused by injecting drugs then referral to a drug clinic may be beneficial in minimizing skin problems in the future by better injecting techniques. Clients may also have long-standing skin infections such as impetigo, infected eczema, and infestations such as scabies and head or body lice. Treatment for these infections should preferably be carried out in the centre. The lack of hygiene facilities and privacy on the streets would prohibit the clients from carrying it out there. Collection, payment and storage of prescription items can also be a problem.

Tuberculosis

The re-emergence of some diseases such as tuberculosis have become a problem for society as a whole, but for the homeless, who are surviving in the very conditions that provide an ideal transmission setting for this disease, the problem is giving great cause for concern.

Detection, treatment and follow-up of cases present unique difficulties. Shelters or drop-in centres for the homeless provide an ideal opportunity to screen, treat and follow up the homeless, and these facilities, whilst not being ideal, should be utilized (Kumar et al 1995). Some areas of the world have devised incentive systems in the form of food vouchers for patients who undergo treatment for tuberculosis. This encourages compliance with treatment and helps to control the transmission.

Medical treatment

The homeless will, just like other people in the community, have underlying medical conditions which may need ongoing treatment, but this continuation of treatment can be problematic. One drop-in clinic in Brighton has encountered problems such as a diabetic patient who was also homeless. The clinic provides refrigerator and storage facilities for his insulin, needles and syringes (Kenny 1999). Clients who are homeless often find keeping to a strict medication regime difficult. Taking insulin when you do not know when and what your next meal will be makes stabilizing diabetes extremely difficult.

This drop-in centre in Brighton, like many others, noticed that clients would only present and discuss minor health complaints once trust and confidence had been established. This was usually due to a prior bad experience with the health service. It can take quite a length of time to build up trust between a client and a health worker. Some larger inner cities have teams working specifically for the homeless and rootless. It is important to work closely with these teams in improving the health of the individual and ensuring the prevention of communicable diseases.

Emergency housing, as previously described, often offers only marginally better facilities than life on the street. The accommodation offered can be overcrowded, damp, run down and may be infested with vermin. A whole family may have only one room in which they all have to live, eat and sleep. Toilet and bathroom facilities being shared by more than one family also increases the risk of gastrointestinal infections being transmitted. Outbreaks of salmonella in bed and breakfast hostels have been reported (Davies 1987). Diet also contributes to the risk of gastrointestinal infections. Where there are limited facilities for correct storage and cooking of food, the conditions may be ideal for the rapid multiplication of bacteria.

Support services

Centres which offer care for homeless people, whether it is overnight accommodation or food kitchens, can all be utilized to provide homeless people with access to health and social care. Used in this way a supportive contact point for accessing mainstream healthcare can be founded. People who are often isolated can be given time to talk and discuss any health problems. Healthchecks can be offered such as tuberculosis screening, immunization advice, and routine cervical and testicular screening.

Information on accessing local services and availability of social and health-related care can be given together with referral, if requested or required.

TRAVELLERS

Travellers include a number of different groups such as gypsies, tinkers, New Age wanderers who all consider themselves different and yet they all share one very important factor, a nomadic lifestyle. Gulland (1997) stated that 'on the road often means off the list for health services'. In 1996, travellers of all groups were thought to number around 66 000 people (Bunce 1996). This figure is likely to have increased since that study was undertaken.

This nomadic lifestyle, along with the distrust, hostility and prejudice that travellers often encounter, can make accessing health and social services very difficult. However, Mathews (1998) argues that socially-excluded minorities such as travellers are not helpless victims and should not be treated as such.

Primary healthcare

Access to primary healthcare is hard. Without an address and postcode travellers cannot register with a general practitioner, except as a temporary resident. Due to the length of time it can take medical records to travel around the system, long-term health planning of any type is extremely difficult. This leads to many children of travellers not completing immunization courses and no opportunity for professionals to give advice about childhood illnesses and infectious diseases.

Some travellers will be staying on official sites where access to basic facilities such as fresh water and toilet/sluice facilities is available. However, these can vary from extremely poor to a good standard and these sites are few in number. Local residents often do not wish a site to be nearby. These reactions may be as a result of distrust and a lack of understanding as to why these people want this kind of lifestyle. Travellers, therefore, set up home on unofficial sites such as lay-bys, roadside encampments and wasteland, where

there are no facilities for fresh water and sanitation. Binnie (1998) stated, 'In these unofficial sites they live in the squalor and type of conditions prevailing in this country a couple of centuries ago. No clean water supply, no sewage disposal, no rubbish collection and totally inadequate education, immunization and medical attention'.

Health-related living conditions

A number of studies (Pahl et al 1986, Hennick 1993) have shown that travellers are more likely to suffer from general poor health including asthma, chest infections, heart disease, alcohol problems, untreated chronic illness and conditions linked to poor sanitation. All these problems have always been linked to overcrowding, poor general living conditions and lack of long-term healthcare.

The lack of education facilities can also mean no opportunity for sex education, or treatment and advice offered through school medical and dental services (Adams 1975). Often, the first opportunity that can arise for advice to be given is if the first child is born in hospital. But yet again, the mother will often only present when in labour and will be discharged soon after the birth.

Lack of sanitation and a fresh water supply can lead to problems with infections and also the control of infection when a problem has occurred.

Infections such as Hepatitis A, food poisoning, viral gastrointestinal illnesses and influenza are the most common encountered.

Vaccination for Hepatitis A, tuberculosis and influenza could control some of these problems. But often travellers have moved on of their own accord or have been forcibly moved on before this can be arranged. Patient-held records would mean that vaccination could be offered to these families on an opportunistic basis. The cards would provide immediate information on their vaccination status.

Gastrointestinal illness

Gastrointestinal illness is widely under-reported in the community generally, therefore unless the person affected is ill enough to require hospitalization then precautions to limit the spread cannot be put into place. This can include bacterial and viral illness.

Travellers' distrust of officialdom can often mean that spread of the infection is already well under way by the time it comes to the attention of the Infection Control Nurse or Consultant for Communicable Disease Control (CCDC). Cases of gastrointestinal illness need prompt investigation to ascertain the infective organism to allow appropriate advice to be given. Whilst specific results are awaited, advice should be given about hygiene, with specific reference to hand hygiene and precautions with water supply. Water should be boiled before being used for any drinks for anyone, especially children.

Giving the appropriate advice is the easy part, but finding practical ways it can be carried out takes more thought. This will depend on the family concerned and finding the best way to advise. A health visitor may be working specifically with travelling families, which is an excellent link for infection control. The health visitor will be able to give information which will allow advice to be tailored for the family or persons concerned.

Health and social services

Community nurses and health visitors are often the key points of contact for many travellers (Gulland 1997), the main thrust of the work being basic public health work, general health and hygiene.

Hawes (1994) concluded from his study that legal, well-serviced sites are an essential prerequisite to the improvement of travellers' health. The health of travellers needs not only a health response but also addressing by social services by looking at the facilities that are available for travellers at any official sites. The lack of legal sites continues to be a hindrance to the health of all travellers and to healthcare work with them. The passing of the Criminal Justice and Public Order Act in 1994 removed the duty of local authorities to provide official sites, and also prevents travellers travelling in groups of more than six vehicles.

REFUGEES AND IMMIGRANTS

Over the last decade the numbers of refugees entering the United Kingdom has continued to increase. Not all refugees are the same. They will have come from a variety of countries and backgrounds and their life experiences will be dependent on their previous lives and what made them leave their homes and native lands.

The Kings Fund produced guidance (Levenson and Coker 1999) for general practitioners on the health of refugees, stating that 'it is all too easy to simplify and stereotype the experiences of men, women and children of all ages and of various ethnic groups'.

Immigrants, unlike refugees, have chosen to leave their country of origin and have not been forced to leave in fear. Refugees all have one thing in common, which is the often-unwanted experience of being uprooted from their country of origin. The guidance defines a refugee simply as 'someone who is unable to return to his or her country of origin for fear of persecution'. The United Nations in 1951 provided a more legalistic definition: 'An asylum seeker is someone who is applying for refugee status. In order to be accepted as a refugee a person must first apply for asylum, each application is examined and if asylum is granted then refugee status is conferred'.

Factors affecting refugee/immigrant health

Most refugees and some immigrants to the United Kingdom have come from poor countries and from countries which are experiencing conflict (Rutter 1996). Factors in their country of origin will affect their health in this country. Many refugees have had employment in their country of origin, such as doctors, lawyers, etc. and not all will be poor rural workers. It must be remembered that they may not speak English and that although translators are available, the sex of the translator may be an issue. Women may prefer a female translator. The use of translation cards is not always appropriate, as they may not read their own language.

It is usual for social structures to break down in countries in conflict. This means that any health-care system in place will undergo changes or disintegrate completely. The longer the conflict continues, the worse the state of chronic health conditions will be, as the provision of medication takes second place to the act of staying alive.

The risks of communicable disease in immigrants and refugees that need to be considered are (Communicable Disease Review 1999):

* The endemic communicable diseases in the country of origin
* The disease present in any countries they have passed through or have been detained in
* The risk of disease from transit camps in which they may have been held for long periods of time. This may also be affected by the season; for example rainy season gives rise to flooding and decrease in sanitation
* Lack of immunization from infectious diseases in the country of origin and the country in which they have been placed.

Possibility of imported diseases

Some of the conditions that are endemic in the country of origin may be uncommon in this country, and there can be delays in diagnosis of some diseases, due to the lack of health professionals' awareness of imported conditions.

Advice on disease prevalence in the country of origin should be sought; this advice is available from the local Consultant for Communicable Disease Control, local travel health clinicians, or the Centre for Communicable Disease Control at Colindale, London.

Some of the communicable diseases that may be present among refugees and asylum seekers are shown in Box 17.2 (Aldous et al 1999).

Reception and health checks

Many immigrants and refugees arrive in the United Kingdom, usually in London. From London the refugees are displaced out to other cities and towns in England, whilst awaiting appeals. Immigrants are usually only passing

---

Box 17.2 Communicable diseases in refugees and asylum seekers

Lice, scabies
Intestinal parasites
Malaria
Leprosy
Tuberculosis
Chronic Hepatitis B
Typhoid
Cholera
HIV/AIDS
Sexually-transmitted diseases

(Aldous et al 1999)

---

through London because of the large airports, and their destination is often a part of the country where they have relatives, friends or there is an established community from their home country.

The initial health screen is undertaken by Port Health at the port of arrival. However, many illnesses may not become apparent until much later.

All immigrants and refugees will be questioned and in some cases examined and X-rayed for signs of tuberculosis. Notification will then be sent to the Communicable Disease Department of the town or city in which the person is intending to settle. Hayward (1998) found that in London, 55% of culture-confirmed cases of tuberculosis occurred in people born outside the United Kingdom. Heathrow Health Control Unit in 1997 found that the prevalence of tuberculosis was significantly higher in refugees and asylum seekers than in other immigrants.

Infection control in UK settlers

Many immigrants and refugees are placed in poor and overcrowded living conditions, especially with shared bathroom and kitchen facilities. This heightens the risks of diseases such as lice, scabies, gastrointestinal diseases and tuberculosis which will easily pass from person to person. There is also great difficulty in controlling the spread of infection once it has become established. The lack of hygiene facilities is an area that needs special attention when dealing with any outbreaks of infection. Due to this lack of facilities, hand hygiene may need to be supplemented by using impregnated hand wipes. It should also be remembered that lavatory and sanitation facilities in other countries differ from ours, in that they may not have been very robust and therefore paper products could not be disposed of in them. Education for the families around what can be disposed of down the toilets may be needed.

The most vulnerable refugees are the children and older people, but it should be remembered that other areas of concern might involve specific problems. Sexual abuse of women, torture of men, women and children may also have taken place. In some races to have been sexually abused or raped is seen as a great disgrace, and may not be acknowledged by the women who have been affected. For this reason sexually-transmitted

diseases may not be detected. There are also refugees from areas of the world where the incidence of HIV is much higher than in the United Kingdom. Questioning about health matters to women refugees must be undertaken with care and compassion. Women in particular may only be happy talking to a female healthcare worker.

Victims of torture may well have suffered sexual abuse as well as beating of a severe nature. This may have inflicted severe mental health issues as well as other physical damage such as sexually-transmitted diseases, scar tissue and internal organ damage.

To address health issues of refugees and immigrants there needs to be a multi-disciplinary approach. It requires social as well as medical intervention.

REFERENCES

Adams B 1975 Gypsies and government policy in England. Heinemann, London

Aldous J, Bardsley M et al 1999 Refugee Health in London. Key issues for public health. The Health of Londoners Project. East London and City Health Authority, London

Binnie G A C 1998 Problem of caring for travellers is British, not just European. British Medical Journal 316: 1825

Bolling K 1994 The Dinamap 8100 calibration study. HMSO, London

Bunce C 1996 A hard road to travel. Nursing Times 92(49): 34–36

Communicable Disease Review 1999 Communicable disease hazards facing refugees from Kosovo. CDR Weekly 23 April, 9(17): 147, 150

Davies P 1987 Health risks for the homeless. Health Service Journal 97: 1069

Department of Health Expert Advisory Group on AIDS and the Advisory Group on Hepatitis 1998 Guidance for Clinical Health Care Workers: Protection Against Infection with Blood-borne Viruses. DoH, London

Department of Health, Welsh Office, Scottish Office, DHSS Northern Ireland 1996 Immunisation against infectious disease. HMSO, London

Dolan K, Hall W, Wodak A 1995 Bleach availability and risk behaviour in prison in New South Wales. Technical report No. 22. Sydney National Drug and Alcohol Centre, Sydney

Drobniewski F 1995 Tuberculosis in prison: the forgotten plague. The Lancet 346: 948–949

Gaze H 1997 Hitting the streets. Nursing Times 93(34): 36–37

Goldberg D, Taylor A, McGregor J et al 1998 A lasting public health response to an outbreak of HIV infection in a Scottish prison. International Journal of STD-AIDS Jan. 1998 9(1): 25

Gulland A 1997 The road less travelled. Nursing Times 93(43): 16

Hawes D J 1994 Delivering health and welfare services to gypsies and travellers. (The effectiveness of organisational working; innovative approaches and the impact of the Criminal Justice and Public Order Act.) NHS Executive (South West) School for Policy Studies, University of Bristol, Bristol

Hayward A 1998 Tuberculosis control in London: the need for change. Report for Thames Regional Directors of Public Health. NHS Executive, London

Hennick M 1993 Primary health care needs of travelling people in Wessex. Department of Social Statistics, Southampton University, Southampton

Hudson B 1989 Down, out and neglected. Health Service Journal 99: 334–335

Hutchinson S J, Goldberg D J, Gore S M et al 1998 Hepatitis B outbreak at Glenochil prison during January to June 1993. Epidemiology and Infection 121(1): 185–191

Kenny C 1999 Open house. Nursing Times 95(3): 44–45

Kumar D, Citron K M, Leese J, Watson J M 1995 Tuberculosis amongst the homeless at a temporary shelter in London. A report of a chest X-ray screening programme. Journal of Epidemiology and Community Health 49: 632–633

Levenson R, Coker N 1999 The Health of Refugees, a Guide for GPs. Kings Fund, London

Levy M 1997 Prison health services should be as good as those for the general community. British Medical Journal 315: 1394

Lowry S 1989 An introduction to housing and health. British Medical Journal 299: 1261–1262

Mason P, Adam S 1992 Breaking into prisons. Health Service Journal 16 January

Mathews Z 1998 The outsiders. Nursing Times 94(37): 26

NHS Executive 1999 The future organisation and delivery of prison healthcare. HSC 1999/077. London

Pahl R, Vaille M 1986 Health and Healthcare among Travellers. Health services research unit, University of Kent, Canterbury

Rotily M, Vernay-Vaisse C et al 1997 Three quarters of one French prison needed immunisation against hepatitis B. British Medical Journal 315: 61

Rutter J 1996 We Left Because We Had To, 2nd edn. Refugee Council, London

Taylor A, Goldberg D, Emslie J et al 1995 Outbreak of HIV in a Scottish Prison. British Medical Journal 310: 289–292

World Health Organization/University of Liverpool 1996 Healthy prisons – a vision for the future. Report of first International Conference on Healthy Prisons. WHO/Liverpool University, Department of Public Health, Liverpool

FURTHER READING

Goldberg D, Taylor A, McGregor J et al 1998 A lasting public health response to an outbreak of HIV infection in a Scottish prison. International Journal of STD-AIDS Jan. 1998 9(1): 25

World Health Organization/University of Liverpool 1996 Healthy prisons – a vision for the future. Report of first International Conference on Healthy Prisons. WHO/Liverpool University, Department of Public Health, Liverpool

18

Travel health and immunization

G. Xavier

INTRODUCTION

The recent figures from the Survey of Travel and Tourism show that UK residents made over 46 million foreign visits in 1997, of which over 5 million were to countries outside Western Europe or North America, an increase of 22% from 1995. Imported infections are an emerging public health issue due to the increasing number of people travelling abroad. The increase in travel includes remote areas.

IMPORTED INFECTIONS

The following factors also increase the risk of imported infections:

- Behaviours abroad which increase the risk of infection. Travellers may fail to take precautions against sexually-transmitted diseases, insect bites or food- and water-borne diseases, especially in wilderness-type holidays.
- Vulnerable travellers, who include pregnant women, very young children and the elderly, as well as those with medical problems such as renal failure and immunosuppression.
- Travellers visiting families abroad. Imported infections affect travellers who make extended visits to families overseas, e.g. those staying with families in the Indian sub-continent are at an increased risk of tuberculosis, and those visiting families often fail to protect themselves against malaria.

- Population movement. Infections imported by refugees and asylum seekers (see Chapter 17) will depend on changing global patterns of war and social upheavals around the world.

There is very little surveillance of imported infections. Although existing data may provide an estimate of the impact of certain infections, for most diseases this is likely to be an underestimate. There have been few recent directed studies of travel-associated infection to supplement routine surveillance data. Infection may be categorized as follows:

- Imported infections which are also endemic in England (Communicable Disease Report 1978). In 1977 laboratory reports in England and Wales indicated that at least 3119 cases of salmonella, 1362 cases of campylobacter, 73 cases of dysentery and 108 cases of legionnaires' disease were acquired abroad.
- Imported infections associated with social contact abroad. In 1998 at least 669 cases of tuberculosis occurred in people who had been born abroad and who had lived in England and Wales for under five years. In the same year 648 people (23% of all newly-reported infections) in the UK were reported as having acquired their human immunodeficiency virus infection from heterosexual exposure abroad.
- Exotic imported infections. In 1997, these included 22 364 cases of malaria, 193 of paratyphoid and 93 cases of typhoid infections, 88 cases of schistosomiasis and 33 cases of cholera. Viral haemorrhagic fever (e.g. Ebola and Lassa fever) remains a constant threat. Constant vigilance is required to combat these.
- Importing antimicrobial resistance. Imported infections may be resistant to antibiotics commonly used in this country, e.g. penicillin-resistant gonorrhoea or chloroquine-resistant malaria.
- Outbreaks of infection. Outbreaks of legionnaires' disease and gastrointestinal disease are now reported with increasing frequency amongst British travellers associated with cruise liners and hotels overseas, particularly those offering all-inclusive holidays.

- Modes of transport. Mosquitoes carried on commercial airlines have been responsible for a number of cases of malaria acquired in people living near airports.
- Emerging infections. A number of important infections developed outside the UK and then were imported, e.g. HIV.

ADVICE AND PREVENTION

Pre-travel advice and care is provided by general practitioners, practice nurses, pharmacists and travel agency clinics. Travellers may also obtain specialist advice from manufacturers or from the primary healthcare team, and prevention may include vaccinations, chemoprophylaxis (for example against malaria) or behavioural advice to prevent sexually-transmitted infections, insect bites and water- or food-borne illness.

Good pre-travel advice must be relevant and accurate. It is important for the primary care professional to give a structured travel consultation to ensure that relevant information is conveyed to the traveller. It is important also to remember that most travel-related illnesses are not preventable with vaccines, and that good management advice may well help to avoid or alleviate 95% of travel-induced illness. The most serious health problems arising with travel are not infections but the consequences of underlying chronic disorders such as myocardial ischaemia, chronic pulmonary disease and cerebrovascular disability, as well as trauma sustained on holiday. Travel consultation advice should cover the aspects given in Box 18.1.

Post-travel advice is also significant as people may feel well at the time of return or entry yet fall ill later. This has implications for the NHS staff,

---

Box 18.1 Travel consultation: aspects to cover

- Advice according to destination/type and duration of travel, including immunizations, preventing gastrointestinal illness and malaria prophylaxis where appropriate
- Advice should take into account the mode of travel
- Individual health problems should be taken into account
- Special situations, such as travelling with children

who need to be alert to the possibility of imported infections. Thus, people may seek advice from the primary care team, Environmental Health, or attend Accident and Emergency Departments. If admitted to hospital they may need expert advice from the hospital infection control team.

Prevention of travel-related infections

Although there is national guidance (DoH 1996) on the general principles to be followed for vaccination and chemoprophylaxis, this is often inadequate to meet the demand for up-to-date information on rapidly changing situations (such as floods in Africa, affecting advice on malaria prophylaxis) or for advising those with complex medical problems (immunosuppressed patients receiving multiple therapies). There are no national data on people who receive vaccinations for travel chemoprophylaxis or on the numbers who receive treatment for imported infections.

Most of the risks travellers face are not vaccine-preventable (Dawood 1993). Emphasis should be on the risks posed by lifestyle and climate change.

General precautions

Health problems in travellers are common. The majority of health problems, however, tend to be relatively minor in their long-term implications. The mode of transmission of any infection in travellers emphasizes the need for generic infection control precautions. The following are covered in this section: gastrointestinal (GI) problems, sexually-transmitted disease, and exposure to blood and body fluids during travel.

Gastrointestinal problems

Many people suffer from gastrointestinal problems on holiday, due to exotic foods consumed and change of routine. Travellers' diarrhoea is usually triggered by the consumption of contaminated food and drink. Travellers' diarrhoea refers to the enteric disease acquired when a person travels from one country to another (Dupont and Khan 1994). Symptoms include passing between three and 10 unformed stools daily, usually for between two and five days. It is also often associated with abdominal pain, cramps, fever and vomiting.

Identifying and understanding the organisms responsible for diarrhoea is crucial in developing appropriate treatments and control measures. The organisms concerned differ greatly in their geographic distribution, as well as the frequency and severity of the diseases they cause. In addition, susceptibility to development of travellers' diarrhoea, and its severity, can be influenced by factors including age, especially very young children; reduced gastric acidity; immunodeficiency disorders; and existing conditions with a predisposition to diarrhoea (Farthing 1995).

The commonest organism associated with travellers' diarrhoea is enterotoxigenic *Escherichia coli*, which may be part of the normal bowel flora of the local population. However, a range of bacteria, viruses and parasites are associated with the condition, including Campylobacter, salmonella, Shigella, and, especially in children, rotavirus. The main parasitic cause is *Giardia lamblia*.

Travellers' diarrhoea, typhoid fever, cholera and Hepatitis A can all be acquired by ingesting contaminated food or water. Travellers can reduce the risk of infection by observing the precautions in Box 18.2.

Generally, all foods consumed should be well cooked, freshly prepared and piping hot.

Box 18.2 Precautions against consuming contaminated food or water

---

- Scrupulous hand hygiene, especially after using the toilet and before handling or eating food
- If the local water is not safe to drink it should be boiled before use for drinking, cleaning teeth, washing salads or making ice cubes
- If a water purifying system is used, the manufacturers' instructions should be followed carefully. It is also advisable to purify only tap water
- If bottled water is consumed it should be from a commercial producer and the cap should be checked to ensure it is properly sealed

Sexually-transmitted disease and travel

HIV and other sexually-transmitted infections are prevalent worldwide. Therefore, random sexual encounters run a high risk of infection with blood-borne viruses and other sexually-transmitted diseases. Gonorrhoea and syphilis may cause serious long-term disability, especially if treatment is delayed. Travellers should be given the following advice:

- Casual sexual intercourse is risky; condoms provide good but not complete protection.
- Drug taking might put the traveller in contact with people who are HIV-positive or have Hepatitis, and should be avoided.
- Needle sharing should be avoided.

Exposure to blood and body fluids during travel

There is also a risk of infection through blood transfusion or by infected instruments used by dentists, chiropodists or tattooists abroad. In most developing countries, blood may not be screened. The risks from blood transfusion in such circumstances are high. Accidents are the commonest reason for needing a blood transfusion. Travellers should be given the following advice:

- Extreme care should be taken when driving on holiday.
- Unless sterility of equipment is guaranteed, skin-damaging procedures such as earpiercing, tattooing and acupuncture should be avoided.
- Travellers to high-risk areas should be advised to carry a sterile equipment pack (containing hypodermic needles and transfusion kits) with them for emergency medical use.

Management of travellers' diarrhoea by the primary care team

Travellers should be advised to go prepared with commercial sachets of replacement sugar and salt, which can be made up with freshly boiled or bottled water if needed. Travellers' diarrhoea is usually a mild disease, though severe fluid and electrolyte disturbance can occur.

A careful history is essential for correct diagnosis and management of travellers' diarrhoea. This should include a travel history; the time elapsed since returning to the UK; and the duration of the diarrhoea. Travellers' diarrhoea usually occurs during travel or very shortly after returning home. The longer the history, the more likely it will be a parasitic cause than a bacterial and viral cause. Malaria also can sometimes present as a diarrhoeal illness.

The travel information should be included in the laboratory request form accompanying stool culture and microscopy.

Management of prophylaxis against malaria by the primary care team

There is no malaria vaccine at present. However, travellers and primary care professionals need to be aware of malaria risk during the planned visit both to select appropriate preventative measures and to ensure prompt medical intervention if malaria occurs in spite of precautions. There have been reported deaths from malaria and these deaths are preventable (Bradley and Warhurst 1977). Most cases occur in those who have failed to take, or comply with, malaria prophylaxis. At particular risk are settled migrants returning to visit relatives abroad; they are often unaware that any natural immunity gained during residence in an endemic area rapidly falls on leaving it.

Many warm climate countries are endemic for malaria and thus pose some risk to travellers. The level of risk may vary enormously between countries, and this will affect the type of prophylaxis recommended. Appropriate chemoprophylaxis combined with prudent behaviour can greatly reduce the risk. Health professionals advising travellers on malaria prophylaxis should be able to offer accurate advice for individual countries, and areas within those countries. The general advice regarding malaria prevention is that:

- Appropriate chemoprophylaxis should be taken. If the drug(s) first recommended cause adverse effects, an alternative should be considered.
- Compliance with chemoprophylaxis is **essential**.

- Any flu-like illness occurring up to one year post-travel should be considered as possibly malaria.
- In addition health professionals also should advise on the use of mosquito repellents and mosquito nets when travelling to malarial regions.

IMMUNIZATION FOR OVERSEAS TRAVEL

Recent developments

Two major changes in travel immunization practice have occurred in recent years. The first has been the reduction in the requirements for international certificates of vaccination – yellow fever is now the only disease for which an international vaccination certificate may be required for entry into a country. The second is the proven range and acceptability of vaccines.

The International Health Regulations (DoH 1995) adopted by the World Health Assembly in 1969 were devised and regularly reviewed to help prevent the international spread of disease and, in the context of international travel, to do so with the minimum of inconvenience to the passenger. However, the regulations are more a public health measure for the receiving country than for the protection of the individual traveller.

Over recent years the emphasis has begun to change and immunization is seen as only part of health advice for travellers. When choosing travel vaccines, the primary care team should assess the disease risk. Some risks may be seasonal, or limited to certain geographical areas, and personal lifestyle or occupation influences the choice.

Immunization schedules for travel

Wherever possible, the recommended intervals between doses and between vaccines should be followed and time allowed for antibody to be produced. In theory, each travel vaccine should be given at least three weeks from another in order to identify the source of any reaction to the vaccine. Live vaccines for travel should be administered at least three weeks apart or on the same day.

However, the two oral vaccines, typhoid and polio, are usually separated by at least two weeks on the theoretical grounds of possible interference in the gut. Live virus vaccines may suppress the tuberculin test and so should be delayed until after the test has been read.

Boxes 18.3 and 18.4 list live and inactivated vaccines.

Inactivated vaccines can be given with any other vaccine, but at a different site. The number given should take into account the comfort of the patient. Courses for most travel vaccines, plus the single dose vaccines, can be administered over a four-week period. The final doses should ideally be completed a little ahead of the departure date to allow immunity to develop. It can take up to four weeks, for instance, for full immunity to develop following Japanese encephalitis vaccine.

More time will be required if a primary course of tetanus, polio or diphtheria is necessary. If the full course cannot be completed before departure, it may be advisable to give the maximum number of doses that the travel departure date allows, completing the course on return.

Box 18.3   Vaccines: live

Measles, Mumps, Rubella and MMR
Oral poliomyelitis
Oral typhoid
BCG (TB)
Yellow fever

Box 18.4   Vaccines: inactivated

Diphtheria toxoid. Tetanus toxoid, Pertussis and combination vaccines
Poliomyelitis (injectable)
Haemophilus influenzae b (Hib)
Influenza
Hepatitis A
Typhoid injectable
Meningococcal vaccine
Japanese encephalitis
Tick-borne encephalitis
Hepatitis B
Rabies
Cholera

SPECIFIC VACCINATIONS FOR TRAVEL

The following vaccines are discussed in detail:

- Hepatitis B
- Hepatitis A
- Typhoid
- Japanese encephalitis
- Meningitis A and C
- Rabies
- Tick-borne encephalitis
- Yellow fever.

Hepatitis B

The World Health Organization has recommended that all countries should include Hepatitis B as part of their childhood immunization programme. At the present time, in the UK Hepatitis B is not offered to infants or adolescents. A selective vaccination policy targets specific at-risk groups. These include:

- healthcare workers
- people with haemophilia
- injecting drug misusers
- practising homosexuals
- people in institutional care, especially those with learning disabilities
- sexual partners of chronic carriers
- babies born to chronic carriers.

This policy does not take into account the vast increase in international travel that has been seen in recent years. However, the Hepatitis B vaccine is recommended for people travelling to areas of high prevalence who intend to seek employment, or those who intend to remain for more than one month.

A second dose should be given one month after the first, while the third dose is given six months after the first dose. An accelerated course may be offered, with the third dose given two months after the initial dose with a booster at 12 months.

Hepatitis A

Hepatitis A infection occurs worldwide but the risk of disease varies widely. All travellers to moderate and high-risk areas should be vaccinated for Hepatitis A. The regimen for people over 16 years is a single dose of Hepatitis A vaccine. This will produce an antibody response persisting for at least one year; offering a booster 6–12 months after the initial dose will give immunity for up to 10 years. Children under 10 years of age tend to develop asymptomatic or very mild disease and gain life-long immunity, therefore Hepatitis A vaccination is not always considered a priority for their personal protection. However, they may excrete the virus and give rise to secondary cases in adults when they return home, and from a public health point of view, the primary care team should consider vaccination.

Some travellers may have immunity to Hepatitis A and, if time allows, it is useful to test for antibody levels in those who have a previous history of jaundice.

Typhoid

Vaccination is recommended for countries where sanitation and hygiene may be poor. This vaccine is not 100% effective; therefore general advice about personal, food and water hygiene should be re-emphasized.

Vi polysaccharide vaccine should be administered in a single intra-muscular injection, with a booster dose every three years for those who remain at risk of infection. Oral Ty 21a vaccine should be administered as a single capsule on alternate days for three days, taken on an empty stomach with a cool drink. The vaccine must be stored in the refrigerator between doses.

Japanese encephalitis

This vaccination is recommended to travellers staying more than one month in South East Asia and the Far East in rural areas where rice growing and pig farming co-exist. The peak season is generally towards the end of the Monsoon season.

Meningococcal A and C

A single dose of the plain polysaccharide A and C immunization is recommended for visitors such as backpackers, people likely to be living in close contact with local populations in sub-Saharan Africa, the area around Delhi, Nepal, Bhutan and Pakistan. It is also recommended for those travelling to Saudi Arabia for the Haj pilgrimage.

Meningococcal A and C should be offered under these circumstances regardless of previous meningococcal C conjugate. Ideally a two-week period should elapse between the meningococcal C conjugate and meningococcal meningitis A and C.

Rabies

Humans may contract rabies from any rabid animal, domestic or wild, but the common cause of human rabies world-wide is the bite of a rabid domestic dog, which may itself have contracted the virus from another dog or cat or from a rabid wild animal. Rabies occurs in most parts of the world, including the main tropical regions. Travellers within rabies-endemic areas should avoid contact with domestic or wild mammals. They should be particularly wary of wild animals that appear tame, for this change in behaviour is a common early sign of rabies in animals.

Rabies vaccination is recommended for those either living or travelling in enzootic areas where they may be exposed. A three-dose course of rabies vaccine on days 0, 7 and 28 is recommended. Travellers planning to spend long periods in remote areas where medical treatment may not be immediately available should be considered for rabies vaccination.

Tick-borne encephalitis

Areas of highest incidence are those where humans have intimate association with large numbers of infected ticks, generally in rural or forested areas, but also in some urban populations. Advice should also be given about covering arms, legs and ankles and the use of insect repellents on outer clothing and socks. Two doses given at a 4–12 week interval will give protection for one year to travellers walking, camping or working in these areas.

Yellow fever

A single dose of vaccine offers 10 years' protection for travellers through or living in infected areas of the world. Many of these countries require an International Certificate of Vaccination for entry into them. As yellow fever is a live attenuated vaccine, consideration should be given if other live vaccines are required. These should either be administered on the same day at different sites, or with a three-week interval between the vaccines. However, this does not apply if polio vaccine is also needed (Moreton 2000).

THE RETURNING TRAVELLER

Primary care professionals should also be prepared to deal with travellers returning from abroad. Patients should be advised that if they feel unwell, particularly with fever, headaches, muscle pain, lethargy and general malaise, it might be wise to have a further check-up in the travel clinic. Such symptoms in patients returning from malarial areas should prompt the suspicion of malaria, and blood should be taken immediately and checked for possible infection. Other blood disorders may take longer to present themselves and may require fuller blood investigation with liver function tests. A post-travel questionnaire is a useful tool to assess the extent of the problem (see Fig. 18.1 for a sample of a post-travel audit questionnaire).

Management of those returning with symptoms depends on the nature of the problem, but many tropical diseases are best handled by a specialized tropical diseases unit where the necessary further investigations can be done and where there is access to a laboratory familiar with the tests involved.

Public health risks can arise from travellers returning with illness, who may infect family members and work or school colleagues. Food-handlers, children and some healthcare workers may have to be excluded until they are clear of infection. In suspected food poisoning or dysentery, stool specimens will be required for laboratory investigation.

Post-Travel Audit Questionnaire

Now that you have just returned from abroad, please complete this questionnaire
and send it to us in the SAE supplied. THANK YOU.

PLEASE PUT A TICK IN THE CORRECT BOX

A   SEX: ☐ MALE   ☐ FEMALE   **B**   YEAR OF BIRTH   19___

C   In which country did you spend the most time? _____

D   Which vaccinations did you receive recently at our clinic?

☐ TETANUS   ☐ POLIO   ☐ TYPHOID   ☐ HEPATITIS
☐ CHOLERA   ☐ OTHER

E   Did you obtain pre-travel health advice?   ☐ YES   ☐ NO
If **yes**, was this from:

☐ DOCTOR   ☐ TRAVEL AGENT
☐ OTHER? (Specify) _____

F   Was this advice   ☐ USEFUL   ☐ NOT VERY USEFUL   ☐ NO HELP?

G   Did you carry medicine with you?   ☐ YES   ☐ NO
If **yes**, was this:

☐ ANTI-MALARIAL TABS?   ☐ ANTIBIOTICS?
☐ ANTI-SICKNESS TABS?   ☐ ANTI-DIARRHOEA TABS?
☐ OTHER? (Specify) _____

H   Did you become ill during travel/stay abroad?   ☐ YES   ☐ NO

I   Did this affect your:
☐ STOMACH & INTESTINES?   ☐ HEART?
☐ CHEST & BREATHING?   ☐ KIDNEYS?
☐ OTHER? (Specify) _____

J   Did the illness:
☐ GET BETTER WITHOUT TREATMENT?
☐ GET BETTER WITH THE REMEDIES YOU HAD WITH YOU?
☐ REQUIRE TREATMENT FROM A DOCTOR ABROAD?
☐ REQUIRE HOSPITAL ADMISSION ABROAD?
☐ REQUIRE ATTENTION OF YOUR GP ON RETURN HOME?

K   Did you have travel insurance cover?   ☐ YES   ☐ NO
If **yes**, did this cover pre-existing illness?   ☐ YES   ☐ NO   ☐ DON'T KNOW

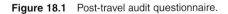

Figure 18.1   Post-travel audit questionnaire.

CONCLUSION

Effective prevention and control of imported infections require an evidence-based risk assessment approach to ensure effective use of NHS resources. The primary care professionals should make every effort:

- to improve the public understanding of the risk factors and trends for imported infections
- to understand the potential threat to public health from imported infections
- to monitor the effectiveness of prevention activities including immunization, chemoprophylaxis and behavioural advice

- to ensure that people with imported infections receive a high standard of primary and secondary care with access to specialist advice when appropriate.

A full understanding of imported infections, their impact, trends and risk factors, needs partnership working between several professional groups including public health professionals, microbiologists, clinicians, occupational health, environmental health and the travel industry.

The emerging public health issue should also be part of the training for public health/community infection control nurses.

REFERENCES

Bartlett C 1999 Prevention and control of imported infections. Unpublished paper for Communicable Disease Strategy Group for Department of Health

Bradley D J, Warhurst D C 1977 Guidelines for the prevention of malaria in travellers from the United Kingdom. CDR Review R137–152

Dawood R 1993 Preparation for travel. British Medical Bulletin 49: 269–284

Department of Health 1995 Health information for overseas travel. HMSO, London

Department of Health 1996 Immunisation against infectious disease. HMSO, London

Dupont H, Khan F 1994 Travellers' diarrhoea; epidemiology, microbiology, prevention and therapy. Journal of Travel Medicine 1(2): 84–92

Farthing M 1995 Travellers' diarrhoea. Gut 35: 1–4

Moreton J 2000 Adolescent and adult immunisation. Overview. Nursing Times 96: 45–46

Office for National Statistics 1996 Travel Trends. HMSO, London

Public Health Laboratory Service 1978 Guideline for the prevention of malaria in travellers from the United Kingdom. CDR Review. PHLS, London

Reed Healthcare Communications 1995 Travel Clinics Manual. Immunisation in General Practice series, Vol. 1. Reed Healthcare Communications, London

19

Documentation and infection control

A. Fuller

INTRODUCTION

As professionals we have an individual responsibility to ensure that we maintain accurate documentation of our actions (UKCC Code of Professional Conduct 1992). The important activity of making and keeping records is an essential and integral part of care. It is a tool of professional practice, and one which should support the care process. Record keeping is not an optional extra to be conducted when circumstances allow.

Records are any permanent form of information recorded about a patient, client, or situation. All records should be regarded as potential legal documents. Consequently, a patient's record of healthcare can provide the most reliable evidence of care or action which has taken place.

To meet legal requirements for documentation and record keeping it is important that written work not only fulfils the UKCC requirements, but reflects current evidence to establish the planning of patient and client care. Furthermore, it provides the structure within which to monitor and evaluate an incident such as an outbreak of infection, and provides documented evidence to support:

- clinical management
- resource management
- self-evaluation
- audit performance
- quality assurance
- research (NHS Training Directorate 1994).

WHY DO WE NEED DOCUMENTATION?

Record keeping is a method which protects the welfare of the patient and client by providing:

- an account in which to evaluate whether patients are being provided with an optimal standard of care
- a foundation on which to assist staff in making new diagnoses, influence treatment, and observe daily progress
- continuity of care
- a basis on which to conduct reflective practice
- the primary source for reference and communication amongst members of the healthcare team
- the written evidence of treatment, care planning and the delivery of that care
- the ability to detect problems at an early stage
- evidence that a service has been delivered, by demonstrating the chronology of events
- the support for standard setting, quality assessment and audit (UKCC 1998).

It is therefore essential that we adopt systematic approaches to documentation, as keeping clear, comprehensive records is part of the duty of care owed to the client. The quality of documentation is paramount, but unfortunately one which is considered by many to be time-consuming. Coldwell and Page (1996) highlight the serious consequences of not documenting accurately and draw attention to the effects this has upon the organization, patients and the individual practitioner.

The approach to record keeping adopted by the law courts is supported by the opinion of Hershey and Lawrence (1986), 'If it is not recorded then you did not do it.' However, Payne (1995) argues that the quality of the document does not always reflect the quality of care delivered. Documentation may not necessarily reflect that the care or procedure was actually delivered, but does indicate that an element of care was omitted. Accurate recording is also important owing to the reliance placed upon patients' records by colleagues or other healthcare workers (see Box 19.1).

To ensure that documentation is accurate and complete, it may be necessary to include the patient's or client's own description of their

---

Box 19.1 Practice Point

In a residential home, a patient develops a rash which is considered to be a reaction to soap. However, there is no further update on the progression of the rash. Three further patients then develop similar symptoms. A diagnosis of scabies is made, and the whole residential home must now be treated. By reviewing the documentation, a situation could have been averted or at least monitored. Good communication is therefore essential.

---

problem. In such cases, quote the patient whenever possible, including refusal of or non-compliance with treatment and education sessions. Documentation must be completed in line with current policy; it is not something to be conducted in isolation (Sullivan 2000).

Litigation

Litigation is a process which has become an inherent part of the new NHS. Meiner (1999) highlights the risk of liability for all healthcare workers, citing a more informed public, changing attitudes towards healthcare service providers and the rapid turnover within healthcare systems for the rising incidence of litigation.

The NHS Training Directorate's manual on record keeping (1994) states that there has been a dramatic increase in the number of legal and professional cases which have involved poor record keeping.

High standards and the keeping of records are of paramount importance. Complaints and legal actions are very difficult to defend where records of the salient events are imprecise, inaccurate or incomplete (Coldwell and Page 1996), even when the healthcare worker believes them to be clear in the detail of the care or decision that has been delivered.

As described by Mandelstam (1998), poor record keeping might make it difficult for the local authority to demonstrate that it has carried out a community care assessment correctly or at all. The Goldsack case (1996) enabled the judge presiding to identify that:

The assessment of needs and the decisions taken about the need for arrangements to provide for them were not formally recorded. There was apparent doubt as to whether the assessment had in fact been conducted at all.

The first step in any clinical negligence case is for a complete set of records to be sent to the plaintiff and statements exchanged on the sequence of events. To prepare for this, it is necessary that a review of the records be undertaken together with a consideration of any relevant clinical guidelines and protocols (Peysner 1998). An example would be the use of the local Infection Control Policy.

Following examination of such documents, an individual may be required to appear as a witness or defendant in a court of law, and if found negligent, to be investigated by their professional bodies. Failure to keep accurate records or to report an incident resulted in the UKCC Professional Conduct Council hearing 455 practice-related issues from April 1997 to March 1998, 19 of which were proven cases leading to a caution or removal from the register (UKCC 1998).

The Health Service Commissioners' Annual Report 1992–1993 (Audit Commission 1995) identified that careful attention to record keeping is not just a matter of good practice but is integral to the delivery and continuity of good care. It is insurance for a member of staff who may later be accused of negligence. However, the report goes on to highlight that case records are often incomplete or lacking in essential detail, including an absence of a record of communication with relatives or carers and subsequent discharge arrangements.

A report (NHS Executive 2000) of an expert group on learning from adverse events in the NHS made ten recommendations. These recommendations were aimed at addressing problems and identifying weaknesses. The report states that 'reporting systems are vital in providing a core of sound representative information on which to base analysis and recommendations'. Documentation is part of representative information.

TYPES OF RECORD KEEPING

Within the sphere of infection control there are many ways in which to record specific details, all of which are subject to local requirements. They are defined as either manually-held records or hard copy computer-held records. The majority of records continue to be manually-held within the community setting.

Patient-held records

Healthcare professionals have recognized the value of patients keeping their own records (Fig. 19.1). Community nurses have used the system of leaving the record of their visit at the patient's house, thus facilitating continuity of care and dialogue between the patient and healthcare provider. Patients and clients are encouraged to become involved in their own care and establish themselves as the owner of their own record. This, in essence, enables the client to be involved in their own care and share the information considered relevant to the assessment and associated care.

Most patients in the community will have a care plan and accompanying notes, which include risk assessment documents. In many cases, there will be a separate set of medical notes at the client's general practice which are not disclosed to the patient. These notes often involve referrals, for example to non-statutory specialists, social workers and housing, all of which generate independent notes. In turn, healthcare professionals will write to each other to keep up-to-date on the patient's progress.

Community nurses need to be aware that the records kept in the patient's home contain all the relevant information. However, the nurse who is required by their employer to keep a set of notes centrally should ensure that these are completed as contemporaneously with current events as possible (Dimond 1997). Loss or damage of records generally occurs when records are kept in the medical records department (Audit Commission 1995) Should they be lost or damaged, a new record needs to be created utilizing information available. However, Dimond (2000) states that should the patient deliberately destroy the record to bring about legal action against the Trust, the burden rests upon the claimant to establish that there has been negligence. Loss of a record would

Care plan

Patient name	
Date	

Nursing Problem/Diagnosis	Pretibial laceration to left leg following a fall in the garden this morning Grade 3 wound measuring 3 cm x 1 cm

Objective	To promote healing

Nursing action		Date and time	Evaluation	Signature
• Assess and map wound • Cleanse using warm sterile saline • Apply iodine-based dressing • Cover with non-adherent dressing and secure with non-allergenic tape (dressing daily) • Advise to elevate leg when sitting • Advise a well-balanced diet • Liaise with general practitioner regarding tetanus status • Advise to contact district nurse/GP should any problems arise (telephone numbers given)		4.6.01 10:40 a.m. 8.6.01 11:20 a.m. 11.6.01 11:50 a.m. 15.6.01 10:30 a.m.	Discussed tetanus status with GP. Booster was given 19.3.98. Wound deterioration noted. Foul smell from wound and pus present. Clinical signs of infection present. Wound swab taken for culture. Swab result demonstrated *Staphylococcus aureus*. Systemic antibiotics commenced. Dressing regime not altered. Wound much improved. Antibiotic course still in progress. Review again in three days.	*B. Bell* *B. Bell* *C. White* *B. Bell*

Assessor's name	
Client agreement to plan of care	

Figure 19.1 Patient-held care plan.

disadvantage the claimant, especially if they were in possession of the record.

Information technology and computer-held records

Information technology has enabled many disciplines to record information, and nursing is no exception. Advantages of using computer-held records include ease of reading by standardizing the content, format and language. These reduce the need for duplication and increase communication across the inter-professional healthcare team (UKCC 1998). The NHS Information Strategy (NHSE 1998) makes a clear commitment to providing lifelong electronic health records for every person in the country. Initially work is being undertaken to develop and implement a first generation of person-based electronic health records, which will provide the basis of lifelong core clinical information with electronic transfer of patient records between general practitioners.

Some district nurses use hand-held computers to record daily information which is subsequently transferred to a central system.

Research and teaching

Patient and client records can be made accessible for use as teaching aids and research. The principles of access and confidentiality apply. However, should a patient/client refuse, then their request must be respected.

All research must be formally directed through the local research ethics committee of a Trust if patient or client records require accessing.

ACCESS TO HEALTH RECORDS

Legislation has provided the individual with a statutory right of access to health records held either in manual form or on computer. The statutory provision for access to health records is categorized into three main areas:

- Data Protection Act 1998
- Access to Medical Reports Act 1988
- Access to Health Records Act 1990.

The Data Protection Act (1998) safeguards the individual. All information is collated for the purpose for which it is intended and the appropriate security measures are taken against unauthorized access to, disclosure of, destruction and alteration of data.

The Medical Report Act (1988) allows an individual access to any medical report issued by a doctor relating to another individual, such as confirmation of health status for employment or insurance purposes. The medical practitioner, however, is not bound to disclose information that in their opinion would cause physical and psychological harm to their client.

The Access to Health Records Act (1990) allowed for the removal of the irregularity whereby the individual had a statutory right of access to their health records when in automated form but not those held in manual form. A health record as defined by Dimond (1997) under the 1990 Act is one which:

- consists of information relating to the physical or mental health of an individual who can be identified from that and other information in the possession of the record
- has been made by or on behalf of a healthcare professional in connection with the care of that individual.

This Act only covers records that are not held in automated form, but prevents overlap between Access to Health Records Act (1990) and the Data Protection Act (1998). Considering that the majority of records held within the community are still held in manual form, the Access to Health Records Act (1990) appears to be the most relevant.

The withholding of information by a registered nurse, midwife or health visitor from a patient or client is in some cases acceptable. This is provided they believe it could cause serious harm to the physical or mental health of the patient or client, or has the potential to breach the confidentiality of another patient or client. If the decision to withhold information is taken, then it must be justified and documented (UKCC 1998). For example, a pregnant woman does not wish her partner to know that she has suffered from a previous sexually-transmitted disease.

OWNERSHIP AND PRESERVATION OF RECORDS

Ownership

NHS-owned records are the property of the statutory authority where the professional was working at the time that they were made. Therefore the Secretary of State, in the case of hospital or community health, delegates control to Health Authorities and NHS Trust boards. Records produced by a general practitioner are the property of the Health Authority and are returned to them should the patient die or be transferred to another practice. This system will at present continue despite implementation of Primary Care Trusts. Those records created following a private visit to the GP, however, are then owned by the practitioner (Dimond 1995). Security, custody and control of the records are the responsibility of the owner and secure storage is in line with the duty of confidentiality (DoH 2001a).

Preservation

Adult health records must be kept for 8 years and those of children and obstetric patients for 25 years. Included within the 8 years are documents pertinent to the management of both patients and the organization. These include local policies, guidelines and teaching aims and objectives, all of which reflect the educational content, evidence base and subsequent adherence to local policy.

QUALITY ASSURANCE OF RECORDS

There are a number of factors that contribute to effective record keeping. The UKCC (1998) clearly sets out the essential elements – documentation should be:

- factual, consistent and accurate
- written as soon as possible after an event has occurred, providing current information on the care and condition of the patient and client
- written legibly and indelibly, signing, dating and timing each entry
- altered if necessary by scoring out with a single line initialled, dated and timed correctly

- updated with the use of dated, timed and signed entries
- exclusive of abbreviation, meaningless phrases and offensive subjective statements
- readable on any photocopies, e.g. in black ink
- written in partnership, where possible (patient-held records), phrased in a manner conclusive to patient/client understanding
- consecutive, and identify problems and any associated actions taken.

Written documentation is required to be factual, providing objective, theoretical information, and does not allow for assumptions or interpretations. The report details must all be relevant, using terms that are common and recognizable to other healthcare workers. Handwriting must be legible with correct spelling and descriptions, which ensures that the report is accurate and that mistakes are preventable. Mistakes or omissions need to be identified within the text. Mistakes should not be erased but identified by a line through the incorrect statement whilst omissions are best added where appropriate or at the bottom of the narrative. The recorded facts are required to describe the relevant situation, including explanations of diversity or changed care planning.

All records must be complete and supported by an accurate date and time of entry and a signature. A healthcare professional responsible for recording, reporting and documentation of information and capable of explaining his/her motives for activity and judgement is considered to be responsible and accountable (Bergman 1981).

During a workshop held for community psychiatric nurses, Dimond (1997) highlights their experiences and delivers essential information on which to question our own practice of record keeping:

- failure to include dates and times
- illegible writing
- use of ambiguous abbreviations
- failure to document caller following a telephone call
- omission of signature
- inaccurate dates and client information
- delays in record keeping up to 24 hours later

- allowing another person to complete the records
- inaccurate patient details including date of birth and address
- unprofessional, ambiguous phrases
- subjective rather than objective assessment.

Applying the above principles to infection control, it is possible to devise a checklist for documentation.

Documentation: checklist

- Is the document legible without concealed errors?
- Is the information concurrent? (e.g. a patient starts with loose stools but there is failure to indicate any further episodes until the following day)
- Are dates and times included (essential to determine incident and outbreak problems)?
- Does the intervention allow for the client/patient to respond (e.g. psychological evaluation following isolation precautions)?
- Has reassuring information been included (use of patient information leaflets, dialogue documented with family member, microbiological results, etc.)?
- Does the information state that infection control input was sought?
- Is a general risk assessment conducted and evaluated (e.g. for drugs, invasive device, underlying illness, etc.)?
- Are there any inappropriate terms? For example abbreviations such as VRE (vancomycin-resistant enterococcus)?
- Is full information included of ward transfers, discharge and admission dates, e.g. from and to hospital, nursing or residential home?
- Are full discharge planning details present, e.g. wound infection and management, other infections, clinical waste collection from the home environment?

PROTOCOL/GUIDELINES

The use of written guidance has a vital role within healthcare practice. The purpose of a

protocol or guideline is to provide a document based on evidence and best practice to perform the particular procedure. Standardizing procedures serves to provide continuity, thus supporting the objective of consistently high standards of care.

According to Elliot Pennels (1997), protocols need to:

- be detailed written documents
- be relevant and designed specifically for the clinical environment where they will be used
- be updated at least annually
- provide clinically relevant information on indications for use
- prioritize patient safety as paramount concern
- ensure relevant skill and knowledge of all involved in using the protocol.

Protocols have more legal connotations as they are meant to be followed exactly through the stages. Consequently there is little allowance for the individual practitioner to display clinical freedom or professional judgement.

Best practice guidelines are defined by Wilson (1996) as the 'systematically developed statements which assist clinicians and patients in making decisions about appropriate treatment of specific conditions'. These are regarded legally in the same way as patient records but are generally used by a defence to show a controlled environment of care. It is important to maintain these documents as they reflect the evidence at that point in time to support current practice. Concurrently they support documented statements highlighting any deviation of care which may follow risk assessment.

AUDITING OF DOCUMENTATION

Auditing existing records establishes whether expected standards have been met, identifies areas for improvement, and highlights any staff development needs. Standards evaluate actual practice. Quality of care delivered can be achieved by marrying clinical judgement with clear national standards.

'Essence of care' (DoH 2001b) introduces bench marking for record keeping. This practical tool kit for nurses and others highlights that there is an overall lack of understanding of components that make up informed infection control care. This is supported by Finn (1997) who concluded from a small study that infection control advice was not being documented by nurses.

Not only is it necessary to audit the content of documentation, but general audit allows the infection control team an opportunity to assess resources and identify strengths and weaknesses of that area and make recommendations for change via detailed reports.

The Audit Commission Report (1995) identified a wide catalogue of record-keeping failings, regarding record keeping to be in general disorganized, poorly structured, illegible, overcrowded and sometimes missing. This original report, and other influential factors, created an agenda in which to review and improve hospital record keeping and focus on improving the quality of what might be described as the fundamental and essential aspects of care. This structured approach allows for sharing and comparing practice in order to identify the best, and subsequent action plans to enhance and correct poor practice. Now that Community Trusts are restructuring to Primary Care Trusts, all aspects of record keeping and audit remain applicable to this environment also.

A follow-up survey conducted by the Audit Commission showed a significant improvement in four years. There was an overall increase in the quality of record keeping: 17 standards were used as an audit tool and overall compliance with these had risen from 78% in 1994/95 to 86% in 1998/99 (Audit Commission 1999).

WHY IS DOCUMENTATION IMPORTANT IN INFECTION CONTROL?

Record keeping enables the Infection Control Nurse Practitioner not only to work through other staff when assessing the chain of events leading to an outbreak, but also to assist in the planning of the most appropriate care for that patient. Furthermore, it allows other healthcare workers the opportunity to assess and evaluate

---

Box 19.2 Documentation points for risk assessment

- Indicate risk assessment, e.g. medication, mobility, underlying illness
- Invasive devices, e.g. urinary catheter, gastrostomy tube
- Change in client's status, e.g. pyrexia, diarrhoea, itching, changes in skin
- Outings, family providing food
- Existing infection or discharges from hospital with infection, e.g. MRSA
- Existing wounds and current treatment
- Information relayed to the patient/family/carer
- Inclusion of existing precautions
- Specimens sent, including date and microbiological examination requested
- Recent travel abroad
- Is the patient immunocompromised?

---

through risk assessment. This can highlight any potential or identified factors that have environmental and cross infection implications (see Box 19.2).

Record keeping identifies strengths and weaknesses within the care and organizational setting. It further identifies the implementation of policies and procedures, communication within multi-disciplinary settings and utilization of current literature and necessary staff training.

Risk management essentially is a process that allows a risk attached to a task or procedure to be identified and management strategies developed to minimize harm. Careful care planning using practical risk assessment documentation provides the tools for appropriate information which raises awareness and highlights the importance of the risks to patients, clients and staff by transferring the information results to written guidance within the care notes (Kingsley 1992, Bowell 1992).

DOCUMENTATION FOLLOWING AN INCIDENT

All reported incidents are monitored through the process of risk management. Once identified, incidents require prompt action, evaluation and an outcome. Incidents are often isolated but may be part of a broader picture. For example, a single

---

Box 19.3 Practice Point 1

Situation
A school nurse is involved with school immunizations, in this instance BCG. The nurse has a room of limited space, but has the necessary equipment to conduct the procedure. A sharps box is close at hand. Unfortunately, at the point following inoculation the child becomes distressed and violently moves her arm. The nurse subsequently sustains a needlestick injury.

Action plan
Adhering to local needlestick/sharps policy what **documentation** is required following this incident?

- Document immediate action, i.e. first aid carried out.
- As soon as possible complete accident form, ensuring no omissions. This should include accurate date and time and be signed.
- Seek medical advice; are risk factors identified, e.g. ethnicity, immigration?
- Document report to line manager (include name).
- Document any consent required to take blood.
- Document if consent is refused by carer/parent, including names, date, time.
- Has the child any known potential exposure to blood-borne illness?
- Ensure the record is sent to appropriate person and retain a copy.

---

needlestick injury may be an isolated incident but through critical review and appraisal identifies a series of similar episodes within the same area. Therefore, documentation is essential as an audit tool but also fulfils health and safety legislation (Health and Safety Commission 1995, 1999a and b; see also Box 19.3).

DOCUMENTATION OF AN OUTBREAK

An outbreak is defined (Horton & Parker 1997) as two or more cases of infection occurring around the same time in residents or carers, or where there is an increase in the number normally observed. It is important to identify potential outbreaks promptly and for control measures to be implemented as soon as possible (see Box 19.4). Therefore, it is important that the local outbreak policy is available to staff (who are aware of its existence) and that there are clear lines of communication with the infection control team.

Box 19.4 Practice Point 2

Situation
A nursing home identifies two residents with diarrhoea and a third resident with one episode of vomiting. When a further four residents begin vomiting the matron realizes that they have a problem. Contact is made with the community infection control team, who make a prompt initial visit.

What **documentation** is necessary to enable an accurate assessment and action plan?

- What information from the symptomatic residents' notes is necessary?
- Who else may be involved?
- How would you collate the information?
- What obstacles may create problems in collating the information?
- How would you disseminate the information and to whom?

Central documentation is essential to establish a clear picture of events. These include date, times and names, symptoms of the individuals and the date of specimens sent. Such information provides clarity and is best presented in a list form (Fig. 19.2). Using such a list enables a chronological presentation of the information.

Problems often occur when there is sparse, inconsistent information or no mention of the individual's symptoms within the case notes. It is therefore important that observation is transferred to the written document as symptoms occur, or as soon as is possible – e.g. frequency and description of symptoms. This contemporaneous documentation should also have a date and time to indicate when the entry was made. Memories fail over time and therefore this type of entry has greater weight in evidence than an entry made later. There must be consecutive and objective accounts for each affected individual. In addition, any staff who present with symptoms need to be included within the overall collated list. This provides an indication of inevitable organizational issues, e.g. staffing levels. Not only residential staff need to be accounted for but also any other nursing or support agencies that may have been involved.

Where advice has been sought, e.g. from Infection Control Nurse, General Practitioner, Consultant for Communicable Disease Control, Environmental Health Officer, etc., document that contact has been made, including date, time and contact details (Fig. 19.3). The information collated provides the baseline of an outbreak plan and demonstrates a responsible, professional attitude utilizing a risk management approach to the identified problem.

An action plan should be developed recording all relevant information. When informing relatives and visitors of an outbreak, a polite notice can be used (Fig. 19.4). This prevents anxiety and allows the person in charge to explain the situation.

DATE	NAME	AGE	DEPT/WARD	STAFF/RESIDENT	SYMPTOMS	ONSET	GP	SPECIMEN	RESULT	COMMENTS

Figure 19.2 Documentation necessary to establish an accurate assessment and action plan.

Greengrass Nursing Home Communication/Information Sheet

Date	Issue	Action	Signature
2.6.01	Seven residents with diarrhoea and/or vomiting	Reported to the community infection control nurse and general practitioners for the clients	
2.6.01	Advised by the infection control team to close the home to activities (i.e. no admissions, discharges or transfers until advised by the infection control team)	• Relatives of clients informed • Staff advised of the infection control guidelines for the duration of the outbreak • Record all client symptoms on individual nursing notes • Cancel tea party for 4.6.01 • Inform podiatry to cancel visits during course of the outbreak	
3.6.01	Client admitted to Grays hospital as an emergency, with severe chest pain. Client not affected with any gastrointestinal symptoms	Admitting ward (35) advised of the situation in the home.	

Figure 19.3 Information collated as baseline of an outbreak plan.

WOULD ALL

VISITORS TO THE HOME

PLEASE REPORT TO THE

NURSE-IN-CHARGE

THANK YOU FOR ASSISTING WITH THIS

INFECTION CONTROL REQUIREMENT

Figure 19.4 Notice to relatives and visitors concerning an outbreak.

CONCLUSION

The important activity of making and keeping records is an essential and integral part of care, providing written evidence of that care. The delivery of safe care requires an adequate and defined knowledge base, and a method of monitoring how community healthcare workers apply this knowledge in practice should be identified.

Accurate, comprehensive record keeping helps staff to care effectively for their patients and clients. As professionals we have an individual responsibility to ensure that we maintain accurate documentation of our actions (UKCC 1992).

REFERENCES

Audit Commission 1995 Setting the Records Straight: a study of hospital medical records. HMSO, London

Audit Commission 1999 Survey of Hospital Medical Records. HMSO, London

Bergman R 1981 Authority, responsibility and accountability in professional nursing. The Nurse Israelo 12: 6–12

Bowell B 1992 Protecting the patient at risk. Nursing Times 88(3): 32–35

Coldwell G, Page S 1996 Just for the record. Nursing Management 2(9): 12–13

Department of Health 2001a Controls Assurance: Record Keeping. DoH, London

Department of Health 2001b Essence of care: patient focused bench marking for health care practitioners. DoH, London

Dimond B 1995 Legal Aspects of Health Care. Health Active Learning. Open Learning Foundation. Churchill Livingstone, Edinburgh

Dimond B 1997 Legal Aspects of Care in the Community. Macmillan, Basingstoke

Dimond B 2000 Legal Issues Arising in Community Nursing 7: Record Keeping. British Journal of Community Nursing 5(6): 297–299

Elliot Pennels C 1997 Protocols. Professional Nurse 13(2): 115–117

Finn L 1997 Nurses' documentation of Infection Control Precautions: 2. British Journal of Nursing 6(12): 678–684

Goldsack 1996 Goldsack: RV Cornwall County Council ex parte (transcript, 28 June 1996) (High Court)

Great Britain 1998 The Data Protection Act 1998. HMSO, London

Health and Safety Commission 1995 Reporting of Injuries, Diseases and Dangerous Occurences Regulations (RIDDOR). HSC, London

Health and Safety Commission 1999a Management of Health and Safety at Work Regulations. HSC, London

Health and Safety Commission 1999b Care of Substances Hazardous to Health Regulations. HSC, London

Hershey N, Lawrence R 1986 The influence of charting upon liability determination. Journal of Nursing Administration 35/37, March/April

Horton R 1993 Introducing high quality infection control in a hospital setting. British Journal of Nursing 2(15): 746–754

Horton R, Parker L 1997 Informed Infection Control Practice. Churchill Livingstone, Edinburgh

Health Service Circular 1999 A First Class Service: Quality in the New NHS. NHS Executive, London

Kingsley A 1992 First step towards a desired outcome: preventing infection by risk recognition. Professional Nurse 7(11): 725–729

Mandlestam, M 1998 An A–Z of Community Care Law. Jessica Kingsley, London

McHale J, Tingle J, Peysner J 1998 Law and Nursing. Butterworth-Heinemann, London

Meiner S E 1999 Nursing Documentation: Legal Focus Across Practice Settings. Sage, Thousand Oaks, CA

NHS Executive 1998 Information for Health. DoH, London

NHS Executive 2000 An Organisation with a Memory. Report of an expert group on learning from adverse events in the NHS chaired by the Chief Medical Officer. The Stationery Office, London

NHS Training Directorate 1994 Keeping the Record Straight. A Guide to Record Keeping for Nurses, Midwives and Health Visitors. DoH, London

Payne C 1995 Audit Methodologies. In: Malby B (ed.) Clinical Audit for Nurses and Therapists. Scutari Press, London

Peysner J 1998 Clinical negligence and nurses: setting the record straight. British Journal of Health Care Management 4: 352

Sullivan G H 2000 Legally speaking: keeping your charting on course. Registered Nurse 63(5): 75–79

UKCC 1992 Code of Professional Conduct for Nurses, Midwives and Health Visitors. UKCC, London

UKCC 1998 Guidelines for Records and Record Keeping. UKCC, London

Wilson J 1996 Integrated Care Management: the path to success. Butterworth-Heinemann, Oxford

20

Antibiotic resistance

A. Smith

INTRODUCTION

The majority of the population will at some time or other in their lifetime take antimicrobial agents, in particular antibiotics. Apart from analgesics, no other drugs are in such widespread use (Standing Medical Advisory Committee (SMAC) 1998).

The Association of Medical Microbiologists reported to the House of Lords that in England alone, General Practitioners (GPs) prescribe 270 million defined daily doses of antibiotics each year – 'enough to treat every man, woman and child in England for five days a year' (House of Lords Select Committee on Science and Technology 1998). Since the initial emergence of antimicrobial chemotherapy in the 1930s, antimicrobial agents have altered the expectations of life and death, transforming the practice of medicine. Some generations still alive will be able to recall the horrors of infection when antibiotics and other antimicrobials were not available. Patients with open pulmonary tuberculosis were placed in isolation hospitals until either they died or the disease healed itself. Even the simplest of cuts and grazes sometimes gave rise to fatal septicaemia, and post-operative wounds were frequently seen to become infected, often with discharging sinuses causing a significant delay in healing, some never healing or with ugly scar tissue.

Antimicrobial agents have enabled interventions that were previously unthinkable, either because the interventions demand or may cause immunosuppression, exposing the patient to possible infection by opportunist pathogens, or because the procedures are so complex that there is a risk of wound contamination (Keighley and Burdon 1979).

There has been a long tradition of treating both external and internal ailments with herbal, animal and other natural medicines. These began to be well understood only in the nineteenth century by chemists and biologists, who had the means to seek or invent more such substances. At this time it also became apparent that the newly discovered causes of infections – micro-organisms – could be attacked in two ways. Firstly, the body's own immune system could be strengthened by using a vaccine. The alternative method was to attack the micro-organisms with a 'bactericide' that was capable of destroying them whilst causing little or no harm to the body (Haeger 1988). This basic principle was named 'antimicrobial chemotherapy'. Antimicrobial agents include antibiotics, antivirals and antifungals.

Unfortunately, the use of antimicrobial chemotherapy in particular antibiotics exerts an inevitable 'Darwinian' selection for resistance. Resistance means that an organism ceases to be killed or inhibited by the drug. Once selected, resistant bacteria can spread, or may transfer resistance genes to other bacteria.

The frequency of resistance in bacteria and the number of drugs to which they are resistant is increasing.

Multi-drug resistance has been a significant marker of the last decade. The result has been erosion of antibiotic efficacy, putting many years of medical progress at risk (Standing Medical Advisory Committee 1998, House of Lords 1998, Levy 1998, Greenwood 1995). At a recent pan-European meeting on antimicrobial resistance, the increasing resistance to antimicrobial agents was described as 'healthcare's version of global warming' (Smith 1998).

Until recently, another agent or a new drug has always been available to treat an infection caused by a resistant organism; however, this is no longer the case. Pharmaceutical companies continue to screen for new products with antimicrobial activity, but compounds suitable for development cease to be found (SMAC 1998, Cohen 1994).

Bacteria possess endless resources to ensure their survival.

Resistance to antimicrobials is not just confined to hospitals but is also seen in community pathogenic organisms, and is gradually increasing (Greenwood 1995).

Although reducing antimicrobial use may not be the answer to reduce rates of resistance, it may reduce the rate at which it accumulates, supported by high standards of infection control, and this is critical in medicine and healthcare (SMAC 1998). The problem of resistance to antibiotics and other anti-infective agents has now become a major concern in medicine throughout the world and is considered to be a major threat to public health and a universal problem requiring universal action to tackle it. The Minister of State for Health in June 2000 endorsed a three-year 'United Kingdom (UK) Antimicrobial Resistance Strategy and Action Plan' (DoH 2000). This strategy identifies a range of activities required to support the control of antimicrobial resistance and the need for commitment from a wide variety of disciplines, including patients and the general population.

INFECTION

The term 'infection' is generally used to mean the deposition and multiplication of bacteria and other micro-organisms in tissues or on the surfaces of the body which are damaged or on mucous membranes, where they can cause adverse effects, often resulting in illness (Lowbury et al 1981).

The pattern of human infection changed significantly between the late 1830s and 1990, a period that began soon after the arrival of Asiatic cholera in Britain in 1831 and towards the close saw the emergence of a new disease, the acquired immune deficiency syndrome (AIDS) in 1981.

Epidemics of cholera in the mid-1800s provided an important stimulus to the campaign to improve the appalling living and working conditions, in particular sanitation conditions, of urban areas. The last cholera epidemic was seen in Britain in 1866 (Office for National Statistics (ONS) 1997b).

Mortality was not seen to decrease until the 1870s and the crude death rate fell from 20 per

1000 to 16 per 1000 in 1901–1905 (ONS 1997a). The fall was in the main attributed to a decrease in deaths from infectious disease, in particular tuberculosis, smallpox, scarlet fever and the gastrointestinal infections: enteric fever, typhus, dysentery and cholera. The fall in gastrointestinal infections was believed to be associated with improvements in sanitation and hygiene. The decrease in deaths from tuberculosis was attributed to an improvement in the general standards of living. The decrease in smallpox was undoubtedly due to the implementation of a wide-spread vaccination programme, and of scarlet fever to the decreased virulence of the causative organism.

However, a similar decline in infant mortality rates was not seen until the period 1911–1951 (ONS 1997a). This decline was achieved following the setting up of maternity, child health and school health services. By the 1960s, infectious diseases were considered to have become an insignificant cause of death, whereas in the middle of the nineteenth century one death in every three was attributed to infectious disease and by the start of the twentieth century, infectious diseases accounted for one death in every five.

As with mortality, morbidity was also seen to decline. The most significant decline was seen after the 1930s. Diseases such as diphtheria, whooping cough and poliomyelitis were controlled by immunization and in the case of smallpox, almost eradicated by immunization. Other infections such as meningococcal disease, pneumococcal infection, streptococcal infection and pulmonary tuberculosis were treatable by newly-discovered antimicrobial chemotherapy. The prognosis for patients with infectious disease was totally transformed. Infection was deemed no longer to be a threat to individual health or the public's health. However, in the 1970s and 1980s, new infections appeared and more significantly a re-emergence of old infections such as tuberculosis.

THE DEVELOPMENT OF ANTIMICROBIAL CHEMOTHERAPY

Treatment against microbial infection, whether the infection is caused by bacteria, viruses or protozoa, is referred to as antimicrobial chemotherapy (SMAC 1998, House of Lords 1998, Greenwood 1995). A German bacteriologist, Paul Ehrlich, was the first to employ the principle of antimicrobial chemotherapy at the turn of the twentieth century. The invading organisms he first studied were not bacteria but the protozoa that cause malaria. In 1910 he discovered salvarsan, the 'magic bullet', a synthetic chemical which was effective in treating syphilis, a spirochaete bacterium (Haeger 1988). In 1908 he shared a Nobel Prize for his discovery. Syphilis was a major cause of mortality: in 1910, 4375 deaths caused by syphilis were reported. This was probably an underestimate, as it was not unknown for physicians to give other diagnoses on the death certificate to minimize offending relations and as a result of the stigma attached to syphilis, a sexually-transmitted disease (ONS 1997a). However, it was penicillin that had the most significant effect in bringing about a decline in deaths caused by syphilis (ONS 1997a, Gray 2001, Haeger 1988).

The next real progress in the treatment of infection came about in the 1930s. A researcher, Gerhard Domagk, whilst studying the antibacterial action of various dyes, found a red dye which was in a sulfonamide that protected mice from the streptococcus bacterium. He subsequently found it was also effective against staphylococcal infection. The drug was patented in 1932 and was known as Prontosil. Prontosil, and its rapidly-multiplying derivatives known as 'sulfa' drugs, proved to be effective against wound infections, pneumonia, urinary tract infections and infections of other organs. Unfortunately, sulfonamide drugs also caused some serious side-effects for the human host, such as damage to the kidneys and white blood cells. Recent advances have significantly improved the safety of these drugs (Haeger 1988).

Penicillin was the first antibiotic identified. In 1928, Alexander Fleming inferred that the mould *Penicillium notatum* contained an antibacterial substance, which he named penicillin. This was the first known antibiotic produced by micro-organisms themselves. However, penicillin did not prove to be truly effective, nor was it made available for use, until the 1940s when Florey and Chain discovered how to purify it and obtain useful amounts (House of Lords 1998, Haeger 1988). Many serious infectious diseases were halted by penicillin, which, unlike sulfonamides, was not harmful to the human host. Various substances related to penicillin have since been produced that are even more effective and are mostly species-specific to fight particular bacteria. Antibiotics received a further boost from Waksman, who became an authority on microbes in the soil. Inspired by Fleming, in 1944 he revealed streptomycin. Streptomycin helped to provide the first real cure for tuberculosis; it also gave surgeons a pre- and post-operative treatment for disease.

Since the 1940s antimicrobial chemotherapy has made huge strides in fighting infections. New drugs are produced by mainly synthetic methods, and by 'engineering' techniques that change the microscopic structure of known drugs to make them more effective (Haeger 1988). The 1950s and 1960s saw the discovery of numerous new classes of antimicrobial agents. From then until the late 1980s only improvements within the classes were seen; since the late 1980s, bacteria have developed resistance faster than new agents can be found to manage them. Micro-organisms are 'getting ahead' and therapeutic options are narrowing (SMAC 1998).

ANTIMICROBIAL RESISTANCE

The main principle of antibiotic resistance is 'survival of the fittest'. Antibacterial agents kill susceptible bacteria but resistant organisms survive to infect patients (SMAC 1998).

Micro-organisms are not sensitive to all antibiotics. The terms sensitive and resistance to antibiotics are used to distinguish between those antibiotics which will or will not destroy a micro-organism. In general terms antimicrobial resistance means that the micro-organism ceases to be killed or inhibited by a drug at the normal dose regimen, and the future treatment of patients with infection caused by that micro-organism is therefore jeopardized (House of Lords 1998). Even where resistance does not cause infections

to become untreatable, it may add cost, both financially and to the patient in undesirable side-effects. Sensitive micro-organisms are killed or inhibited by the drug at its normal concentration and dose regimen.

The most resistant bacterium can be killed by a sufficiently high concentration of antibiotic. Patients, however, would not be able to tolerate the high concentration required, and this is known as clinical resistance (Hawkey 1998). The concept of resistance has been described as one in which the type of infecting bacterium, its location in the body, the distribution of the antibiotic in the body, its concentration at the site of infection, and the immune status of the patient all interact.

During the development of penicillin in the 1930s-40s, the enzyme that could destroy it was isolated and it was predicted that penicillin resistance would become a problem (Haeger 1988).

All antibiotic resistance has a genetic basis. The origins of antibiotic-resistant genes are obscure because at the time that antibiotics were introduced the biochemical and molecular basis of resistance had not been discovered. Bacteria collected up to 1950 were later found to be completely sensitive to antibiotics. They did, however, contain a range of plasmids capable of conjugative transfer (Hughes and Datta 1983). Sulfonamide resistance was reported in the early 1940s in streptococci and gonococci. The introduction of streptomycin for treating tuberculosis was thwarted by the rapid development of resistance by mutation of genes.

Resistance in bacteria can be intrinsic or acquired. Intrinsic resistance arises as a result of selection during exposure to antibacterial drugs of inherently resistant species. Acquired resistance occurs when a bacterium that has been sensitive to antibiotics develops resistance. This may happen by mutation or by the acquisition of new genes determining resistance from other bacteria.

Acquired resistance

Mutation

This involves spontaneous genetic changes, arising randomly, which may be passed vertically within the species. Resistance may be demonstrated by various mechanisms:

- increasing destruction of the antimicrobial agent
- reducing drug uptake
- increasing drug excretion
- altering the antimicrobial agent target
- activating an alternative metabolic pathway that bypasses the target.

Once a resistant mutant emerges it may rapidly become predominant in the bacterial population (SMAC 1998, Hawkey 1998).

Gene transfer

This involves the horizontal transfer of genes determining resistance from one organism to another: genetic material is most frequently transferred as plasmids which are self-replicating loops of deoxyribonucleic acid (DNA), which encode their transfer by replication into another bacterial strain or species. Transposons (jumping genes) are discrete segments of DNA, capable of transfer from one plasmid to another, and are able to spread resistance across boundaries where plasmid spread may be restricted. The resistant gene found in methicillin-resistant *Staphylococcus aureus* (MRSA) may have been acquired through the transfer of transposons. When bacteria die, they release DNA, which can be taken up by competent bacteria and inserted into their own chromosomes. This process is known as transformation and is increasingly recognized as important for a few species such as *Streptococcus pneumoniae*, *Neisseria meningitidis* and *Neisseria gonorrhoeae* who use the resulting 'mosaic' genes for the main route of spread of resistance (Drug and Therapeutics Bulletin (DTB) 1999, SMAC 1998, Hawkey 1998). Bacteriophages, which are viruses that infect bacteria, may transfer resistance by inserting resistant genes directly in the bacterial chromosome.

Resistance may pass between species, including from pathogens to commensals and vice versa. Organisms may have multi-resistance, which results from the acquisition of plasmids encoding multiple resistance mechanisms, or from the cumulative acquisition of resistances through several mechanisms (Hawkey 1998).

The importance of those processes for antibiotic resistance in man or animals is that, by whichever process genes for resistance have been acquired, the presence of an antibiotic in the environment of the bacterium imposes 'selection pressure' and encourages resistance to spread. The antibiotic kills all susceptible bacteria, thereby 'selecting out', and the resistant organisms become dominant. The speed at which antibiotic resistance emerges and the nature of geographical spread may vary. However, it cannot be disputed that the continued circle of development of resistance to new antibiotics has led to the reduction in value or often loss in value of their use to medicine (Keighley and Burdon 1979).

Viruses can also become resistant to the drugs used in their treatment. This takes place inside the cells of the patient, within which the virus multiples. Although encoded, drug resistance has been demonstrated against the majority of antiviral treatments; such resistance is also known to have a genetic basis (Pillay and Zambon 1998).

Antibiotics used against pathogens may also select resistance in the commensal bacterial flora, with the resultant emergence of future opportunistic micro-organisms. The gut is the main site for selection of resistance in the commensal flora because it contains a huge density of organisms. Selection may also occur on the skin, and it has been demonstrated that some antibiotics (quinolones) may be excreted in human sweat. This may explain some of the resistance seen in staphylococci (SMAC 1998, House of Lords 1998, Levy 1998).

EPIDEMIOLOGY OF ANTIMICROBIAL RESISTANCE

The epidemiology of resistance has been defined by data from a variety of sources, including prospective and retrospective studies, outbreak investigations and small amounts of surveillance. In addition, analytical epidemiology using case control and cohort studies has identified many of the risk factors associated with resistant infections. These include:

- the use of broad-spectrum antibiotics
- an increase in the number of susceptible hosts
- societal and technological changes leading to increased risk of exposure to resistant organisms
- high-pressure healthcare systems
- a breakdown in hygiene and infection control practices.

(House of Lords 1998, Pillay and Zambon 1998, Breathnach et al 1998, Cohen 1992, 1994).

This has been disputed, however, and it is argued that the incidence of antibiotic resistance is poorly and sporadically reported and that from a therapeutic perspective, data on outcomes are so rare that the clinical impact of infections caused by resistant strains is often unknown (Finch 1998). This argument is supported by the fact that there are few papers reporting on prevalence, incidence and outcomes in relation to antibiotic-resistant organisms. The suggestion is made that selective cross-sectional surveys or 'spotter' units in the community may provide opportunities to enhance epidemiological data (Finch 1998).

Surveillance is essential for controlling and understanding antimicrobial resistance and for supporting the decision-making processes around treatments and practice.

When studying patterns of antimicrobial resistance, organisms are frequently divided into hospital-acquired (HAI) or nosocomial and community-acquired (CAI) pathogens. This is not to suggest that antimicrobial-resistant organisms cannot be transmitted from hospitals to the community and vice versa, as many of the risk factors and pressures for the emergence, persistence or transmission of resistance exist in both environments.

Hospital-acquired infection (HAI)

Resistant and multi-resistant organisms are particularly important as a cause of HAI, especially in the immunocompromised, debilitated or elderly patients for whom they can pose a serious threat to life (Drug and Therapeutics Bulletin (DTB) 1999). Four groups of organisms are of particular concern: staphylococci, enterococci, Gram-negative organisms and *Mycobacterium tuberculosis*. All are demonstrating an increasing frequency of resistance (Cohen 1994). Vancomycin-resistant enterococci have proved to be untreatable in some cases (Williams and Ryan 1998, Leclercq et al 1992). MRSA has spread rapidly through our healthcare settings (House of Lords 1998, Cohen 1994). The resistant Gram-negative organisms such as Klebsiella and Pseudomonas have created many problems for intensive care units (House of Lords 1998, Drug and Therapeutics Bulletin 1999).

Community-acquired infection (CAI)

Infection with *Streptococcus pneumoniae* is the biggest cause of CAIs such as pneumonia, meningitis, otitis media and sinusitis (Goosens and Sprenger 1993). This pathogen has evolved to reach unexpected levels of resistance to antibiotics. Prior to the 1990s most pneumococci isolated in Britain were susceptible to penicillin. Since then resistance has increased substantially, with prevalence rates of 5%–10%. In some countries such as Spain and France resistant strains are already dominant, with reports of prevalence rates of 45% and 25% respectively (Pradier et al 1997, Jacoby 1994, Goosens and Sprenger 1993). Risk factors for the development of penicillin resistance in communities include (Friedland and McCracken 1994):

- patients who have been treated with frequent courses of antibiotics
- poor compliance with treatment regimens
- poor housing
- overcrowding in communities.

Few options are available for treating meningitis caused by resistant strains, and in some poorer countries treatments have effectively become unavailable. Thus antimicrobial resistance in pneumococci has emerged as a serious global problem which is likely to continue to grow.

MRSA is not solely a problem in hospitals, as many patients with MRSA are seen in the community, both in their own home and in residential and nursing homes. Treatment of serious MRSA infection includes the use of the antibiotics teicoplanin and vancomycin. Vancomycin-resistant strains have now been isolated and are termed 'VISA'. These appear to have occurred due to patients receiving vancomycin therapy or as a result of cross infection (Hiramatsu 1998).

The emergence of antimicrobial resistance in the community micro-organisms *Neisseria meningitidis* and *Streptococcus pyogenes* would pose important public health problems. Subtle increases in the minimum inhibitory concentration for penicillin for *N. meningitidis* and the emergence of plasmid-mediated resistance to erythromycin in *Streptococcus pyogenes* suggests potential development of resistance (Pillay and Zambon 1998, Pradier et al 1997, Jacoby 1994, Cohen 1994).

Salmonellosis is caused by over 2200 different serotypes. Most resistance has been concentrated in *Salmonella typhimurium*, one of the most important serotypes that can transfer disease from animals to humans. Since the 1960s there has been a series of recorded epidemics in humans and animals due to *S. typhimurium*. Following an extensive epidemic with a multi-resistant strain, an expert committee recommended that certain antibacterial agents should only be available on prescription for veterinary purposes. Since this period, however, epidemics have continued and multi-drug resistance has extended to new antimicrobial agents (SMAC 1998). Reports of resistance in other Gram-negative bacteria are increasing, such as resistance to trimethoprim in urinary tract infections caused by *Escherichia coli*.

From these few examples it is clear that the emergence of organisms resistant to various antimicrobial agents is gaining pace, resulting in increasing morbidity, mortality and treatment costs. Antimicrobial resistance poses an important and increasing public health threat and must be addressed if the human population does not want to be faced with the very real prospect of a return to the pre-antibiotic era where there will be no treatment for both serious and common infectious diseases (SMAC 1998, House of Lords 1998).

ANTIBIOTIC PRESCRIBING AND USE IN THE COMMUNITY

In order to reduce the use of antimicrobials, it is essential to identify where the use occurs. In the United Kingdom about 50% of use is in man and 50% in veterinary medicine and animal farming. The majority of use in the UK is in the community (80%). Of all the antibiotics prescribed in the community, 80% are oral antibiotics. The majority of prescribing is carried out by GPs, but dentists account for 7% of community prescriptions (SMAC 1998). The world market for antibiotics was $17 billion (£10.6 bn) of which $12 bn was for community use (Carbon and Bax 1998).

In the Audit Commission's Report 'A Prescription for Improvement' (1994), it was found that seven out of every ten consultations by a GP result in the issue of a prescription. Antibiotics accounted for over 10% of prescribed medicines and were the seventh most common group of drugs that had repeat prescriptions issued. Inappropriate prescribing was identified, with one of the most common areas being antibiotics prescribed for viral infections such as colds and influenza.

In 1989 the British Society for Antimicrobial Chemotherapy established a working party to look at the use of antibiotics. Included in this working party was a GP group whose remit was to identify usage of antibiotics in General Practice (Davey et al 1996). Over the period 1980–93, there was a steady annual increase in the number of prescriptions for antibiotics in England, the greatest of which was for quinolones (22% increase). The overall increase in the number of prescriptions for antibiotics in England was 45.8% from 1980–91, yet the incidence of infection had not altered over a similar time period. It was suggested that the main reason for an increase in prescribing was due to an overall increase in antibiotic prescribing for respiratory symptoms.

Fifty per cent of the community use of antibiotics is for respiratory tract infection, with the next most common reason being for urinary tract infection. Data from the UK Primary Care Database demonstrates that from 1995–97, there were 221 000 prescriptions per year for amoxycillin, and that respiratory symptoms accounted for over 70% of prescribing of amoxycillin (9 million community prescriptions per annum). In 1997 the world-wide figure was 818 billion prescriptions for respiratory tract infection (Carbon and Bax 1998).

Macfarlane et al (1997) found that 115 GPs prescribed antibiotics to 75% of patients presenting with respiratory symptoms. The reasons for GPs prescribing were not solely based on clinical factors. Other factors influencing their decision to prescribe include patient pressure, social factors, GP work pressure, and previous experience of the individual patient.

Time constraints can be a significant factor in influencing prescribing. It is usually quicker to prescribe, which may serve as a useful signal to the patient that the consultation is at an end. On average, GPs who allow 10 minutes or more per consultation prescribe fewer antibiotics (Audit Commission 1994). Good interpersonal communications between patients and the GP are important. Time will facilitate this and will enable the GP to fully understand the patient's expectations. However, many GPs will prescribe to foster good relations, even though they are aware of the evidence of effectiveness for clinical conditions such as sore throats (Butler et al 1998). Sore throats should not be treated with antibiotics unless there is good evidence that they are caused by *Streptococcus pyogenes*. Routine prescribing of antibiotics for self-limiting conditions may encourage patient dependence and re-consultation with the GP, taking up valuable time. In addition, there are the financial costs to the GP surgery and health service. In addition, costs to the patient cannot be ruled out, such as side-effects and allergy (Madden 1997, Little and Williamson 1994, Webb and Lloyd 1994, Bradley 1992a). The costs of such prescribing are likely to outweigh the benefits. The issue of doctor–patient relationship and the influence it has on the decision to prescribe is reinforced in many studies (Webb 1994, Bradley 1992b).

The age of a patient may influence prescribing decisions, with GPs more likely to prescribe for the elderly and children (Carbon and Bax 1998, Bradley 1992b).

The Audit Commission (1994) and SMAC (1998) reported similar findings, suggesting 'patients expected a prescription as part of the consultation process' and that 'excessive prescribing of antibacterial agents for trivial and non-bacterial infections in primary care partly reflects consumer pressure'.

Local antibiotic prescribing policies will lend support to prescribing practice. Any national or international developments in treatment or emergence in resistance patterns should be reflected in both these policies and infection control policies. Education regarding prescribing or anti-microbial use should be provided for those who prescribe and are involved in clinical practice.

Patient behaviour

Working adults have been described as having the poorest compliance record with antibiotic treatment (Branthwaite and Pechere 1996). Reasons for stopping medication were given as feeling better, forgetting, disliking the taste and believing that part of the course could be saved and used on another occasion. A patient prescribed antibiotics may not be compliant with the treatment regimen at all. Antibiotic prescriptions are one of the most common prescriptions not submitted to the pharmacy for dispensing, and also for partial courses being returned or discarded (Buckinghamshire HA unpublished 1998, Carbon and Bax 1998).

Antibacterial agents can be bought openly without prescription in many countries outside the UK. The tablets can be bought singly or in any multiple, with differing (usually low) potency. This can result in significant selection for resistance.

All of these factors may have an influence on antibiotic resistance and highlight the need for education of the patient, the public and the healthcare professional as an important part of the overall strategy to reduce antibiotic resistance and the threat to public health.

SPECIFIC ANTIBIOTIC-RESISTANT ORGANISMS

Two specific antibiotic-resistant organisms have received much attention from the media in recent years: MRSA, which is increasing in incidence and is a significant challenge for minimizing cross infection, and multi-drug resistant tuberculosis (MDRTB) which is seen as a major public health problem.

Methicillin-resistant *Staphylococcus aureus* (MRSA)

Staphylococcus aureus is carried as a skin commensal by approximately 30% of the population, usually in moist sites such as the nose, axilla and perineum. It is capable of surviving for long periods on dry surfaces, including hands and equipment. *S. aureus* is capable of causing a range of infections and is the primary pathogen in wound infections.

Since the early 1960s, *S. aureus* has demonstrated a remarkable ability to adapt to the presence of beta-lactamase antibiotics in their environment by developing resistance. These resistant strains are termed MRSA. The incidence of MRSA increased until the 1970s and was responsible for many serious outbreaks of infection in hospitals. In the late 1970s gentamicin resistance had emerged; subsequently a series of epidemic strains (EMRSA) have evolved and spread widely. The incidence of MRSA continued to increase through the 1980s and by the end of the 1990s MRSA affected most healthcare settings, including the community in the UK. The two epidemic strains most prevalent in the UK are EMRSA 15 and EMRSA 16. Recent reports indicate that vancomycin intermediate resistant strains (VISA) have been identified. These strains are resistant to all available antibacterial agents and appear to have considerable pathogenicity for patients who are not already severely immunocompromised (SMAC 1998, Hiramatsu 1998). MRSA is not a notifiable disease; however, MRSA bacteraemias are part of a national surveillance programme.

MRSA is generally considered to be a problem of cross infection rather than one of repeated evolution of resistance. MRSA, in particular

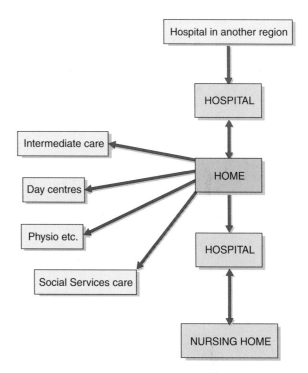

Figure 20.1 Possible routes of spread of MRSA between healthcare settings.

EMRSA, has the ability to spread easily and rapidly. Spread of MRSA from one healthcare setting to another has been aided where patients are moved at short notice and with inadequate communication and preparation (Fig. 20.1). Effective control of MRSA is dependent on high standards of infection control and hygiene practice, especially hand hygiene and environmental control of dust, together with patient risk assessment (Fig. 20.2), and on-going education of healthcare workers and carers. It has never been more important to ensure appropriate clinical care than with the current transfer of more dependent patients into the community, particularly to nursing homes with the development of intermediate care (Duckworth and Heathcock 1995, Cox et al 1995). Table 20.1 summarizes the precautions/actions required in Community and Primary Care.

Definitions

- *Colonization*: *Staphylococcus aureus* can normally be found on the skin, skin folds, anterior

INFECTION ASSESSMENT AND CARE PLAN

NAME .... CARE OF (GP/CONS) ....

LOCATION/ADDRESS ....

....

(Delete as appropriate)

PROBLEM   * COLONIZATION OF BODY SITES?   YES/NO

* INFECTION (Wound, Respiratory, Urinary, Other)   YES/NO

OUTCOME   To inhibit further colonization/infection and to minimize potential cross infection and environmental contamination.

NURSING ASSESSMENT ACTION (Delete as appropriate)

ENVIRONMENT	Single room	Main ward	• Own home • Nursing home • Residential home • Group home
ELIMINATION	Own toilet	Own commode	Shared toilet
HAND WASHING	Liquid soap	Chlorhexidine liquid hand wash	Alcohol rub
GLOVES (disposable)	Latex disposable	Vinyl disposable	Other (please state)
PLASTIC APRONS	**DISPOSABLE SINGLE USE ONLY**		
CLINICAL WASTE	YELLOW WASTE BAG (follow Waste Policy)		
LAUNDRY	MACHINE WASH Follow laundry guidance for colour For hand washing as hot as possible		
EQUIPMENT (State type in use, e.g. beds/baths)			
SPILLAGE	Follow policy in infection control manual		
INFORMATION TO PATIENT	YES	NO	UNABLE TO UNDERSTAND
INFORMATION TO RELATIVES	YES	NO	NO RELATIVE
WOUND CARE	YES	NO	TOPICAL TO WOUND
SKIN CARE	YES	NO	• BODY WASHES • NASAL CREAM • SKIN CREAMS • POWDER

Figure 20.2 Patient infection assessment and care plan.

SPECIMENS

DATE	RESULT	COMMENT
....		
....		
....		
....		
....		
....		
....		

GENERAL COMMENTS

....

....

ASSESSED BY .... DATE ....

FORM COMPLETED BY .... DATE ....

Figure 20.2   (*continued*).

Table 20.1   Key principles for nursing patients with MRSA in community

	Recommendations	Comment
In residential/nursing home	Single room preferable	Can share with another resident with MRSA. If already sharing, ensure separate toilets, etc.
Own home	No isolation in patient's own home	Socialize as normal
GP practice	Universal infection control precautions	End of list for dressings, etc.
Crockery and cutlery	No special precautions needed	
Domestic services	Damp dust and vacuum daily Clean bath after use – as normal	
Hand washing	After giving personal care After bed making After removing protective clothing	Should have a hand washing sink in the room if in a residential home
Hand washing products	Liquid soap Alcohol hand rub	
Laundry	No need to segregate if wash temperature 60°C or more, but wash separately if washed at a temperature below 60°C	Wash at the highest temperature if the fabric allows
Dressings	Areas of broken skin must be covered with an occlusive dressing	Advice on MRSA colonization in wound from Community IC Nurse and Microbiologist
Protective clothing	Disposable gloves and aprons	Use when giving personal care Use when making bed Wash hands after removal
Personal hygiene	Encourage hand and personal hygiene	
Social activities	No need for restriction	
Staff with skin disorders	Ensure skin lesions are covered	E.g. eczema, psoriasis Advice from CICN
Swabbing	On advice from Microbiologist	
Visitors	No restrictions	
Waste	Dispose as domestic waste unless categorized as clinical waste	

nares, perineum and umbilicus. It survives in these areas but does not cause infection.

- *Infection*: Bacteria deposit themselves or enter the body and multiply rapidly in the tissues. There will be signs and symptoms of infection present, i.e. inflammation, redness, swelling, pain, and pyrexia. Pus may also be present at the affected site.

Swabs and screening

Routine screening is not essential. Any screening required must be assessed on an individual basis. Screening may be required during an outbreak or when the infection control team advises to do so.

Transfers/admissions/discharges

Communication regarding infection or colonization must be included in the information to all other providers of healthcare. A copy of a treatment/care plan is useful (Fig. 20.2).

Multi-drug resistant tuberculosis (MDRTB)

In recent years, MDRTB has become an important public health problem (House of Lords 1998, Breathnach et al 1998, Mendez et al 1998, Frieden et al 1993). It has emerged partly as a result of the breakdown in the public health infrastructure such as homelessness, non-compliance with therapy, immigration, overcrowding and HIV disease. MDRTB has been associated with important hospital outbreaks, but is not just a problem for hospitals but also the community. In 1998 a report for the World Health Organisation concluded that MDRTB threatens all efforts to control tuberculosis. Resistance to the four first-line drugs was found in all 35 countries surveyed, suggesting that MDRTB is a global problem (WHO 1998). All forms of tuberculosis are compulsorily notifiable under the Public Health (Control of Disease) Act 1984. (See Chapter 4.)

The incidence of MDRTB is rising and the management of this illness is both complex and difficult. MDRTB should be seen as a warning for what might happen with other infections as resistance develops and spreads. MDRTB has been found to be directly associated with poor compliance with treatment (House of Lords 1998, Breathnach et al 1998, Mendez et al 1998, Frieden et al 1993).

MDRTB is considered to be one of the most serious resistance problems and a major public health threat. Tuberculosis is caused by *Mycobacterium tuberculosis*. It is a chronic, progressive infection that most commonly affects the lungs (pulmonary TB) but may affect other organs and tissues such as the kidney, intestine and bone. Unusually for bacterial infections, *Mycobacterium tuberculosis* infections require treatment with combinations of three or four drugs for at least six months. The relevant drugs include (Joint Tuberculosis Committee of the British Thoracic Society 2000):

- Isoniazid
- Rifampicin
- Pyrazinamide
- Ethambutol.

Resistant TB is defined as when the bacteria are resistant to one or more of the first line antituberculous drugs. Resistance was first recognized when streptomycin became available. Therefore a combination of antibiotics is used to reduce the risk of resistance to individual drugs.

Drug-resistant organisms initially emerge as a result of inadequate treatment of drug-sensitive disease, either through incorrect prescribing, poor absorption of the drugs or poor compliance with treatment. They are more likely where there are greater numbers of bacteria, such as in extensive or cavitating disease (see Box 20.1).

The greatest treatment problem relates to treatment of individuals with multi-drug resistant TB (MDRTB). MDRTB is defined as isolates resistant to both rifampicin and isoniazid with or without other resistances. Mortality from MDRTB is high,

---

Box 20.1 MDRTB: factors to consider

- Previous drug treatment for tuberculosis
- Contact with a case of known MDRTB
- HIV infection
- Failure of clinical response on treatment
- Prolonged sputum smear or culture positive while on treatment (smear positivity at 4 months or culture positivity at 5 months)

44% in HIV-negative patients and as high as 80% in HIV-positive patients (SMAC 1998, House of Lords 1998, Breathnach et al 1998, Mendez et al 1998, Frieden et al 1993). Treatment for MDRTB usually consists of a five-drug regimen. The alternative drugs available tend to be more commonly associated with adverse reactions, are less effective, and the treatment needs to be for a longer period of time. Inappropriate treatment may result in the creation of further drug resistance. Rapid detection of resistance is essential to

reduce the risk of transmission to others and is also vital to the health of the individual.

Transmission of TB occurs through person-to-person spread, almost exclusively by the respiratory route. Close continuous contact is usually required for transmission to occur. The reduction of spread through appropriate infection control measures is a crucial aspect of TB management, including respiratory protection measures and isolation facilities and precautions particularly for MDRTB (Fig. 20.3). Tracing, investigating and

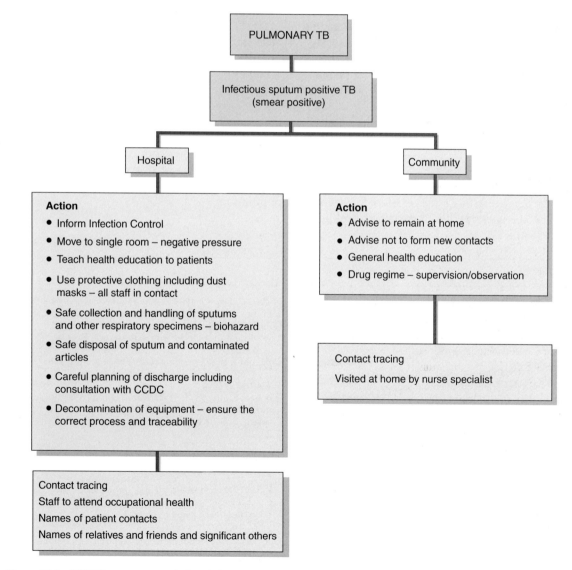

Figure 20.3 MDRTB: management in hospital and the community.

Box 20.2 Achieving control of antimicrobial resistance: the three elements (DoH 2000)

- *Surveillance:* to monitor how we are doing and provide data on resistant organisms, illness due to them, and antimicrobial usage necessary to inform action.
- *Prudent antimicrobial use*: to reduce the 'pressure for resistance' by reducing unnecessary and inappropriate exposure of micro-organisms to

antimicrobial agents in clinical practice, veterinary practice, animal husbandry, agriculture and horticulture.
- *Infection control*; to reduce the spread of infection in general (and thus some of the need for antimicrobial agents) and of antimicrobial-resistant micro-organisms in particular.

---

managing the contacts of an infectious case is an essential part of TB control as it may identify additional cases (Interdepartmental Working Group on Tuberculosis 1998). Directly-observed treatment (DOT), where compliance with treatment is observed, is recommended for all patients who cannot be relied upon to comply with treatment regimens, for patients with a history of non-compliance and for patients with drug-resistant TB (the latter for at least the initial phase of treatment).

SUMMARY

Antimicrobial resistance has existed for several decades. However, the increasing problems

associated with resistance are considered to be a major threat to public health.

The Department of Health in its strategy for the basis of control of antimicrobial resistance states that there are three key, inter-related elements to achieve control, as set out in Box 20.2.

Each of these elements needs to be supported by the provision of information, policy, guidelines, education, communication, research, evaluation of effectiveness of interventions, resources and organizational support. Communication and education should not stop at healthcare workers but should include patients and the general population.

REFERENCES

Audit Commission 1994 A Prescription for Improvement. Towards More Rational Prescribing in General Practice. HMSO, London

Bradley C P 1992a Uncomfortable prescribing decisions: a critical incident study. British Medical Journal 304: 294–296

Bradley C P 1992b Factors which influence the decision whether to prescribe: the dilemma facing general practitioners. British Journal of General Practice 42: 454–458

Branthwaite A, Pechere J C 1996 Pan-European survey of patients' attitudes to antibiotics and antibiotic use. Journal of International Medical Research 24: 229–238

Breathnach A S, deRuiter A, Holdsworth G M C et al 1998 An outbreak of multi-drug resistant tuberculosis in a London Teaching Hospital. Journal of Hospital Infection 39: 111–117

Buckinghamshire Health Authority 1998 Money to Burn? Unpublished

Butler C C, Rollnick S, Pill R, Maggs-Rapport F, Stott N 1998 Understanding the culture of prescribing: qualitative study of general practitioners' and patients' perceptions of antibiotics for sore throats. British Medical Journal 317: 637–642

Carbon C, Bax R P 1998 Regulating the use of antibiotics in the community. British Medical Journal 317: 663–665

Cohen M L 1992 Epidemiology of drug resistance: implication for a post antimicrobial era. Science 257: 1050–1055

Cohen M L 1994 Emerging problems of antimicrobial resistance. Annals of Emergency Medicine 24(3): 454–457

Cox R A, Conquest C, Mallaghan C, King J 1995 Epidemic methicillin resistant *Staphylococcus aureus*: controlling the spread outside hospital. Journal of Hospital Infection 29: 107–119

Davey P G, Bax R P, Newey J et al 1996 Growth in the use of antibiotics in the community in England and Scotland in 1980–93. British Medical Journal 312: 61

Department of Health 2000 UK Antimicrobial Resistance Strategy and Action Plan. DoH, London

Drug and Therapeutics Bulletin 1999 Tackling Antimicrobial Resistance. DTB 37(2): 9–16. Consumers Association, Hertford

Duckworth G, Heathcock R 1995 Report of a Combined Working Party of the British Society for Anti-microbial Chemotherapy and the Hospital Infection Society. Guidelines on the Control of Methicillin-resistant

Staphylococcus aureus in the Community. Journal of Hospital Infection 31: 1–12

Finch R G 1998 Antibiotic resistance. Journal of Antimicrobial Chemotherapy 42: 125–128

Frieden T R, Sterling T, Pablos-Mendez A 1993 The emergence of drug resistant tuberculosis in New York City. New England Journal of Medicine 328: 521–526

Friedland I R, McCracken G H 1994 Management of infections caused by antibiotic-resistant *Streptococcus pneumoniae*. New England Journal of Medicine 331: 377–382

Goosens H, Sprenger M J W 1998 Community Acquired Infections and Bacterial Resistance. British Medical Journal 317: 654–657

Gray A 2001 Mortality and morbidity: causes and determinants. In: Gray A (ed.) World Health and Disease, 2nd edn. Open University Press, Buckingham

Greenwood D 1995 Sixty years on: antimicrobial resistance comes of age. Lancet 346, Suppl 1

Haeger K 1988 The world of modern surgery. In: Knut H The Illustrated History of Surgery. AB Nordbook, Gothenburg

Hawkey P M 1998 The origins and molecular basis of antibiotic resistance. British Medical Journal 317: 657–660

Hiramatsu K 1998 Vancomycin resistance in Staphylococcus. Drug Resistance Updates 1: 135–150

House of Lords Select Committee on Science and Technology 1998 Resistance to Antibiotics and other Antimicrobial Agents. HMSO, London

Hughes V M, Datta N 1983 Conjugative plasmids in bacteria of the pre-antibiotic era. Nature 302: 725–726

Interdepartmental Working Group on Tuberculosis 1998. The Prevention and Control of Tuberculosis in the United Kingdom: UK Guidance on the Prevention and Control of Transmission of Drug-Resistant, including Multiple Drug Resistant, Tuberculosis. DoH, London

Jacoby G A 1994 Prevalence and resistance mechanisms of common bacterial respiratory pathogens. Clinical Infectious Disease 18: 951–957

Joint Tuberculosis Committee of the British Thoracic Society 2000. Control and Prevention of Tuberculosis in the United Kingdom: Code of Practice 2000. Thorax 55: 887–901

Keighley M R B, Burdon D W B 1979 Antimicrobial Chemoprophylaxis in Surgery. Pitman Medical, London

Leclercq R, Dukta-Malen S, Brisson-Noel A 1992 Resistance of enterococci to aminoglycosides and glycopeptides. Clinical Infectious Disease 15: 651–660

Levy S B 1998 Multidrug resistance – A sign of the times. Editorial. New England Journal of Medicine 338: 1376–1378

Little P, Williamson I 1994 Are antibiotics appropriate for sore throats? British Medical Journal 309: 1010–1011

Lowbury E J L, Ayliffe G A, Geddes A M, Williams J D 1981 Introduction. In: Control of Hospital Infection. A Practical Handbook, 2nd edn. Chapman & Hall, London

Macfarlane J, Lewis S A, Macfarlane R, Holmes W 1997 Contemporary use of antibiotics in 1809 adults presenting with acute lower respiratory tract illness in general practice in the UK: implications for developing management guidelines. Respiratory Medicine 91: 427–434

Madden T A 1977 Adverse penicillin reactions in the records of general practice. Journal of the Royal College of General Practitioners 27: 73–77

Mendez A P, Laszlo A, Binkin N et al 1998 Global surveillance for Antituberculosis-Drug Resistance 1994–1997. WHO/The New England Journal of Medicine 338(23): 1641–1690

Office for National Statistics 1997a Trends in all cause mortality 1841–1994. In: The Health of Adult Britain 1841–1994, Vol. 1. HMSO, London

Office for National Statistics 1997b Infection in England and Wales 1838–1993. In: The Health of Adult Britain 1841–1994, Vol. 2. HMSO, London

Pillay D, Zambon M 1998 Antiviral drug resistance. British Medical Journal 317: 660–662

Pradier C, Dunais B, Carsenti-Etesse H, Dellamonica P 1997 Pneumococcal resistance in Europe. European Journal of Clinical Microbiology Infectious Disease 16: 644–647

Smith R 1998 Action on antimicrobial resistance. Editorial. British Medical Journal 317: 764–770

Standing Medical Advisory Committee 1998 The Path of Least Resistance. DoH, London

Webb S, Lloyd M 1994 Prescribing and referral in general practice: a study of patients' expectations and doctors' actions. British Journal of General Practice 44: 165–169

Williams R J, Ryan J 1998 Surveillance of antimicrobial resistance – an international perspective. British Medical Journal 317: 651–660

World Health Organization 1998 World Health Organization Resolution WHA51.17 Emerging and other communicable diseases: antimicrobial resistance. In: Fifty First World Health Assembly Resolutions and Decisions Annexe. World Health Organization, Geneva

21

Tattooing and body piercing

K. Gunn

INTRODUCTION

'Special treatments' is a portmanteau term taking in many treatments and procedures ranging from tattooing, skin piercing and beauty therapies to laser treatments and massage. For the purpose of this chapter the main focus will be upon procedures identified in the Local Government (Miscellaneous Provisions) Act 1982 (HMSO 1982). These include tattooing, acupuncture, ear piercing and electrolysis. Body piercing is not specifically identified in the Act at present; nevertheless the risk of infection following such procedures warrants specific address.

The surveillance, investigation, prevention and control of communicable disease in the population is an important task for all public health departments. These functions are usually the responsibility of the Consultant in Communicable Disease Control (CCDC), who with varying degrees of support will lead and co-ordinate outbreak management and infection control advice within the given population. The CCDC will usually be the designated Proper Officer of the Local Authority and as such is 'notified' formally of persons being diagnosed as suffering or suspected to be suffering from one of thirty notifiable communicable diseases. (See also Chapter 3.) Viral hepatitis is one such disease which is statutorily notifiable to the Proper Officer under the Public Health (Infectious Diseases) Regulations 1988 (HMSO 1988).

The first documented evidence of the spread of blood-borne infection (Hepatitis B virus) associated with poor infection control practice in a tattoo studio was reported in 1950 in Panama. An outbreak of Hepatitis B reported in 1979 in the UK involved 34 cases, with 26% of cases admitted to hospital. Following this particular incident clinicians involved in the management of the outbreak produced hygiene guidelines for use in tattooing practice (Noah 1993).

Despite this guidance and the advent of certain laws, serious infections, including bloodborne infections, still occur following tattooing, skin piercing and alternative therapy treatments. Such infections are preventable if strict attention is given to the basic principles of infection control.

HISTORY AND BACKGROUND OF TATTOOING AND SKIN PIERCING

Various cultures worldwide have performed tattooing for thousands of years; it was introduced into Europe in the 1770s by mariners who had visited the Polynesian Islands. The popularity of tattoos increased in Britain during the nineteenth century, which was partly attributable to the invention of the electric tattoo machine in the 1890s. More recently there has been a surge of interest among the general population, including females as well as males, teenagers and school children. Tattoos may also be used for medical or cosmetic reasons, for instance to camouflage burns by micro-pigmentation (MPI) and to create permanent dots as markers during radiation therapy.

Body piercing is also not new: historically it was a sign of virility and courage. Egyptian pharaohs underwent rites of passage by piercing their navels, Mayans pierced their tongues and Roman soldiers wore nipple rings to secure their capes as a sign of manhood. These customs appear to have religious, sexual, tribal or marital significance. With the exception of ear piercing, body piercing did not become generally fashionable throughout Europe until recently. Whilst no figures exist in relation to piercing in the UK, a booming industry in books, magazines and videos would suggest an increasing interest.

THE LAW RELATING TO THESE ACTIVITIES

The relevant laws are listed in Box 21.1.

The Local Government (Miscellaneous Provisions) Act 1982 is the current legislation which relates to the practice of tattooing, acupuncture, ear piercing and electrolysis in England and Wales. This Act provides that local authorities may make bye-laws to secure certain standards. A breach of the bye-laws is an offence which may lead to the magistrates imposing a fine and/or suspending or cancelling registration.

The Act states that the activities listed may only be undertaken by a person in premises registered by the Local Authority (except for occasional visits elsewhere); therefore both the individual and the premises need to be registered. The Act is not applicable when any of the activities are carried out by, or under the supervision of, a registered medical practitioner or, in the case of acupuncture, if carried out by a registered dental practitioner. Tattooists working from studios are regulated by local government bye-laws, with studios being subject to regular inspection. The Health and Safety at Work Act 1974 also governs their practice. Unfortunately 'scratchers', who tattoo outside business premises on an informal basis, also exist. The quality of their work is often inferior and their equipment is not subject to any inspection.

In the event of young persons requesting tattoos, practitioners must be satisfied that the person is 18 years of age as it is an offence under

---

Box 21.1 Laws relating to tattooing and skin piercing. Publisher: HMSO, London

Health and Safety at Work Act 1974
Tattooing of Minors Act 1969
Prohibition of Female Circumcision Act 1985
Local Government (Miscellaneous Provisions) Act 1982
Greater London Council (General Powers) Act 1981
London Local Authorities Act 1991
Control of Substances Hazardous to Health Regulations 1994 (ISBN 07176 08190)

the Tattooing of Minors Act 1969 to carry out the procedure on an under aged person. Similar issues arise around cosmetic body piercing. There are reports of severe blood loss and other major injuries in relation to body piercing which have called into question whether such practices should be classed as cosmetic treatments or whether they are closer to surgical procedures. This would make a difference to the allocation of enforcement responsibility under the Health and Safety at Work Act.

Alarmingly, some studios in the UK are willing to carry out genital piercing on women although under British laws designed to prohibit female genital mutilation, cutting, piercing or otherwise surgically modifying genitalia for non-medical reasons is an offence (HMSO 1985).

Local authorities within the London area have two other Acts under which they may regulate tattooing/skin piercing practice: the Greater London Council (General Powers) Act 1981 (HMSO 1981) and the London Local Authorities Act 1991 (HMSO 1991). There are anomalies in relation to the licensing of piercing practices when considering the UK position; presently all cosmetic piercing is included in the legislation relating to London, but only ear-piercing is covered in the Local Government (Miscellaneous Provisions) Act 1982 which enables local authorities outside London to make bye-laws. This gives specific regulating powers to the Local Authorities in London, which are not available to the rest of the UK.

INFECTION RISKS ASSOCIATED WITH TATTOOING AND SKIN PIERCING

The risk of acquiring a blood-borne infectious disease is inherent in tattooing, as the loss of serosanguinous fluid always follows the repetitive puncturing of the skin with electrically-driven tattoo needles. Although the last case of syphilis spread by tattooing was reported more than 100 years ago, the association of tattoos with syphilis was so well known in the nineteenth and early twentieth century that some suggested that a tattoo was an almost certain sign of a positive Wasserman test for syphilis!

In modern skin piercing practice, if infection control procedures are adhered to, the spread of infection by tattooing and skin piercing should be a rare occurrence. The consequences of a lapse in such practice and procedures, however, continue to be serious. Large outbreaks of infection have occurred. Thirty seven people were diagnosed as having acute Hepatitis B infection following acupuncture in 1988 (Kent et al 1988) and more recently there were eight confirmed cases of acute Hepatitis B following clients undergoing autohaemotherapy at an alternative therapy centre (Vickers et al 1994). The transmission of Hepatitis C following cosmetic tattooing of the eyelids and eyebrows is reported (Dian-Xing et al 1996) and case control studies not associated with outbreaks also showed a significant association with tattooing, ear piercing and Hepatitis C (Mele et al 1995). The only cases of possible transmission of Human Immuno-deficiency Virus (HIV) infection reported from tattoos were of two men who received tattoos in prison.

The evidence relating to the spread of infections and communicable disease associated with skin piercing is well documented (Long and Rickman 1994, Wright 1995). Local bacterial infections, gangrene, amputation and even death are documented following skin piercing procedures. Other risks may include secondary bacterial infections, localized severe swelling and scarring at the site of the piercing, allergic reactions to skin antiseptics, ointments and jewellery. Jewellery which may become embedded in the soft tissue surrounding the piercing can also create problems.

Nasal piercing also poses risks of infection because of the staphylococcal organisms in the nose, and cases of endocarditis have resulted from a nose piercing (Wright 1995).

Many infections and complications of piercings will go unreported as those performing piercings may be reluctant to report adverse reactions for fear of legal consequences. Those receiving them may also be reluctant to report negative consequences, particularly where piercings are of an intimate nature.

PROCEDURES

Tattooing procedures

The tattooing procedure begins with the selection of a design. The art work and designs of tattoos are very important, with many clients travelling to visit specific tattooists because of their reputation for 'good art work' and original designs.

Figures 21.1, 21.2 and 21.3 illustrate the tattooing process.

The skin to be tattooed is sprayed with an antiseptic solution and may be shaved. The design is drawn or stencilled on, and a thin layer of petroleum jelly or similar is spread over the site. With the exception of Japan, where professional tattooing is still done by hand, most professional tattooists in developed countries today use electric tattoo guns. A tattoo gun consists of a rotating motor in a handle connected to a bar that runs through a shaft to the needles. One to fourteen solid-bore needles are used, depending on the thickness of the line or shading desired. The needle or needles protrude from the end of the shaft about 2–3 mm when the motor is activated. The needles move up and down 50 to 3000 times per minute.

The tattooist holds the tattoo gun at a constant level over the client's skin. The needles are repeatedly dipped into the ink prior to the gun being run over the skin, rapidly puncturing and inserting the pigment through the epidermis into the dermis. Excess ink and blood that oozes from the site are repeatedly wiped away.

The process can take from 15 minutes to several hours, with some being completed over a course of months depending on the size and complexity of the tattoo.

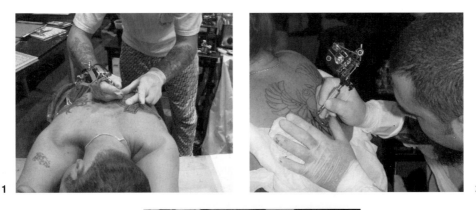

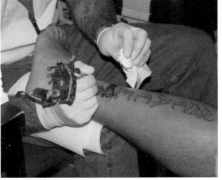

Figures 21.1, 21.2, 21.3 The tattooing process. Reproduced by kind permission of Hippozone Limited.

Skin piercing procedures

Body piercing is primarily carried out for sexual or aesthetic reasons, although some people say it has spiritual benefits.

Various items of medical equipment are used to pierce skin and create holes for body jewellery. Ear piercing guns, surgical clamps, forceps and large gauge hollow needles are the instruments most commonly used. It is important to note that piercing guns designed for piercing ears should not be used on other areas of the body as their design may lead to damage of cartilage and soft tissue. Studio piercers should not administer local anaesthetics unless medically qualified. There are documented risks associated with the use of topical anaesthetics which are not recommended for use in skin piercing practice. Many practitioners do use topical anaesthetics, and serious consideration should be given to health risks associated with the use of these preparations, such as 'frost bite' following use of ethyl chloride. Appropriate documentation should be in place if topical anaesthetics are administered.

The procedure begins with the skin being marked to guide the needle path. The skin is held taut by forceps and the opening made with a hollow needle similar to a needle and thread action. Once the hole is made, the jewellery is quickly pulled through the piercing site. As a small to moderate amount of bleeding may occur following the procedure, manual pressure is applied to the site. The oral procedure is typically carried out using a medical cutting catheter and the insertion of a temporary device, which allows for the inevitable swelling that occurs over the 3–5 week healing period. Thereafter the permanent jewellery is placed and worn constantly to prevent the perforation from closing spontaneously.

The style of jewellery ranges from small to wide hoops to ear or barbell type studs. The jewellery needs to be in place at all times to keep the hole patent. Usual cosmetic items used for ears should not be used for other body areas because ear wires are usually stainless steel or gold plated. The latter wears off easily, leaving the exposed brass foundation which may cause skin reactions. Surgical quality stainless steel or

14 and 18 carat gold should be used. Additionally nobium, platinum or titanium with no rough edges are also acceptable.

While different healing times are predicted by the piercers, the average healing times depend on the site and may range from 1 to 5 months or longer. Facial piercings, eyebrows, noses and lips are open to the air and therefore tend to heal faster. Tongues also heal quickly owing to the vascular nature of the site.

Written and verbal information on aftercare of tattoos and piercings should always be provided following each procedure. The practitioner should describe the procedure in detail and provide written information to be carried away with the client, giving advice on the daily routines for aftercare of the site.

RECORD KEEPING AND REPORTING

It is important for practitioners of tattooing/skin piercing to keep records of their clients (Box 21.2). Detailed records will prove invaluable if there is any question of infection linked to premises which would be indicative of need for a 'look back' exercise. Records should be kept for a minimum of two years.

INFECTION CONTROL RISK ASSESSMENT IN STUDIOS AND GUIDANCE FOR 'BEST PRACTICE'

An assessment of infection control procedures in tattooing and skin piercing studios (Dawson

---

Box 21.2 Records required about all tattooing/skin piercing procedures

- Date of procedure
- Client name, contact address and telephone number
- The procedure carried out
- Record of type of body jewellery used if applicable
- Relevant medical history
- Any previous piercings/tattoos carried out by the practitioner
- A consent form to be signed by all clients undergoing procedures

---

Box 21.3 Commonly identified problems found in tattooing/skin piercing studios following infection control assessment (Dawson 1998)

Hand hygiene
- Poor hand washing facilities
- No liquid/bar soap
- Cotton hand towels in use for hand drying
- Small water boilers supplying water to hand washing sink

Practices
- No disposable plastic aprons available
- No eye protection available
- Poor understanding of spills procedure
- Wide range of skin disinfectants in use, varying dilutions, spray bottles unlabelled
- Multi-use ointments and creams in use
- Using products against manufacturer's instructions
- Inappropriate use of spray/topical anaesthetics

Environment
- Working from wooden surfaces not easily cleaned
- Poor, permeable, ill-fitting floor coverings
- Non-intact, damaged couches and chairs

Waste and sharps disposal
- No written waste guidelines
- No appropriate waste collection service
- Unaware of inoculation injury procedure

Chemicals
- Non-adherence to COSHH regulations
- Inappropriate use of glutaraldehyde (Cidex) to decontaminate equipment, soak needles in and as a surface disinfectant
- Practitioners unaware of the hazards and legislation pertaining to the use of such chemicals
- Proprietary brands of detergents and disinfectants diluted against manufacturer's instructions

Equipment
- Single use equipment being reused
- Sterilizers not used in accordance with HTM 2010 (HMSO 1994)
- UVA light boxes used as a method of sterilization
- No maintenance contracts for sterilizing equipment in use

Box 21.4 Accepted best practice for infection control in tattooing/skin piercing establishments

- Hands will be washed correctly using a cleansing agent at the facilities available, to reduce cross-infection.
- Tattooing/skin piercing practices will reflect Local Authority Guidelines, Bye-Laws and best practice to reduce the risk of cross infection to clients whilst providing appropriate protection to operators.
- The studio environment will be appropriately maintained to negate the risk of cross infection.
- Waste will be disposed of without risk of contamination or injury and within current guidelines.
- Sharps will be handled safely in order to negate the risk of sharps injury and in accordance with current guidelines.
- Appropriate detergents/disinfectants and antiseptics are used correctly to negate the risk of infection.
- Equipment will be decontaminated appropriately and stored correctly in order to negate the risk of cross infection.

---

the risk of the spread of infection in tattooing/skin piercing studios. The infection control assessment document used (Dawson 1998) was adapted from an infection control audit tool developed by the West Midlands Regional Group of the Infection Control Nurses Association (ICNA). The 'best practice' statements (Box 21.4) for each section of the assessment document were derived from the Local Authority's bye-laws, the most up-to-date legislation, evidence in the literature and accepted best practice for the control of infection. Each section of the assessment document has a 'best practice' statement and varying numbers of practice points to be observed.

It should be noted that the 'best practice' statements and practice points are intended for use by the practitioners themselves, they are written in user-friendly terms and do not address infection control practice and procedure in the depth expected of healthcare establishments. The practice points can be audited, and this will be a useful measure of infection control practice and procedure for the inspection officers of Local Authorities on routine inspection visits. Seven 'best practice' statements are detailed and the list is by no means exhaustive.

1998) identified elements of practice which give cause for concern (Box 21.3). Many health and local authorities have guidelines or policy documents available for use in tattoo/skin piercing studios (nationally agreed guidance is still awaited at time of going to press). The local guidelines will support safe working and provide guidance to practitioners.

The following section describes points for safe working and accepted best practice in reducing

Practice points for each of the seven 'best practice' statements

*Hands will be washed correctly using a
cleansing agent at the facilities available,
to reduce cross infection* (Box 21.5)

Hand washing is the single most important
means of preventing the spread of infection (Box
21.5). An intact skin is an efficient waterproof
barrier; practitioners should look after their skin
and cover all lesions with a waterproof dressing (ICNA 1993). Thorough hand washing, using
a good technique with soap and running water
at an appropriate temperature, is particularly
important:

- before and after tattooing/skin piercing
  procedures
- if hands are accidentally contaminated with
  blood, body fluids or secretions
- after removing gloves
- after visiting the toilet
- before handling food and drinks.

*Tattooing/skin piercing practices will reflect
Local Authority Guidance, Bye-Laws and best
practice to reduce the risk of cross infection to
clients, whilst providing appropriate protection
to operators* (Box 21.6)

Appropriate personal protective clothing should
be available at all times for use in the studio.

*The studio environment will be appropriately
maintained to negate the risk of
cross infection* (Box 21.7)

All surfaces liable to become contaminated with
blood/body fluids must be protected with an

intact water-repellent cover/surface. Effective infection control measures are aided and simplified by using a strict system of zoning, that is, designated clean and dirty work areas zoning one way from clean to dirty with no reintroduction of used items into the clean zone, as described in Chapter 11 and Figure 11.1.

Waste will be disposed of without risk of contamination or injury and within current guidelines (Box 21.8)

Box 21.8 Practice points: waste disposal

The studio has written instructions on the safe disposal of waste.
Foot-operational bins are in working order in practice areas.
Appropriate yellow bags are used for disposal of clinical waste.
Clinical waste and domestic waste is correctly segregated.
Waste bags are less than three quarters full and securely tied.
Clinical waste is stored in a designated area prior to disposal.
The storage area is locked and inaccessible to unauthorized persons and pests.
The storage area is cleaned at least weekly, and immediately following a spill.
Bags are labelled with source (Studio Name) – in accordance with the Duty of Care (HMSO 1990).
Protective clothing, e.g. gloves and aprons, is available to staff handling clinical waste.
Collection of clinical waste is undertaken at least weekly with a registered company and waste is disposed of by incineration.

Box 21.9 Practice points: sharps disposal

Sharps boxes are available for use.
Sharps boxes conform with British Standard BS7320/UN3291.
The box is less than three-quarters full with no protruding sharps.
The sharps box is assembled correctly – check lid is secure.
The sharps box is labelled with name of the premises.
Practitioners are aware of inoculation injury policy and procedure to take in case of accident.
Sharps boxes are stored above floor level and safely out of reach of children and visitors.
Sharps boxes are disposed of appropriately in accordance with the Duty of Care.

Sharps will be handled safely in order to negate the risk of sharps injury and in accordance with current guidelines (Box 21.9)

'Inoculation risk' is a term used when referring to certain infections which can be transmitted when blood or some other tissue or body fluid from an infected person comes into contact with tissues/body fluids of another person. Inoculation injuries are the most likely route for the transmission of blood-borne viral and other infections in tattooing/skin piercing practice. Great care must be taken when handling and disposing of ALL sharps.

As defined in previous chapters regarding other clinical situations, a sharps/inoculation injury may be defined as:

- sticking or stabbing with a used needle or other sharp instrument
- splashes of blood/body fluid into the eyes, mucous membranes or open lesions on the skin surface
- cuts with used equipment
- bites or scratches inflicted by clients.

In the event of a sharps injury:

- **DO NOT SUCK** the wound
- Make it bleed
- Wash it with soap and running water and cover with a waterproof dressing
- Splashes into the eyes or mouth should be rinsed out with copious amounts of water
- Report to your GP or accident and emergency department for further assessment.

Inoculation injuries involving **known or highly suspected HIV clients** must be referred to the A&E Department immediately for further advice. (Treatment may be advised which must be started as soon as possible.)

Appropriate detergents/disinfectants and antiseptics are used correctly to negate the risk of infection (Box 21.10)

Chapter 5 gives full details of cleaning, disinfection and sterilization processes.

- *Cleaning*: the removal of dirt, dust and some micro-organisms by washing with detergent and hot water and thorough drying.

Box 21.10 Practice points: cleaning the studio

Disinfectants are used at the correct dilution and appropriately.
Chemical disinfectants are used only for heat-labile equipment.
A deep sink is available for washing items separate from hand washing facilities.
Data sheets are available on products in conjunction with COSHH.
Environmental surfaces are cleaned appropriately between clients.
Environmental surfaces are protected with disposable paper towelling between clients.

Box 21.11 Practice points: equipment and sterilizing

There is no evidence of single use equipment being reused.
Sterilizing equipment is maintained on a quality maintenance programme in accordance with HTM 2010 (HMSO 1994).
Sterilizing equipment cycle is checked and recorded daily/sessionally.
Sterilizing equipment is checked weekly in accordance with HTM 2010.
Sterilizing equipment is clean and in a good state of repair.
Instruments are unwrapped and not in pouches unless the sterilizer incorporates a pre-sterilizing vacuum cycle.
Water boilers are not used for instruments requiring sterilizing.
Used contaminated equipment is stored safely out of client areas after use.
A system is in place to accommodate breakdown and repair of equipment (autoclaves/ultrasonic cleaning machines, etc.).
Ultrasonic cleaners are emptied daily and kept dry overnight.
Dye containers are single use only and are appropriately disposed of following use.
Sterile disposable needles are single use only.
If needles are reused they are appropriately decontaminated between use (washed in an ultrasonic cleaner, dried and autoclaved (NOT IN POUCHES).
Water boilers, hot air ovens and UVA light boxes are not effective methods of sterilizing tattooing/skin piercing equipment and must not be used (Health Technical Memorandum 2010) (HMSO 1994).

- *Disinfection*: a reduction in the number of micro-organisms (not usually spores) by the use of heat or chemicals, for example by dish-washers, washing machines, bleach.
- *Sterilization*: the killing of all micro-organisms including spores by the use of heat under pressure (most common method in tattoo/skin piercing studios).

Thorough cleaning of equipment and the environment is essential and removes the majority of micro-organisms. Therefore the purposes for which disinfectants are used in the studio/practice should be few and limited to those of proven value. The disinfectants available in the studio/practice should be restricted to a preparatory skin disinfectant and an appropriate product to enable the safe clearing up of spills of blood/body fluids.

N.B. *Equipment and surfaces must be cleaned before applying a disinfectant as this will remove organic matter and ensure penetration of the disinfectant.*

Equipment will be decontaminated appropriately and stored correctly to negate the risk of cross infection (Box 21.11)

All instruments and equipment likely to be contaminated must be decontaminated between client use. Instruments which may breach intact skin are considered 'high risk' and should be sterile for use. All needles, needle bars and needle tubes whenever possible should be sterilized immediately before use or as near to the procedure as possible and stored in a sealed container.

All equipment must be thoroughly cleaned before sterilization and all visible deposits must be removed. Ultrasonic cleaners are recommended wherever possible for small items.

Gloves (heavy duty 'kitchen' type), protective eye wear and disposable plastic aprons should be worn whilst cleaning equipment and instruments prior to sterilization. The equipment/instruments should be scrubbed in a designated deep sink using water and general purpose detergent such as Fairy liquid.

Great care should be taken to avoid inoculation (sharps) injury while cleaning equipment/instruments.

NOTES ON ACUPUNCTURE AND ELECTROLYSIS

As with any 'alternative' therapies or beauty treatments where the operator may come into contact with the blood or other body fluid of a client, the safe working practice points described above should be adhered to at all times. Acupuncture needles and electrolysis needles must be sterile, single client use and always discarded following use into an appropriate sharps container.

REFERENCES

Dawson J K 1998 An assessment of infection control practice and procedures in tattooing/skin piercing studios registered with the Local Authorities in North Staffordshire. Dissertation. Birmingham University, Birmingham

Dian-Xing Sun, Fu-Guang Zhang, Yun-Quin Geng, De-Sheng Xi 1996 Hepatitis C transmission by cosmetic tattooing in women (letter). Lancet 347: 541

Health and Safety Executive 1989, 1994, 1999 Control of Substances Hazardous to Health Regulations. HSE Books, Sudbury (ISBN 07176 08190).

HMSO 1969 Tattooing of Minors Act 1969. HMSO, London

HMSO 1974 Health and Safety at Work Act 1974. HMSO, London

HMSO 1981 Greater London Council (General Powers) Act 1981. HMSO, London

HMSO 1982 Local Government (Miscellaneous Provisions) Act 1982. HMSO, London

HMSO 1985 Prohibition of Female Circumcision Act 1985. HMSO, London

HMSO 1988 Public Health (Infectious Diseases) Regulations, SI 1988 No. 1546. HMSO, London

HMSO 1990 Environmental Protection Act 1990. HMSO, London

HMSO 1991 London Local Authorities Act 1991. HMSO, London

HMSO 1994 Health Technical Memorandum 2010. HMSO, London

Infection Control Nurses Association 1997 Guidelines for Hand Hygiene. ICNA, Bathgate

Kent G P, Brondum J, Keenlyside R A, LaFazia L M, Scott H A D 1988 A large outbreak of acupuncture-associated hepatitis B. American Journal of Epidemiology 127: 591–598

Long C E, Rickman L S 1994 Infectious complications of tattoos. Review article. Clinical Infectious Diseases 18(4): 610–619

Mele A, Corona R, Tosti M E et al 1995 Beauty treatments and risk of parenterally transmitted hepatitis: results from the hepatitis surveillance system in Italy. Scandinavian Journal of Infectious Diseases 27(5): 441–444

Noah N 1993 A guide to hygienic skin piercing. PHLS, London (ISBN 0-901144-10 – updated 1997 not yet in press – personal communication).

Vickers J, Painter M J, Heptonstall J, Yusof J H M, Craske J 1994 Hepatitis B outbreak in a drugs trials unit: investigation and recommendations. CDR Review 1994, Vol. 4: Review No 1, 1–5

Wright J 1995 Modifying the body: piercing and tattoos. Nursing Standard 10(11): 27–30

Appendices

Appendix A

Internet resources on evidence-based healthcare

M. Briggs

USEFUL WEB PAGES

ACP Journal Club http://www.acponline.org/journals/acpjc/jcmenu American College of Physicians – American Society of Internal Medicine. ACP Journal Club's general purpose is to select from the biomedical literature those articles reporting studies and reviews that warrant immediate attention by physicians attempting to keep pace with important advances in internal medicine. These articles are summarized in 'value added' abstracts commented on by clinical experts.

Bandolier http://www.jr2.ox.ac.uk:80/Bandolier-

British Medical Journal http://www.bmj.org

Centre for Evidence-based Nursing http:// www.york.ac.uk/depts/hstttd/centres/evidence/ev-intro Based at York University, the Centre for Evidence-based Nursing works with nurses in practice, management, research and education to identify evidence-based practice.

Centre for Reviews and Dissemination http://www.york.ac.uk/inst/crd The NHS Centre for Reviews and Dissemination is a facility commissioned by the NHS R&D division to produce and disseminate reviews concerning the effectiveness and cost-effectiveness of healthcare interventions.

Cochrane Collaboration http://www.cochrane.org This is a world-wide collaboration, which exists to create, review, maintain and disseminate systematic reviews of the available healthcare literature. This web page houses the Cochrane

Library and the abstracts of all reviews and pro-tocol are available free on the net. This provides access to:

1. Cochrane Database of systematic reviews – regularly updated reviews of the effects of healthcare.

2. Database of Abstracts of Reviews of Effectiveness – critical assessment and structured abstracts of good systematic reviews published elsewhere.

3. Cochrane controlled trials register – bibliographic information on controlled trials.

Critical Appraisal Skills Programme http://www.phru.org/casp/rct CASP is a UK pro-ject that aims to help health service decision-makers develop skills to find, critically appraise and change practice in line with evidence of effectiveness.

DARE database (Database of Reviews of Effectiveness) Produced by the Centre for Reviews and Dissemination (CRD), this is available on the Cochrane Library or via the CRD web site.

Effectiveness Matters Effectiveness Matters provides updates on the effectiveness of impor-tant health interventions for practitioners and decision-makers in the NHS. Topics covered to date include aspirin and myocardial infection and influenza vaccination. Effectiveness Matters is available from CRD http://www.york/ac.uk/inst/crd/dissem.htm#em

Effective Health Care Bulletin Effective Health Care is a bi-monthly bulletin that aims to assist decision-makers by examining the effectiveness of various healthcare interventions. The bulletins are based on a systematic review of the clinical effectiveness, cost-effectiveness and acceptability of interventions. A research team conduct the reviews with help from a panel of clinical experts. The full texts of bulletins are available via the web. http://www.york.ac.uk/inst/crd/ehcb.htm

NEED, NHS Economic Evaluations Database Produced by the NHS Centre for Reviews and Dissemination (CRD), NEED is available via CRD web site.

NHS R&D Programme/NHS HTA Programme The HTA programme funded health services research in the UK. It covers primary research and systematic reviews. The programme has a useful web site detailing its research activity (past, present and future priorities), http://www.soton.ac.uk/~hta

National Guideline-clearing House The national guideline-clearing House (NGC) is a comprehen-sive database of evidence-based clinical practice guidelines and related documents produced by the Agency for Health Care Policy and Research (AHCPR) in partnership with the American Medical Association (AMA) and the American Association of Health Plans (AAHP). The NGC mission is to provide clinicians with an acces-sible mechanism to obtain detailed clinical guide-lines. Web address http://www.guidelines.gov/index.asp

National Institute for Clinical Excellence NICE systematically appraises health interventions. The aim is to offer clinicians and managers clear guidance on which treatments work best for patients. http://www.nice.org.uk/

OPAC 97 British Lending Library, Boston Spa: http://www.opac97.bl.uk

Primary Care National Electronic Library for Health – provides a search facility which allows you to search Cochrane, Bandolier, Evidence-based Medicine, NICE, and Effectiveness Matters at the same time. http://www.nelh-pc.nhs.uk

Royal College of Nursing – Research Society The RCN Research Society provides useful infor-mation about all aspects of research related to nursing. http://www.man.ac.uk/rcn

School of Health and Related Research (ScHARR), University of Sheffield. This health services research department has a number of web-based resources for finding and appraising evidence. For example:

Scharr–Lock's Guide to the Evidence, http://www.shef.ac.uk/uniacademic/RZ/scharr/ir/netting.html This is a guide to printed sources of evidence – not published in journals (grey literature), for example government reports.

ScHARR site for netting the evidence, http://www.shef.ac.uk/~scharr/ir/netting

TRIP searchable database of a group of evidence-based sites. This resource hosted by the Centre of Research Support in Wales aims to support those working in primary care. The database has 8000 links covering resources at 28 different centres and allows both Boolean searching (AND OR NOT) and truncation. http://www.ceres. uwcm. ac.uk-

OTHER USEFUL INTERNET INFORMATION

www.rcn.org.uk The Royal College of Nursing's site. Comprehensive centre for various information, including the library.

www.doh.gov.uk The Department of Health. This can be used to download government reports and documents.

www.hea.org.uk The Health Education Authority. Information on all aspects relating to health promotion.

www.asmusa.org American Society for Microbiology.

www.amm.co.uk Association of Medical Microbiologists.

www.apic.org/index.html (USA) Association for Professionals in Infection Control and Epidemiology.

www.cdc.gov Centers for Disease Control in Atlanta, USA.

www.his.org.uk The Hospital Infection Society.

www.icna.co.uk The Infection Control Nurses' Association.

www.harcourt-international.com/journals/jhin/default.cfm?/mainmenu.htm Journal of Hospital Infection.

www.phls.co.uk Public Health Laboratory Service.

www.riphh.org.uk Royal Institute of Public Health and Hygiene.

www.Virtual Library: Microbiology and Virology http://microbiol. org/vlmicro/index. htm

www.nhs.uk Homepage of the NHS Website. Connects to local services and provides national information.

www.nhs.uk/nelh Health electronic library for health professionals. Gives best practice information on diagnosis and treatment.

www.woundcaresociety.org The Wound Care Society in the UK.

www.tvs.org.uk The Tissue Viability Society in the UK.

www.immunisation.org.uk For health professionals and the general public: information on various vaccines and immunization.

The URLs quoted were correct at the time of going to press, however, information on the internet, including URLs, are subject to constant change.

Appendix B

Infectious disease notifications: action to be taken

Disease	Incubation period	Period of communicability	Action to be taken
Acute encephalitis	Unknown	Unknown	Monitor for clusters; seek cause if possible
Acute meningitis	Variable	Variable	Prophylaxis to household contacts of confirmed or probable cases of meningococcal disease Follow CDR guidelines on management of clusters in educational establishments
Acute polio	7–14 days	7 days prior to onset and 7 days post onset	**URGENT** Investigate source; seek contacts Immunize – major outbreak procedure Inform DoH, CDSC, PHLS, RDPH/RE
Anthrax	<7 days	During illness until lesions stop discharging	**URGENT** Investigate source; major outbreak procedure Inform DoH, CDSC, PHLS, RDPH/RE, DEFRA
Cholera	Few hours to 5 days	Upto 14 days, carrier state possible	**URGENT** Investigate source; inform DoH, CDSC, PHLS, RDPH; if local source possible – major outbreak procedure
Diphtheria	2–5 days	2–3 weeks. Carrier state possible	Investigate source; seek contacts, immunize Inform DoH, CDSC, PHLS, RDPH/RE Major outbreak procedure
Amoebic dysentery	3 days to months	During illness until bacteriological clearance	Cases – Enteric precautions until treatment is complete. Screen household contacts microbiologically to detect excreters. Late follow-up to detect chronic carriage
Food poisoning	Half-hour to several days	Depends on organism or toxin	All cases of gastroenteritis should be regarded as infectious. Faecal specimen required. Enteric precautions
Hepatitis A	15–50 days	7 days prior and 7 days post onset	Isolate for 1st week; focus on hygiene; consider Gamma globulin; investigate source
Hepatitis B	45–60 days	Unknown	Investigate source; give advice about routes of infection
Legionnaires' disease	2–10 days	Not transmissible from person to person	**URGENT** – Look for overseas travel. A single case locally acquired needs to be investigated. EHOs have a major role in identifying source. RE, CDSC, DoH, PHLS
Leptospirosis	4–10 days	During illness until urine clear	Investigate source; disinfect urine; consider rodent control; discuss with DEFRA/PHLS
Leprosy	Unknown	Varies	Investigate source; ensure appropriate treatment; ensure entry on CDSC register
Malaria	Up to 14 days or longer	Requires vector	Investigate source; if UK source discuss with CDSC
Measles	7–14 days	From onset to 5 days after rash	Check sibling immunization; check individual immunization
Ophthalmia neonatorum	36–48 hours	As long as eyes are discharging	Ensure proper treatment; advise treatment of mother and significant other(s)

(continued)

Disease	Incubation period	Period of communicability	Action to be taken
Paratyphoid fever	1–10 days	As long as bacteria in faeces	Investigate. Household contacts and contacts outside the home in risk groups must be tested. Follow-up stools examinations advisable for all cases and mandatory for food handlers
Plague	3–6 days	Pneumonic form, highly communicable	**URGENT** Investigate source Major outbreak procedure; inform DoH, CDSC, PHLS, RDPH/RE
Rabies	2–52 weeks	3–5 days prior to onset until death	**URGENT** Person bitten by an animal suspected to have rabies may need post-exposure prophylaxis. Inform PHLS
Relapsing fever	3–12 days	Not communicable person to person	Investigate source; inform DoH, CDSC, PHLS, RDPH/RE
Rubella	14–21 days	7 days prior to and 5 days post rash	Check immunization history; keep away from pregnant women
Scarlet fever	2–5 days	10–21 days	Check occupation; if midwife, theatre nurse, milk handler, consider exclusion
Tetanus	4–21 days	Not communicable person to person	Check immunization history; check source of infection
Tuberculosis	Unknown	Until bacteriological clearance	Inform Chest Clinic; liaise with chest physician on contacts and BCG
Typhoid fever	7–21 days	Until bacteriological clearance	Investigate. Household contacts and contacts outside the home in risk groups must be tested. Follow-up stools examinations advisable for all cases and mandatory for food handlers
Whooping cough	7–10 days	7 days prior to and 21 days after onset	Check immunization history; immunize siblings as needed
Yellow fever	3–6 days	2 days prior to and 4 days post onset	Investigate source; inform DoH, CDSC, PHLS, RDPH/RE
Viral haemorrhagic fever	Variable	Caused by several agents	Investigate source; inform DoH, CDSC, PHLS, RE

DoH   – Department of Health.
CDR   – Communicable Disease Report.
RE   – Regional Epidemiologist.
CDSC   – Communicable Disease Surveillance Centre.
PHLS   – Public Health Laboratory Service.
RDPH   – Regional Director of Public Health.
EHO   – Environmental Health Officer.
DEFRA   – Department of Environment, Food and Rural Affairs.

Infectious Disease Control – the legislation

The legislation covers the key areas in Infectious Disease Control:

(1) The Notification System
(2) Disease Control Measures
(3) Port Health

KEY ACTS

The Public Health Act 1936
The Public Health Act 1961
The Public Health (Control of Diseases) Act 1984
The Public Health (Infectious Diseases) Regulations 1988
Supplementary legislation includes:

(a) The Port Health Authorities (England) Order 1974
(b) The Port Health Authorities (Wales) Order 1974
(c) The Public Health (Aircraft) Regulations 1979
(d) The Public Health (Ships) Regulations 1979
(e) The Immigration Act 1971
(f) The Prevention of Damage By Pests Act 1949
(g) All Food Regulation legislation and regulations:
— Food Safety Act 1990. HMSO
— Food handlers' fitness to work – guidance for food businesses, enforcement officers and health professionals. DoH 1995
— EEC Council Directive 93/43/EEC 14.6.93. Food safety (general food hygiene) regulations 1995
— Food safety (temperature control) regulations 1995 S1:2200

— Management of food hygiene and food services in the NHS. NHS Executive 1996 HSG(96):20

— Product-specific regulations, e.g. The fresh meat (hygiene and inspection) regulations 1995, Ref 51:539. [These reflect products of specific concern and cover dairy, poultry, molluscs/fish eggs, wild game, fresh meat and meat preparation]

(h) Health and Safety Law plus relevant regulations and Codes of Practice

(i) All Animal Law

(j) Health and Safety Legislation.

The Public Health (Control of Disease) Act 1984 together with corresponding regulations particularly The Public Health (Infectious Diseases) Regulations 1988 consolidated previous legislation from the late 19th and early 20th century. Some go back as far as the Sanitary laws of 1870.

PUBLIC INFORMATION BOOKLETS

(a) Food safety: A guide from HM Government.

(b) The Food Safety Act 1990 and You – A guide for the food industry. Food Sense, London, SE99 7TT.

(c) Food Sense MAFF guidance.

(d) The guide to good hygiene. Lever Industrial, PO Box 100, Runcorn, Cheshire WA7 3JZ.

Glossary

Abscess   a localized collection of pus

Acquired immunity   immunity which develops in response to a stimulus, such as an infection

Aerobe   a microbe that grows in the presence of oxygen. A strict aerobe requires oxygen

Allergy   an undesirable immune response due to hypersensitivity

Anaerobe   a microbe that grows in the absence of oxygen. A strict anaerobe will not grow in the presence of oxygen. A facultative anaerobe can grow in the presence or absence of oxygen

Antibiotic   a substance which is toxic for certain micro-organisms, that either kills or inhibits their growth

Antibody   an immunoglobulin (Ig) which adheres to a specific antigen and whose production is activated by the presence of the antigen

Antigen   a substance which can induce an immune response

Antimicrobial   a substance which is inhibitory or lethal to micro-organisms. May be synthetic or produced naturally

Antiseptic   a chemical used to kill numbers of microbes on body surfaces

Aseptic technique   a practice/procedure designed to ensure freedom from microbial contamination, e.g. wound dressings, catheterization

Autoclave   a machine in which materials are exposed to steam under pressure and therefore at a temperature higher than that of boiling water

Autolytic debridement   removal of non-viable tissue through natural cellular activity, e.g. phagocytosis may be assisted through using hydrogels to hydrate non-viable tissue

Bactericide   a chemical or physical agent that rapidly kills vegetative (non-sporing) bacteria

Bacteriophage   a virus that infects bacterial cells

Bacteriuria   the presence of micro-organisms in the bladder with no signs or symptoms of infection

Benchtop sterilizer   a small autoclave, either non-vacuum or vacuum type, used in clinics and general practices and other community premises requiring devices to be sterilized

Binary fission   division of one cell into two daughter cells, the usual method of bacterial reproduction

Biofilm   a film of proteins and micro-organisms that forms over the surface of foreign material when it is in contact with tissue

Carrier   a person without symptoms who has excreted pathogenic organisms in faeces or urine either continuously or intermittently for more than 12 months

Case   a person with symptoms

Cell-mediated   immunity resulting from the action of T lymphocytes against foreign or infected cells

CJD   Creutzfeldt–Jakob disease. A prion disease in humans which causes a spongiform encephalopathy associated with the destruction of brain tissue

Commensals   a commensal organism lives in association with another, without harming or benefiting it. Many members of the gut flora appear to be commensals. Commensals may be pathogenic if the host is immunocompromised

Communicable   any disease that is transmitted from one person to another is communicable

Complement   a complex of enzyme proteins found in plasma, which triggers or enhances immune function

Conjugation   the transfer of genetic material from one bacterial cell to another by cell-to-cell contact

Contact   a person who may have been exposed to infection from a person already infected

Contamination the soiling of inanimate objects or living material with harmful, potentially infectious or unwanted matter

COSHH Control of Substances Hazardous to Health Regulations requiring employers to assess the risk to health from the use of substances that may be hazardous

Cross infection the transmission of infection between persons infected with pathogenic micro-organisms

Cytopathic having the capacity to destroy cells, e.g. toxin or virus affecting tissue

Cytotoxic toxic or destructive to cells

Disinfection a process that is intended to kill or remove pathogenic micro-organisms but which cannot usually kill bacterial spores

DOT (Directly observed therapy) compliance with treatment is observed e.g. with anti-tubercular therapy

Ectoparasite a parasite that lives on the outer surface of the host, e.g. ticks, lice

Ectoparasitic relating to parasites which live on the outer surface of the host, e.g. ticks, lice

Endontic relating to root canal therapy. Removing infected or damaged tissue from inside a tooth

Endotoxins lipopolysaccharides in outer membrane of Gram-negative cells. When cells are lysed these are released and can cause severe systemic symptoms (endotoxic shock)

Epidemic when an unusually high incidence of an endemic infection occurs, or occurrence of an infection not usually seen in that population

Epidemiology the study of how various states of health are distributed in the population and the study of disease causation

Episome DNA which is additional to, or outside, the nuclear DNA

Excretor a person without symptoms but excreting pathogenic organisms in faeces or urine for less than 12 months. This can apply to someone recovered from an infection or someone who had asymptomatic infection

Exotoxins proteins secreted by bacteria, which damage host tissues

Family outbreak two or more cases within the same household

Fibrin formed by fibrinogen during blood clotting, a protein that meshes together to repair damaged blood vessels

Fomites inanimate objects, other than food, that may harbour and transmit micro-organisms

Gastro-enteritis diarrhoea present for seven days or less, with or without vomiting, where no other cause has been identified

General outbreak two or more cases associated in place or time but not within the same household

Handpiece a device used to attach all types of dental drills

Hangtime the time recommended for feeds used in enteral feeding to be delivered whilst in room temperature

Heat-labile a device or material which is unable to be sterilized/disinfected at high temperatures

Histamine a molecule released by mast cells; it causes increased permeability of blood vessels, and is responsible for the signs of inflammation; excess is associated with hay fever, asthma, etc.

Hospital-acquired infection infection acquired by a patient whilst in hospital or by a member of hospital staff

Humoral immunity immunity mediated by antibodies circulating in the blood

Immunization the use of a vaccine to produce an immune response in an individual to particular diseases

Immunocompromised an individual with impaired immunity due to disease or treatment

Immunoglobulin (Ig) see **antibody**

Impervious   not allowing the passage of fluids, e.g. dressings

Incidence   the number of new events or episodes of a disease that occur in a population in a given time period

Incubation period   period between infection and onset of signs of illness

Index case   a person who first has symptoms of a disease when defining an outbreak of infection

Intravenous   the insertion of a catheter/cannula into a vein

Light curing unit   a curing unit which produces a visible white light which initiates polymerization of light-activated dental materials such as composite resins, bonding agents, adhesive primers and pit and fissure sealants

Lymphocytes   white blood cells also found in the lymphatic system, which play a major role in the immune system, specifically the cell-mediated immune response

Lymphokines   chemicals released by lymphocytes which can contribute to antigen destruction

Macrophages   large mononuclear phagocytic cells

Maternal antibodies   antibodies transferred from mother to baby via the placenta offering short-term protection

MDRTB   Multi-Drug Resistant Tuberculosis. Resistant to the first-line drugs used in the treatment of tuberculosis

Microbiological clearance   the reduction of the number of pathogenic organisms in a specimen below that detectable by conventional means

Micro-organism   an organism too small to be seen by the naked eye, requiring a microscope to become visible. This includes bacteria, fungi, protozoa, viruses and some algae

Modular feed   a feed which is pre-prepared and presented in cans or bottles for decanting or bags ready to hang

Morbidity   a reduced state of health (symptoms of disease)

Mortality   death

MRSA   Methicillin-resistant *Staphylococcus aureus*. A strain of *S. aureus* resistant to methicillin and a spectrum of resistance to other agents

Mutation   a change in the sequence of DNA nucleotides, which can occur spontaneously or under the influence of external factors

Mycoses   infections caused by fungi

Obligate organism   an organism restricted to a particular way of life: e.g. an obligate parasite cannot live free without a host, an obligate aerobe cannot live without oxygen

Opsonization   the coating of cells by antibodies to enhance phagocytosis

Parasite   an organism that lives in or on another creature, e.g. lice, scabies

Pasteurization   a process that kills non-sporing micro-organisms by hot water or steam at 65–100°C

Pathogen   a micro-organism with the ability to cause disease

Puerperal infection   an infection occurring in a woman following childbirth

Phagocytosis   ingestion of foreign matter by phagocytic cells

Pili   present on many Gram-negative bacteria, which enable the organism to adhere to specific host cells, e.g. *Escherichia coli* in urinary tract infections. Some are called sex pili, used to join two cells together allowing them to exchange genetic information

Plasma   fluid portion of the blood containing proteins, lipids, electrolytes, hormones, vitamins and carbohydrates

Plasmid   a double-stranded circle of DNA, which may be present in the cytoplasm of a microbial cell. Plasmids often carry genes for antibiotic resistance

Polymorphonuclear neutrophil phagocytic lymphocyte with a multi-lobed nucleus

Prevalence the total number of cases of a specific disease present in a defined population at a point in time

Prophylaxis a means used to prevent a disease, such as giving antibiotics without evidence of infection being present or incubating, e.g. pre-operative

Protozoa microscopic single-celled eukaryotic microbes; some are free-living, others are important parasites, e.g. *Entamoeba histolytica*

Replication the synthesis of copies of a DNA molecule or a virus

Rickettsiae very small bacteria that cannot grow outside the cells of their host. Transmitted by insects, except for Q fever, e.g. typhus

Rubber dam a device placed in the mouth which provides a reduction in micro-organisms escaping from the mouth in aerosol or 'spatter'

Sensitivity the susceptibility of certain organisms to specific agents, e.g. antibiotics

Septicaemia bacteria present in the bloodstream accompanied by signs and symptoms of infection with no other recognized cause

Single use a device intended to be used during a single procedure and then discarded

Skin flora the community of microbes that colonize a body surface without harming the host

Specific immunity acts against specific antigens

Sporadic case a single case not associated with other cases, carriers or excretors

Spores resistant casings that some bacteria use to enclose their cells in adverse environmental conditions. Spores germinate when conditions improve and the cell recommences multiplication, e.g. tetanus

Strain a sub-group of a given bacterial species whose individual organisms are genetically similar

Strikethrough the appearance of wound exudate which has soaked through to the outside of the dressing

Symbiosis an obligate association between two species in which there is mutual benefit

Thermocouple a device used to check the efficient working of a sterilizer, e.g. temperature and holding temperature

Toxin poison released by a pathogen

Traceability systems a system employed to enable instruments and equipment used for surgical and other interventions to be traced over a period of time

Transmission the means by which an infection is spread, e.g. airborne spread, ingestion, inoculation

Transposon a 'jumping gene', a segment of DNA which can move from one DNA molecule to another, or from one site to another in the same DNA molecule

TSE Transmissible spongiform encephalopathy (see CJD)

Ultrasonic cleaner a machine used for efficient cleaning of instruments by immersing in a tank

Vaccine a preparation of killed or inactivated microbes, inactivated microbial toxins or microbial antigens used to induce immunity

Index